Vinko V. Dolenc (ed.)

The Cavernous Sinus

A Multidisciplinary Approach to Vascular and Tumorous Lesions

Springer-Verlag Wien GmbH

Vinko V. Dolenc, M.D.
Professor, Department of Neurosurgery
University Medical Center, Ljubljana
Yugoslavia

Originally published by Springer-Verlag/Wien in 1987

With 195 Figures

ISBN 978-3-7091-7460-9 ISBN 978-3-7091-6982-7 (eBook)
DOI 10.1007/978-3-7091-6982-7

Foreword

The management of vascular and tumorous lesions of the parasellar region still remains one of the most demanding tasks in neurosurgery. It is only a short time ago that the major concepts of the anatomy of the so-called cavernous sinus were described in detail. Surgical interventions in this region are very complex, they are time-consuming and require an extensive background of experience in surgery of the cranial base.

Pioneer anatomical studies of the parasellar region done by Taptas, and the daring direct operative approach introduced by Parkinson promoted the development of modern neuroradiological intervention procedures, which were initiated by Serbinenko and further refined by Debrun, Viñuela and others. The technique of the detachable balloon catheter stimulated surgeons to proceed with the direct operative approach to lesions of the parasellar region. Today, it is hard to imagine a successful management of vascular pathologies of this region without a complementary use of the two techniques.

Similar, yet considerably different, is the situation in the treatment of parasellar tumors. Modern neuroradiological diagnostic procedures and neurophysiological tests employed prior to surgery can supply many valuable data which are indispensable for the surgeon who wishes to devise optimal treatment strategies for each case separately. Preoperative embolization of the tumor vessels and peroperative monitoring of the function of cranial nerves III through VI enable the surgeon to plan a more radical excision, and provide for greater safety of the procedure. In the entire treatment of parasellar tumors, though benign, which are not amenable to complete excision, radiotherapy should be considered as an adjuvant therapeutic modality.

Complete removal of the lesion with preservation of function of all vascular and nerve structures remains the ultimate solution to the problem of vascular and tumorous lesions of the parasellar region. We believe that this volume will be of use to all surgeons concerned with those problems, and that it will motivate them to use a team approach, which, in our opinion, is the only guarantee of a successful management of these lesions.

Ljubljana, August 1987 *V. V. Dolenc*

Contents

Historical review and pioneer work

Anatomy

Diagnostic procedures

Occlusion techniques

Surgery of vascular lesions

Tumor surgery

Historical review and pioneer work

Carotid cavernous fistula. History and anatomy

D. PARKINSON

University of Manitoba, Winnipeg, Manitoba, Canada

History

The parasellar compartment commonly known as the "cavernous sinus" contains a more compact complexity of gross anatomy than any other structure, a veritable anatomic jewel box. The orbit, a much larger cavity, would be its closest rival. The orbit literature fills many library shelves whereas its poorer back door neighbour barely rates and address in the library catalogue. Its printed papers over the centuries would fill no more than one small text. The discrepancy reflects the relative visibility, accessibility, and number of clinical syndromes involved. Virtually all disturbances of the "cavernous sinus" are manifested first and foremost by its prominent front door neighbour the orbit and hence described under such titles. We can be reasonably certain that the classical syndrome resulting from the carotid cavernous fistula (CCF) was noticed long before first described by Bartholow [4]. "Evil Eye Fleegle" of comic book fame [17] was unlikely the first to inspire belief that the owner of a pulsating, protruding, engorged eye (or eyes) possessed supernatural powers, evil or otherwise.

It is recognized that some cases of CCF cause no eye signs and many cases of pulsating exophthalmos are caused by conditions other than CCF but it is rare that the combination of, bruit, pulsating exophthalmos and venous engorgement are caused by anything else [56].

Medical progress is additive. Our present understanding of the "cavernous sinus" is based on a multitude of previous observations, some antedating Hippocrates. Attempting to list the significant firsts invites the perils of inadvertant ommission.

For a more complete history one should read Hamby [39]. Long before mankind was aware of the „cavernous sinus" he was experimenting with tubes to catheterize bladders. Egyptian priest physicians more than 3,000 years ago relieved distended bladders with bronze catheters. The Chinese used hollow leaves of Illium fistulosum. Hippocrates is alleged to have advocated a silver tube attached to a sow's bladder filled with milk to irrigate the womb, "best inserted by the women herself as she knows where to place it". In 1952 Ben Franklin invented a flexible silver catheter for his brother. Then in 1860 Napoleon's physician Nelaton introduced rubber catheters as well as sounds with which he probed for the bullet that wounded Garibaldi. (The same Nelaton [70] later drew an accurate picture of a carotid cavernous fistula). In 1844 Claude Bernard tried to measure the temperatures in horses' heart by introducing urologists's sounds through carotid arteries and jugular veins. In 1905 Bleichroeder catheterized his own right atrium [64]. Thus the stage was set for the entrance of Seljeskog and Serbinenko [111, 112] and their spectacular development of the therapeutic and diagnostic use of guided catheters and detachable balloons!

Not all medical knowledge pertaining to the "cavernous sinus" has been additive. Galen's [32] authoritative error was monumentally subtractive. He dissected lower animals, accurately described their "rete mirable", then mistakenly assigned the same anatomy to humans where it rested unchallenged until corrected by Vesalius [127] in 1543. Many of Galen's errors persisted long after corrected by Vesalius. Some academicans in high places resented any questioning of the world of Galen. Possibly Winslow [129] was looking at Calve's retia when he coined the term, "cavernous sinus", thinking it resembled the corpus cavernous of the penis. He should have known better as the two serve no similar purpose and nature does nothing in vain.

Harvey's demonstration of arteries and veins and Malphighi's [62] demonstration of the capillaries set the stage for William Hunter [49] to understand and describe an arterio venous fistula in 1762. Then Travers [123] recognized and successfully treated a carotid CCF in 1811; daring to ligate the common carotid (Fig. 1), having witnessed Cooper [18] in 1808 perform the first carotid ligation. Both were indebted to Ambroise Pare [75] who in 1552 first used a ligature to control hemorrhage. As interest in the cerebral circulation progressed awareness of the collateral function of the circle of Willis drew attention [97]. The ophthalmic artery was recognized as a potential collateral to the hemisphere [120] (Fig. 1 a, b). More significantly back in 1893 Elschnig [30] found that the collateral to the eye from the external system was sufficient to preserve vision with the ophthalmic occluded. As with many original observations this had to be rediscovered several times.

Twichell [124] in 1807 noticed that the open internal carotid would bleed from either direction and in 1855 Blackman [10] stated that after ligation of the common carotid the internal carotid becomes a branch of the external. (Sweet ultimately measured such pressures in 1948 [117]). The significance of these seemingly self evident facts were missed by very astute observed for years to come. Retrograde flow in any artery comes from collaterals and reduces the perfusion to the bypassed designated organ; a phenomenon known as "steal". Occluding the retrograde flow can only improve the perfusion pressure to the organ, eye or cerebral hemisphere in these instances (eventually beautifully described by Hoyt [48, 106] for the eye). Dandy [24] and Adson [1], as astute and perceptive as any surgeons alive failed to grasp this fact while virtually describing it.

The art of trephining remained static for thousands of years. The pioneering of advances of MacEwan [59], Horsley [47] and Cushing [21] rapidly brought craniotomy skills to the level where supraclinoid clipping of the carotid could be considered. Cushing's clips [22], Gigli's [33] and Bovie's cautery [23] along with anesthesia and asepsis played major roles. Kocher's [55] admonition to Cushing to intensify his studies and limit his interests to one field of surgery may be an example more of the shadow than of the substance of history.

Gardner [40] had ligated the supraclinoid carotid in 1933. Dandy [24] recognized that carotid backflow perpetuated some fistulae (Fig. 1 a). Eventually he clipped this while expressing hopefully the safety of the procedure, stating tolerance had been demonstrated in the patient by previous cervical ligation of the carotid! Dandy [24] also recognized the retrograde ophthalmic artery flow contribution to the otherwise trapped fistula but avoided clipping it in order to preserve sight (Fig. 1 b)! Nafziger [69] in discussion of Dandy's paper also missed this. Adson in 1942 also recognized the backflow from the ophthalmic perpetuating an otherwise trapped fistula and expressed relief when sight was not lost after he clipped the ophthalmic!

Mont [67] in discussion of Dandy's paper advocated resection and ligation of the supraorbital vein and even suggested scouring the lumen with a small test tube brush soaked in 50% glucose. Singleton [113] in 1939, may have heard Mont and either or both of them may have been aware of Brainerd's [13] attempt in 1953 to cure an, "erectile tumor of the orbit" by retrograde injection of lactate of iron yet in 1975 Peterson [101] credits Mullan [68] with the suggestion for his first retrograde venous passage of a wire for the purpose of electro coagulation with a cure of a CCF.

Thus experience, knowledge and occassionally logic are passed from one brillant investigator like an olympic torch to the next mind capable of grasping and carrying the precious commodity on to its next destination. Some had a firmer grip and a more certain knowledge of destiny than others.

At any rate by 1940 there was no excuse for not recognizing that with a large fistula it was safer to expose the carotid in the neck then, occlude the ophthalmic artery, next the supraclinoid carotid and finally the internal in the neck (Fig. 1 b). Altering this technique could result in monocular blindness from the temporarily aggravated ophthalmic steal. Yet this fundamental physiologic principal continued to the overlooked as late as 1965 [99].

Scarcely noted in 1931 was the startling announcement by Brooks [15], that he had cured a fistula by floating a muscle embolus up the carotid. Eleven years later Jaeger [51] more prudently floated emboli up the carotid after supra clinoid occlusion. In 1937 Browder [16] had stuffed some muscle through a stab wound in the roof of the sinus a reported cure of a fistula.

Thus by the mid-20th century the additive knowledge of many developments, courageous and innovative, enable Gardner, Hamby [40] and Dohn [42] to "standardize" the treatment of large fistulae by first exposing the carotid in the neck, next clipping the ophthalmic, then the supraclinoid carotid then introducing a marked muscle embolus [40] via the opened external to wash up the internal which was then ligated. Isamat [50] in 1970 ingeniously embolized the fistula and preserved the patency of the carotid using a metal clip on a muscle embolus guided by a magnet [2].

Arterial anatomy

Still the persistance of some fistula so treated meant there had to be an available collateral to the otherwise isolated carotid segment (Fig. 1 c). As a result of such observations we began in the 1950's to look for the normal collateral canals available to the parasellar carotid. We reasoned that such canals must be normally present as the existence of a fistula cannot cause new vessels to grow into or out of the wall of a major artery such as the carotid. The normal presence of such anastomotic canals was readily

---

Fig. 1. 1811: **a** Common carotid ligated. Both eyes and hemispheres dependent on collateral from opposite common. Minimal reduction of pressure to fistula which is able to steal from all sources. Retina at minimal peril. **b** Internal carotid ligated ispilateral hemisphere and eye dependent on collateral. Greater reduction of pressure to fistula still stealing from all sources. Retina at greater peril. 1933: **c** Supraclinoid carotid additionally clipped. Hemisphere and eye dependent on collateral. Great reduction in pressure to fistula which still is able to steal from the ophthalmic artery. Retina at maximal peril. 1942: **d** Ophthalmic also clipped. Eye dependent on collateral. Retina protected from moment ophthalmic clipped. Fistula theoretically completely trapped. 1963: **e** Fistula perpetuated in some instances by collaterals from ipsilateral external and contralateral internal and external carotids. **f** Close up of type II CCF. Tear in parasellar branches capable of bleeding from either direction. Reprinted with permission from Parkinson D (1972) In: Vinken PJ, Bruyn GW (eds) Handbook of Clinical Neurology. North Holland, Amsterdam, pp 18–23, Fig. 14

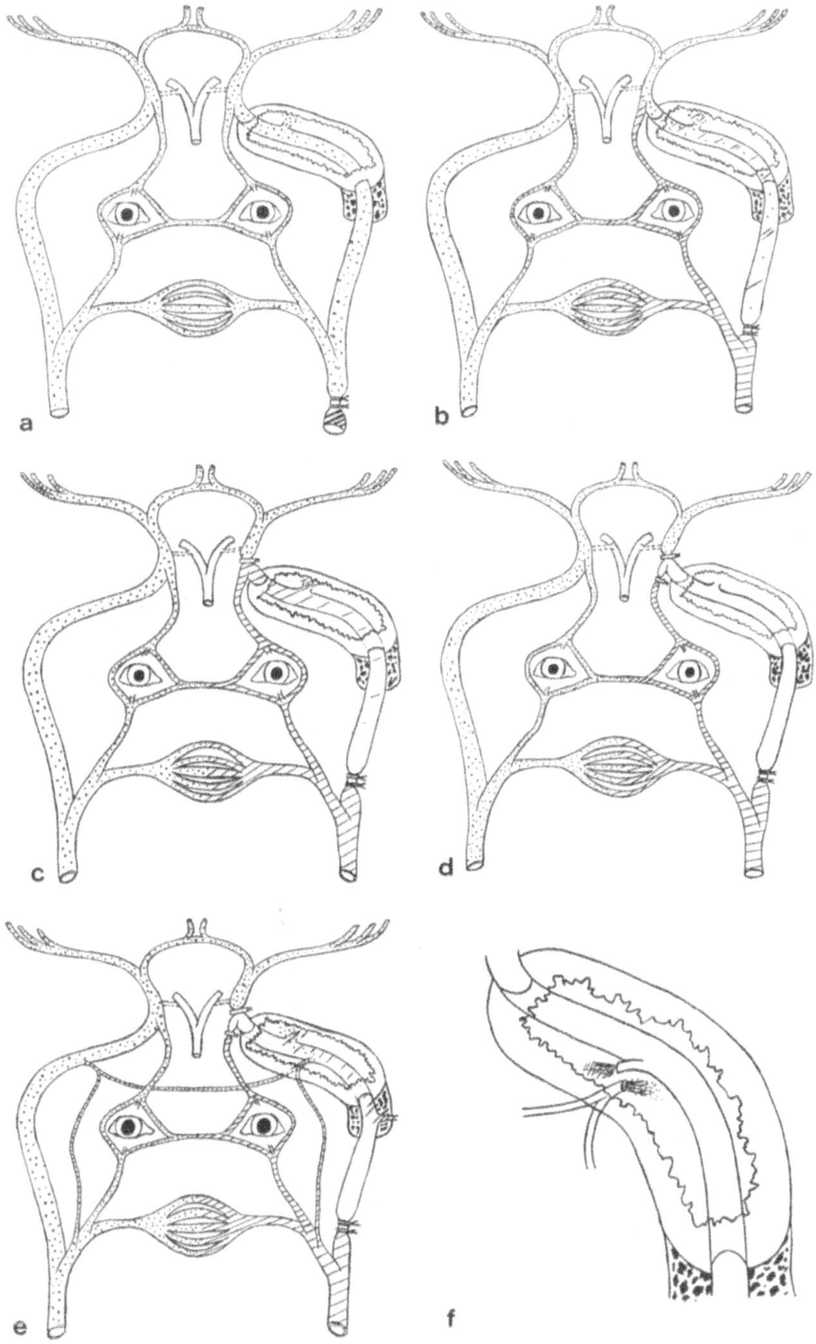
a
b
c
d
e
f

demonstrated with the simple autopsy cadaver experiment in Fig. 2. Finding the vessels wasn't quite to easy. In fresh cadavers the vessels are so thin walled as to be transparent remembling fine arachnoid adhesions (Fig. 3) (or trabeculae?). When fixed and/or injected they become easier to find especially after one knows where a how to look. Fig. 4 presents the artists composite of the average location and connections of these vessels which provide a small caliber but short and hence very effective collateral between the two internal carotids and the internal and externals bilaterally. Dorcas Paget [74] generously reviewed our findings. She thought the meningo hypophyseal might be the remnant of assimilation of the maxillary artery and the artery to Rathke's pouch.

Branches of the parasellar carotid are mentioned as early as 1863 (Power [103]), but today's standard texts still picture the carotid as a smooth non-branching tube from the bifurcation in the neck to the departure of the ophthalmic [19, 20, 45, 100, 115]. Singleton [113] in 1939 mentioned that there might possibly be collaterals in parasellar region but not significant as compared to the ophthalmic artery. Harrison and Hearn [43] in 1961 also postulated a possible partial collateral via such vessels but did not describe their presence. Then within one decade the definitive normal anastomotic pathways in the parasellar region were determined [60, 108, 77]. It was gratifying to find that independently and simultaneously Schnurer and Stattin [108] 1963 found vasculature virtually identical to that found by us the same year [77] except for the occassional different take off of the inferior hypophyseal artery. We found the arteries tend to adhere to the wall of the carotid giving the appearance of departing at some distance from the common trunk, occassionally even branching in the adventitia (Fig. 3). Understandably they chose different terminology. We used terms that described the destination as much as possible. Wallace [128] 1967 demonstrated all these vessels angiographically except the capsular arteries and created a nice chart comparing the terminology.

Coincidental findings are not at all surprising as the levels of knowledge, clinical challenges etc. are common world wide. Sometimes a significant original source is buried and forgotten under a misleading title. Sometimes a worker is unaware of his own source of current knowledge, honestly but mistakenly believing his ideas are original forgetting that he heard or read of a similar concept before.

However, it is more than suprising when 10 or more years later authors copied the drawings without reference [111]: use identical terminology, refer to another aspect of the original work (thus obviously aware of it) but not to the vascular findings [31, 104] and then in a later publication refer only to their own work for this anatomy [130] or publish without reference a word for word copy of the original description [118].

Whereas the carotid floats free of contact with bone throughout most of

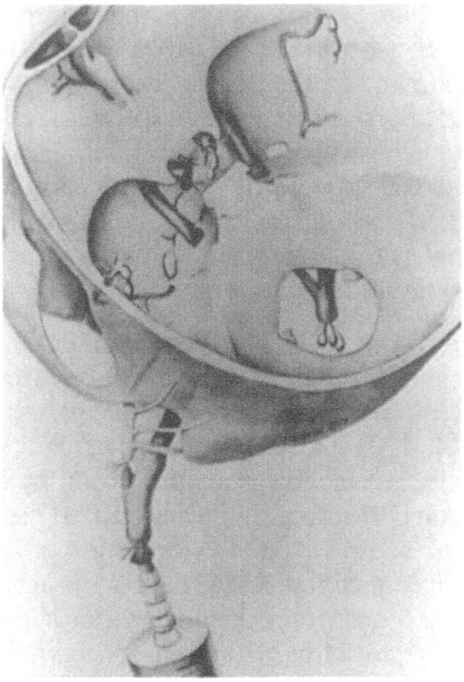

Fig. 2. Cadaver experiment with left external, ophthalmic and supraclinoid carotid ligated. Water injected into left common carotid appears instantly at cut ends of opposite carotids and both middle meningeals. Reprinted with permission from Parkinson D (1964) Can J Surg 7: 251–268, Fig. 1

its parasellar course (usually in contact only medially and anteriorly for a small space at the point of curving upward to pierce the dura) the branches come into intimate contact with bone shortly after leaving this carotid and hence possibly are more susceptible to tear with fractures.

Finding a route into these vessels was the next problem. Anatomy texts were less then helpful with different spacings of the cranial nerves pictured from text to text, one [45] stating that the relationship is, "actually of no clinical importance as the nerves are grouped so closely that a lesion is apt to affect all together", ignoring Jefferson's [52] observations. Examination of a series of cadavers confirmed that posteriorly cranial nerves three and four enter the dura via a groove between the anterior and posterior clinoid attachments of the tentorium while five and six enter posteriorly much lower down leaving a triangular space [78] as they all converge at the superior orbital fissure. Posteriorly the space is widest and deepest as the dura of the dorsum slopes laterally and upward to form the under surface of the tentorium on the way is the medial wall of the cavity commonly called "cavernous sinus" (Figs. 4 and 5). An incision in this triangle with retraction provided an exposure of the carotid and its lateral and posterior branches without damage to the cranial nerves [78, 79] (Fig. 5). No one should attempt this approach without first verifying these landmarks on cadavers. This approach was first used to obliterate a fistula that persisted after occlusion of all the "standard" collaterals, and next used on similar case [83] with marked emboli floated through to lodge in the parasellar space (and the lung! [116]). Complete circulatory arrest was used with profound hypothermia and bypass pump.

The venous findings in these two cases convinced us that the normal anatomy was not a trabeculated venous cavity through which ran the carotid artery and its branches, but rather a plexus of veins as others suspected [5, 12, 14, 120]. In long-standing cases arterilized veins were adherant to and indistinguishable in texture from the carotid. A fistula as illustrated by Nelaton [70] with a single arterialized venous outflow via the superior orbital vein, would be cured by occlusion of such a vein anywhere between the carotid connection and the first branch of the vein just as certainly as clamping a persistent ductus arteriosus cures that condition.

We realized that we could be within the space known as the cavernous sinus yet outside the venous canals [83, 86, 88]. Encouraged by Norman Dott [29] we decided that we would approach any subsequent fresh case with the objective of preserving the carotid. Emil Holman [46] in 1923 recognized the futility of attacking entering and leaving vessels as recommended by Hunter [49] in 1762 and proposed block resection for fistulae of extremities; not feasible for a CCF. Our objective was to close the fistula. We avoided temporarily clipping the carotid for fear of intimal damage and operated the next case as the two previous ones with circulatory arrest under profound hypothermia with the excellent anesthetic and vascular team of W. Syslak, L. Whytehead and A. Downs [83, 86]. We used increments of total arrest up to 50 minutes at a time. Elevating the head and draining the venous blood helped clear the field rapidly.

Mannitol and lumbar puncture drainage were used at first but it soon become evident that they were not necessary as the combination of

---

Fig. 3. a Dissection left parasellar carotid. Note how tentorial artery (*T*) and inferior hypophyseal artery (*IH*) are adherent to wall of carotid appearing to leave as separate vessels. Pituitary gland (*PIT*). Dorsal meningeal artery (*DM*). Cranial nerve (*VI*). Note the delicate adhesions as the carotid is pulled away from the contact with the underlying soft tissue. **b** Looking down on left parasellar carotid with dorsum broken off. *m* Meningo-hypophyseal artery and its early branches and just beyond the broken off stub of artery to the inferior cavernous sinus (*c*). Reprinted with permission from Parkinson D (1964) Can J Surg 7: 251–268, Fig. 1

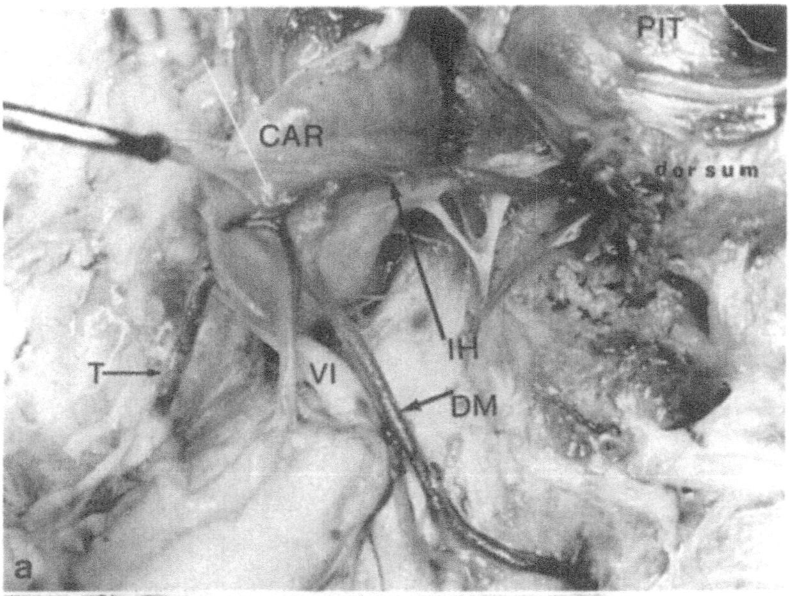
PIT
CAR
dorsum
IH
T
VI
DM
a

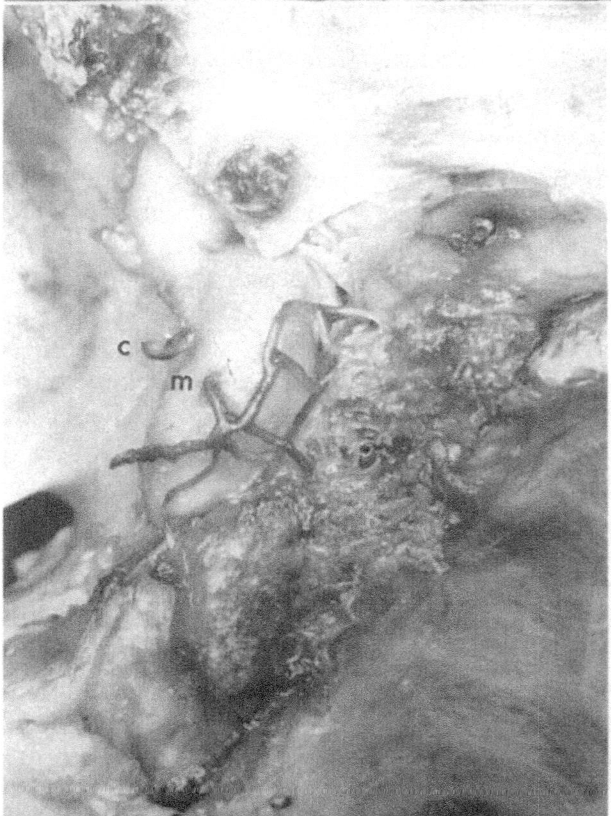
c
m
b

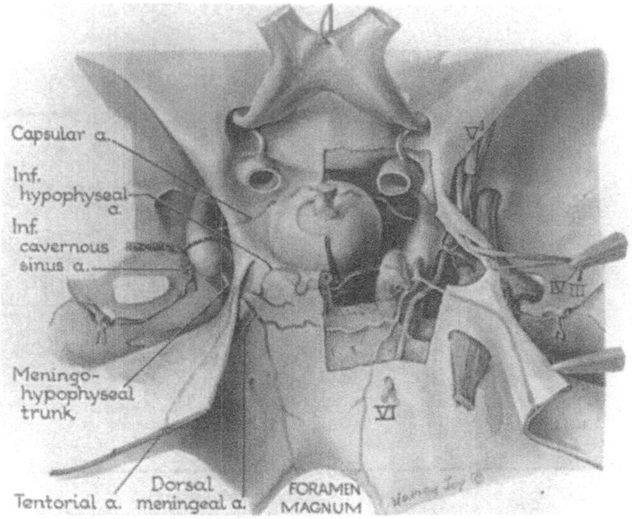

Fig. 4. Artists composite drawing of parasellar collaterals in average arrangements. Note also positions of nerves III and IV entering above and nerves V and VI entering below. Reprinted with permission from Parkinson D (1964) Can J Surg 7: 251–268, Fig. 1

hypothermia and drainage of the venous blood provided adequate dry exposure with minimal retraction. In the next thirty-six cases [86, 87, 88] using this method we were able to preserve the carotid and spare the cranial nerves. However, we had five deaths, much too high a mortality rate for what is essentially a benign lesion.

During these years it was the author's great privilege to visit Moscow as the guest of Serbinenko [112] and see at first hand the marvelous work he was pioneering with his fine balloon catheters making our procedure then obsolete.

Venous anatomy

Although occassionally pictured as a plexus of veins [100, 115] in the texts it is called a "cavernous sinus". The French on occasion use the delightful term "plexus caverneus la loge cavernuse". Our casts revealed an enormous [84, 92, 93, 95, 96] variation in the parasellar venous anatomy. Consistently there were multiple canals separating and coalescing, incompletely surrounding the artery leaving bare areas of the carotid wall. The most constant feature was the total lack of similarity from specimen to specimen and even from side to side in the same specimen. Unlike any of the standard intracranial sinuses there was no lateral edge or boundary; the venous

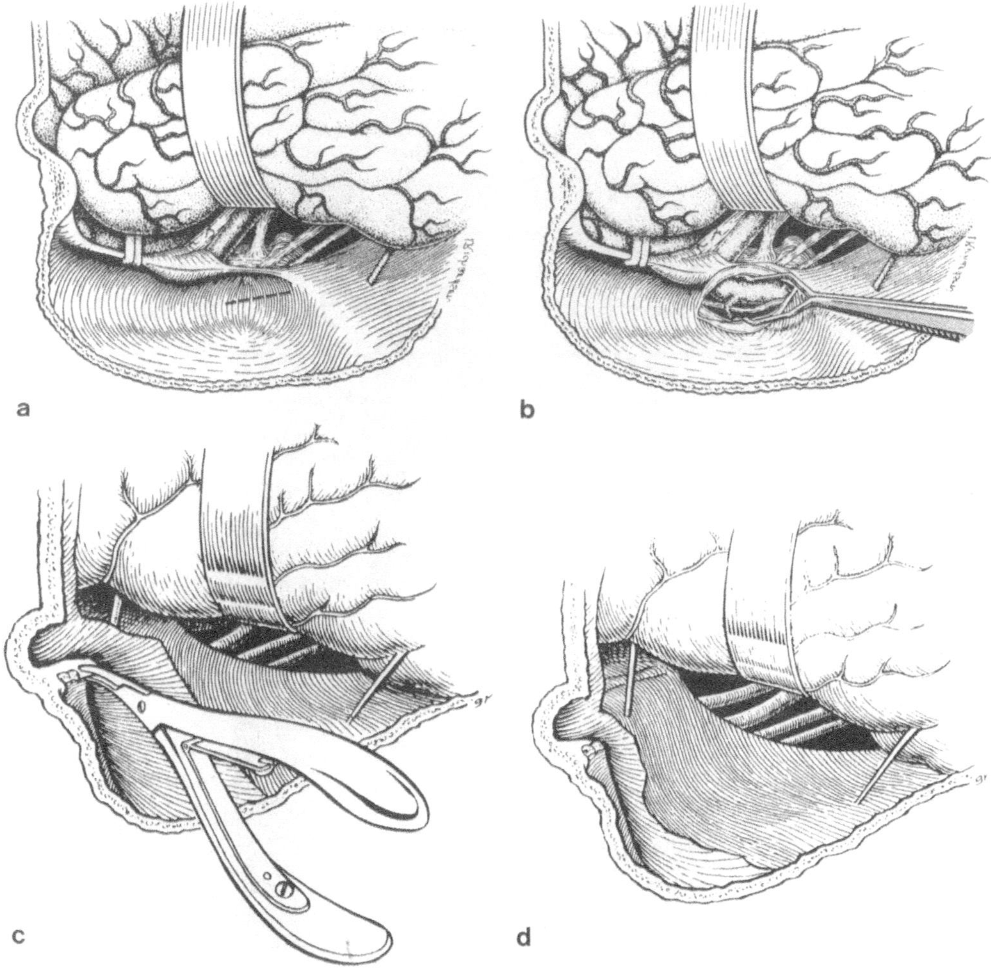

Fig. 5. **a** Incision outlined with dotted line. Note the "shelving" limiting anterior exposure. **b** Extradural removal of lesser wing of sphenoid and anterior clinoid increase available space and releases tethering of the Sylvian veins. Reprinted with permission from Parkinson D (1982) In: Youmans JR (ed) Neurological Surgery. Saunders, Philadelphia, p 3019, Figs. 15 a, b

plexus extended in continuity with the veins of the dura in the floor of the middle fossa (Fig. 6) like a road map with the national boundaries erased. The fat we found between some of the venous canals we thought was an original observation but it wasn't [11].

Kubic [57] described four venous canals in cross section with none interposed between the bone and the carotid. His illustration shows a partial interposition. An almost identical cross section of our shows a complete

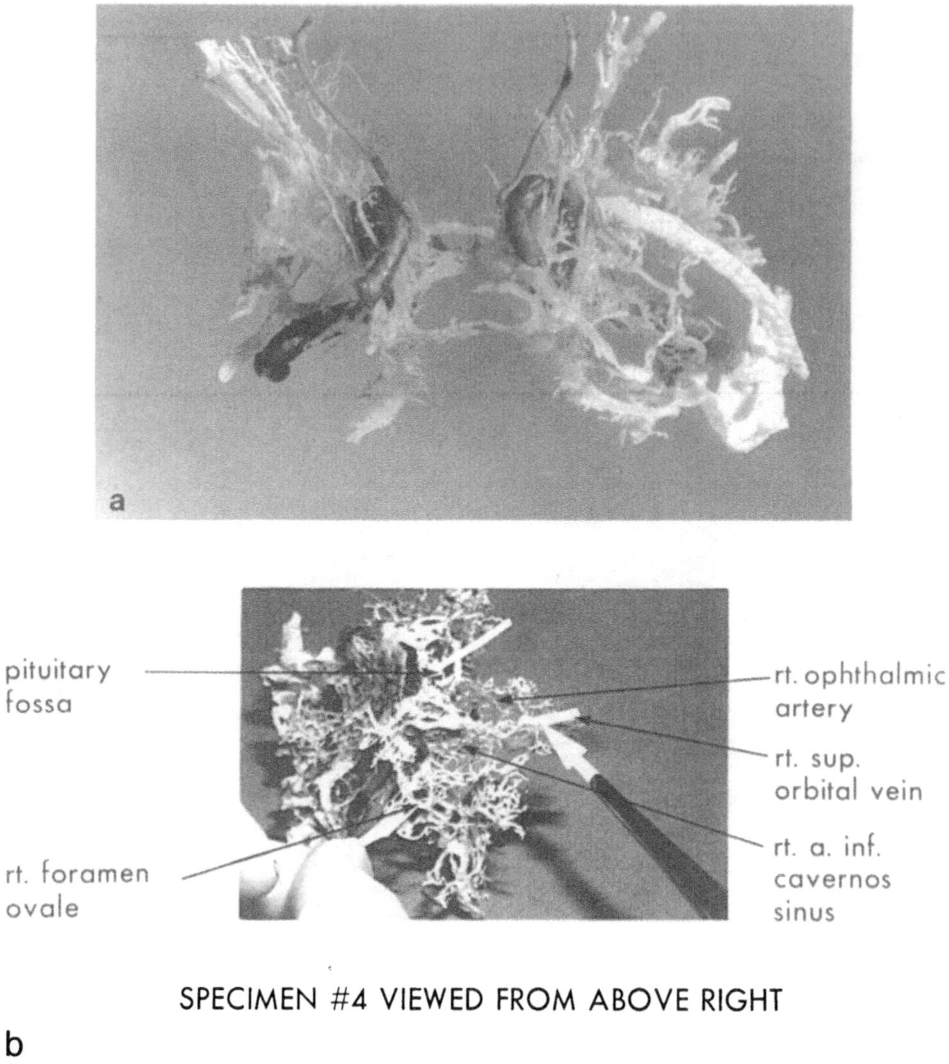

Fig. 6. a Arteries dark, veins light, ophthalmic arteries and superior orbital veins extending upward. Note incomplete covering of parasellar carotid by plexus of converging and separating veins without distinct lateral boundaries such as seen in the sphenoid sinus on the right. **b** Note continuity of parasellar veins with the veins along the floor of the middle fossa without change in character. Reprinted with permission from Parkinson D (1979) In: Pia HW, Langmaid C, Zierski J (eds) Cerebral aneurysms. Springer, Berlin Heidelberg New York, p 66, Fig. 3

interposition of a vein (Fig. 7). Schnitzlein [107] found a canal through the dorsum connecting the two sides in 76% of his cases. None of our casts revealed evidence of trabeculae but could not exclude their presence. There must have been something seen therein for so many competent observers to report even a few trabeculae [54, 104, 105, 107, 125]. One explanation for all the different findings is that different authors are looking at different specimens [6, 58]. Drawing any conclusion on the basis of one or two specimens is hazardous. Many specimens in our series have multiple, short, thin-walled veins. Adjacent walls would appear as wide trabeculae or short septae in cross section. We also found when the dural space is stretched some of the thin walls of the larger veins tend to fenestrate. Some specimens have a fairly large vein superiorly. On opening into this we have consistently found, "trabeculae" which on section have proved to be arteries. Along with the sympathetic fibers known to be in the region (see below) this may explain some of the "trabeculae".

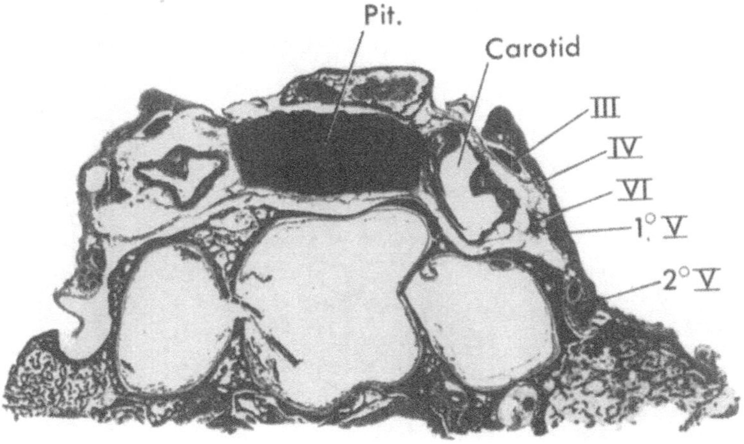

Fig. 7. Cross section through the center of the pituitary gland. Note just medial to and below the IV nerve on the right a small collection of fat cells. Note large venous canal on left extending from below the second vision of the V across the midline beneath the pituitary and just above this another canal extending also beneath the pituitary. The separating walls might appear as, "trabeculae". Note carotid on left completely separated from the pituitary by venous canals and not on the right. Reprinted with permission from Parkinson D (1972) In: Smith L (ed) Neuroophthalmology. Mosby, St. Louis, pp 98, Fig. 20

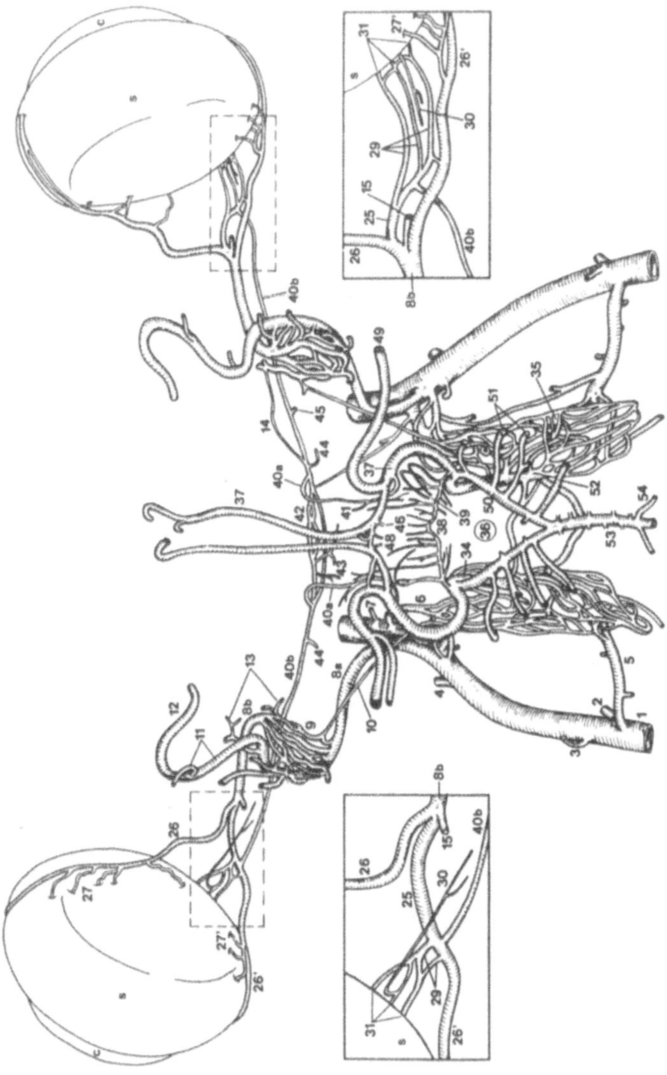

Fig. 8. Showing parasellar retia (*35*) and ophthalmic (*9*) of sheep. Note internal carotid (*34*) formed by coalescing of arteries of rete in turn made up of maxillary artery (*1*) and its caudal branch (*5*) with rostral branch (*6*). External ophthalmic artery disperses to form ophthalmic rete (*9*) which regathers to form continuing external ophthalmic artery (*8b*). *49* middle cerebral artery, (*53*) basilar artery. Reprinted with permission from Simoens P, Choshal NG (1981) J Anat 133: 481–497, Fig. 4

Solasol [114] found a plexus in infants and makes no mention of trabeculae. Interestingly in the Hunterian museum in London, specimens K-391-2 and K-427-2 casts of a still born, show the parasellar carotid branches and specimen K-429-1 shows a venous parasellar patterns similar to ours, *i.e.* multiple separating and coalescing venous canals without any demarcation laterally. In the Welcome Museum K-429 the venous casts look like ours (there is a persistant trigeminal artery [83] in this not noted by the curator) specimen S-228 beautifully demonstrates the triangular space between the nerves. Although it seems well established that the venous anatomy in the parasellar region is a greatly variable plexus of veins it is not proven that some of the veins do not contain some trabeculae in some individuals, we just haven't found such other than small arteries and sympathetic nerve fibers. Could trabeculae be remnants of the retia never found in humans [61, 85] but normally found in lower animals up to the size of the eland and the orix [121] (Fig. 8) and thought to be related to heat control [34, 35, 36, 37, 122]? Goshal [34–37] a world authority who has done an enormous amount of fascinating work on the retia finds them to be bathed in venous blood which connects across the midline as in humans (Fig. 8). If, however, the retia are a secondary development as believed by Tandler [119] rather than an embryologic development then any "trabeculae" in humans could not be a "remnant", of retia, but if related at all would be from later erroneous developmental attempts. Our work on the venous anatomy in the parasellar region is continuing. The finding of trabeculae in the posterior part of the superior sagittal sinus in 10% of autopsies by Berquist [8] is most interesting.

This while the parasellar venous canals are neither singular nor cavernous, rarely, if ever trabeculated nor, except that they are within the dural leaves, a "sinus" in the sense that the sigmoid, petrosal etc. are sinuses with distinct lateral edges, the term "cavernous sinus" will probably wrongfully endure. Whatever terminology the veins are a surgical problem only when arterialized. Anyone old enough to remember tic doloreux surgery on the sensory root recalls that the veins of the "cavernous sinus" can be troublesome as they are held open by the rigid dural walls, but the bleeding is easily controlled by pledgets of cottonoid etc. In case of any mass within this space the venous canals are obliterated and the surgical problem is solely one of the mass, its own vasculature and its environment of cranial nerves.

Saccular aneurysms [109] are a "mass" in this region as far as the veins are concerned and we have been able to open directly into them and repair the normal continuity of the lumen [92, 95] (Fig. 9). Although we used circulatory arrest this could be accomplished just as well with temporary trapping. We have never seen an aneurysm in this location with a neck to

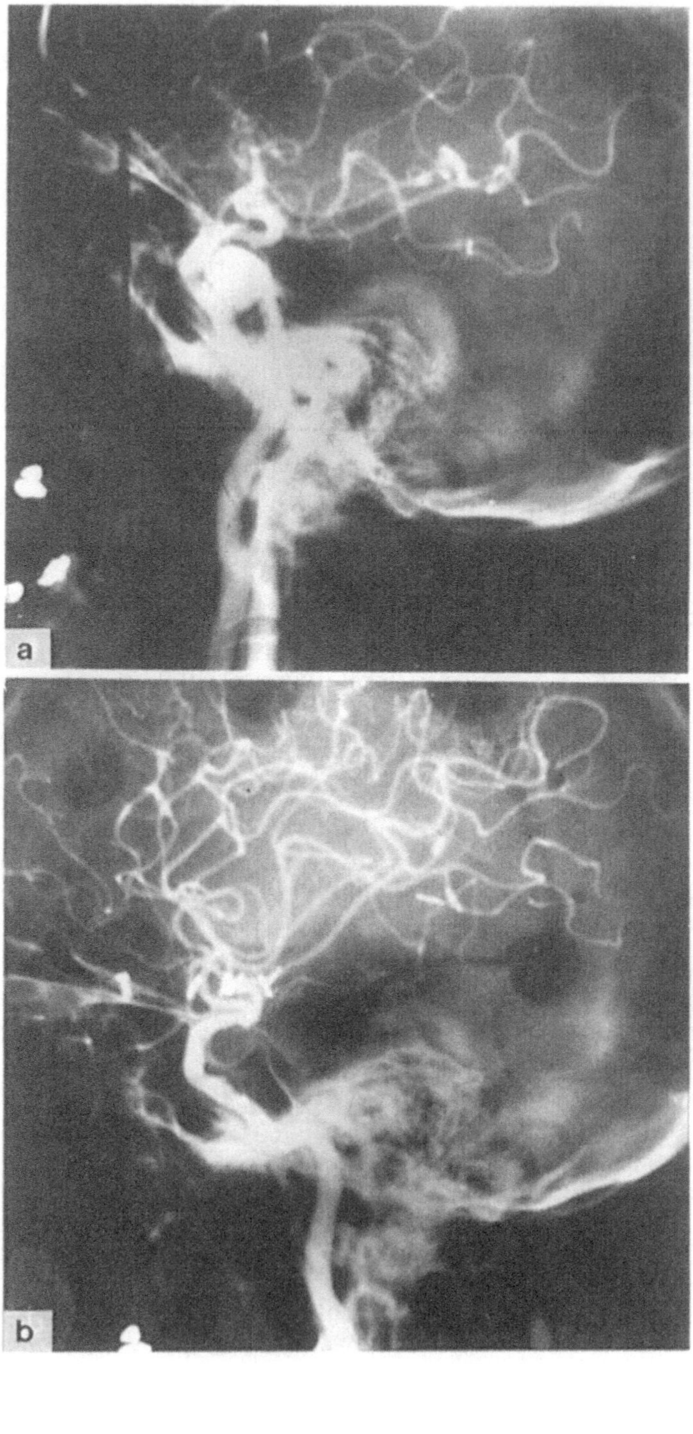
a
b

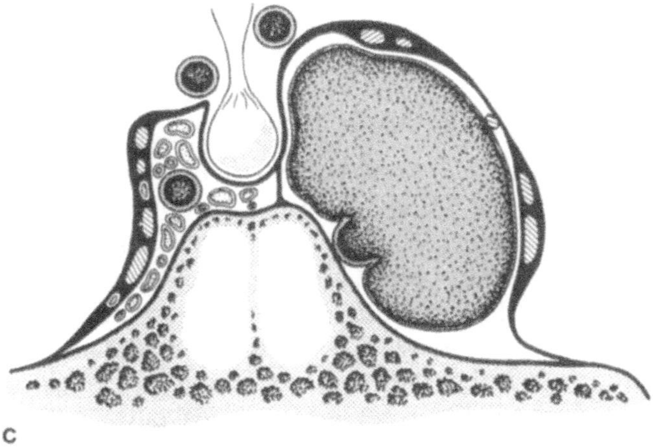

c

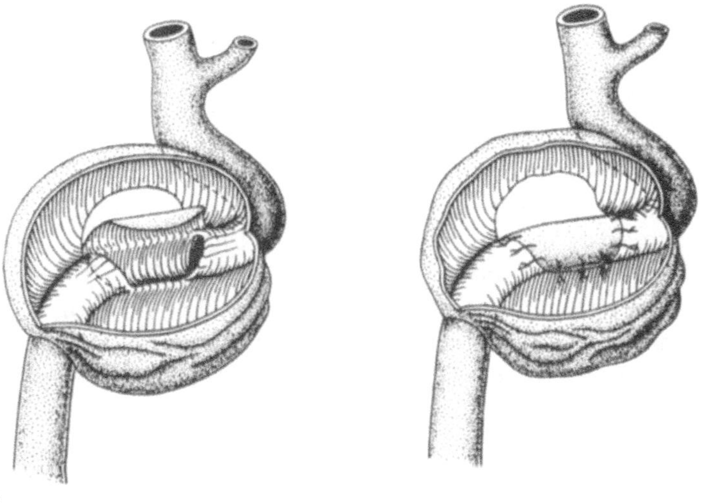

d

Fig. 9. **a** Saccular aneurysm of parasellar carotid; **b** After repair; **c** Mass of aneurysm obliterates venous canals and widens space between IV and VI cranial nerves; **d** Method of repair. Reprinted with permission from Parkinson D (1981) In: Youmans JR (ed) Neurological Surgery, vol 5. Saunders, Philadelphia, p 3020 which a clip could be applied, all have lumen expansions as illustrated. No doubt some do exist with clippable necks and the approach would require no circulatory interruption, only the assurance that the cranial nerves were brushed safely aside.

Sympathetic anatomy

While working in this space we found the carotid sympathetic joining the sixth nerve; an original observation until we found that Monro [66] published the same connection in 1732. Later we found that when this connection is made all the connecting fibers later leave the sixth to join the first devision of the fifth [98, 99] and postulated that the sympathetic supply to the arteries and other structures comes from the carotid nerve(s) as elsewhere in the body rather than that a plexus of the carotid artery give off branches to the pupil etc. If correct this would leave two as yet unrecognized syndromes (Figs. 10 and 11).

Surgical aids

1. Intraoperative serial angiography [89, 91] has been the single greatest assistance enabling instant evaluation of the lesion at any time without disturbing the operative field (Fig. 12).

2. In cases with extreme "shelving" restricting the space anteriorly rongeuring away the sphenoid ridge including the anterior clinoid extradurally enormously improves the exposure (Fig. 5).

3. Brushing across the course of the fith cranial nerve with the handle of a scalpel enables one to feel and often to see the first division of the fifth if other landmarks are obliterated. If in doubt always go a bit lower as it is better to split a few fibers of the fifth than to disturb the fourth.

4. After starting the incision posteriorly in the triangular space it is safely extended forward by "plowing" the edges apart with a blunt hook.

5. An enormous aid in localizing the definitive fistula opening in difficult cases is obtained by using gentle suction once the veins are opened and noticing the supraclinoid arterial collapse and reexpansion or "flutter" and the increase of this phenomenon as the suction nears the fistula.

The foregoing may in part have set the stage for the brillant, innovative advance recorded in the chapters to follow but no amount of documentation, demonstration or teaching can endow the almost superhuman technical skills of Dolenc [26, 27] or Isamat [50].

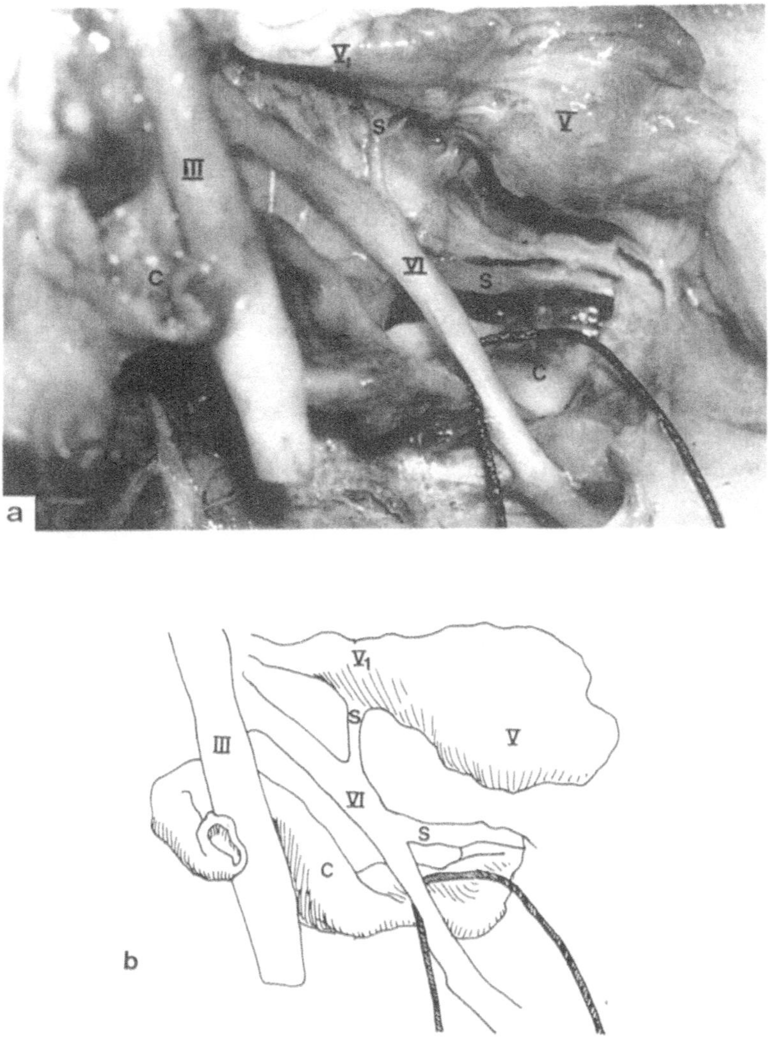

Fig. 10. a Dissection of right parasellar structures viewed from above and lateral V and VI. Gasserian ganglion and first division of V nerve turned down and out. *VI* Sixth nerve; *S* Sympathetic nerve joining VI nerve and leaving to join first division of V; *C* Carotid; *III* Third nerve. **b** Diagram of **a**

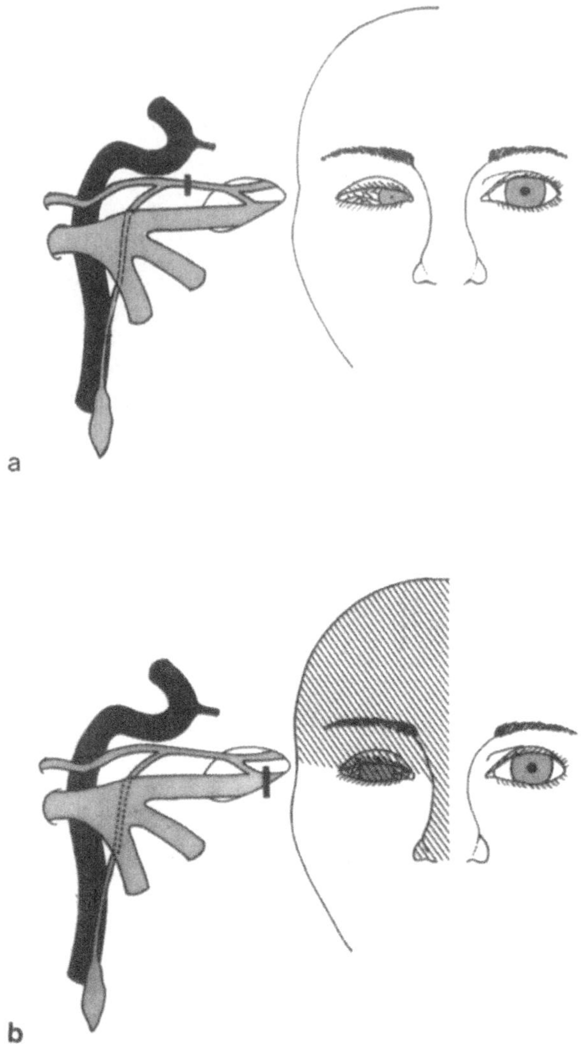

Fig. 11. a Syndrome that theoretically should result from a lesion (black bar) of VI cranial nerve proximal to supraorbital fissure: the eye signs of Horners plus a VI nerve palsy. Might also have vascular nad sudomotor changes in forehead. **b** Syndrome that theoretically should result from lesion (black bar) along first division of V cranial nerve at or beyond supraorbital fissure: eye signs of Horners and sensory disturbance in first division of V cranial nerve. Might also have sudomotor in vascular changes in forehead. Reprinted with permission from Parkinson D et al. (1979) Surg Neurol 11: 223

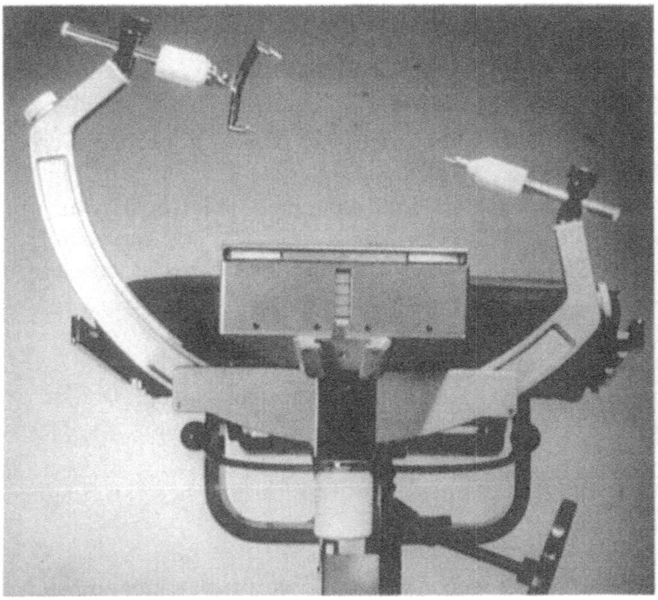

Fig. 12. Head holder for intraoperative serial angiography. Multipose C arm of sufficient diameter to accommodate automatic cassette changer which holds six cassettes. Reprinted with permission from Parkinson D et al. (1978) J Neurosurg 48: 1038–1041

References

1. Adson AW (1942) Surgical treatment of vascular diseases altering the function of the eyes. J Am Acad Ophthalmol 46: 95–111
2. Alksne JF, Fingerhut AG, R and RW (1966) Magnetically controlled focal intra-vascular thrombosis in dogs. JNS 25: 516
3. Baker MA, Hayward JN (1967) Carotid rete and brain temperature in the cat. Nature 216: 139–141
4. Bartholow R (1872) Aneurysms of the arteries of the base of the brain—their symptomatology diagnosis and treatment. Ann J Med Sci 64: 375–386
5. Bedford MA (1966) Cavernous sinus. Br J Ophthalmol 52: 41–46
6. Bergland MA, Ray BS, Tarack RM (1968) Anatomic deviations in the pituitary gland and adjacent strictures in 225 human autopsy cases. JNS 28: 93–99
7. Bernasconi V, Casserini V (1957) Caratteristiche angiografiche dei meningeomi del tentorio. Radiol Med 43: 1015–1026
8. Berquist E, Willen R (1974) Cavernous nodules in the dural sinuses. JNS 40: 330–335

9. Birley JL, Trotter W (1918) Traumatic aneurysm of the intracranial portion of the internal carotid artery. Brain 51: 184–208
10. Blackman GC (1848) Ligature of both primitive carotids. Am J Med Sci 75: 357–359
11. Bol'Shakow OP (1964) Macroscopical structural of the cavernous sinus. Fed Proc [Transl Suppl] 23: 308
12. Bonnet P (1953) Physiologie pathologique de l'exophthalmos pulsatile. Arch Ophthalmol 13: 233–251
13. Brainerd P (1985) A case of erectile tumor of the orbit: cured by infiltration of lactate of ion and puncture with hot needles after carotid ligation had failed. Lancet 2: 162–164
14. Brihaye J (1976) Pathogenesis and symptomatology of the carotid cavernous fistula. Third postgraduate course in neurosurgery. Pécs, July 1976
15. Brooks B (1931) Discussion Noland L and Taylor AS. J S Surg 43: 176–177
16. Browder J (1937) Treatment of carotid artery cavernous sinus fistula. Arch Ophthalmol 18: 95–102
17. Capp Al (1965) Personal communication
18. Cooper A (1908) A second case of carotid aneurysm. J Med Chir Soc Edinburg 1: 222
19. Cunningham DHJ, Romanes GJ (ed) (1981) Textbook of anatomy, 12th edn. Oxford University Press, London, p 907–909
20. Cunningham DHJ, Brash JC (ed) (1956) Textbook of anatomy, 9th edn. Oxford University Press, London, p 824
21. Cushing H (1905) The special field of neurological surgery. Bull Johns Hopkins Hospital 16: 168
22. Cushing H (1911) The control of bleeding in operations for brain tumors. Ann Surg 54: 1–19
23. Cushing H (1931) Electrosurgery as an aid to the removal of intra-cranial surgery. SGO 52: 129
24. Dandy WE (1935) The treatment of carotid cavernous a.v. aneurysms. Ann Surg 102: 916–210
25. Delens E (1870) De la communication de la carotide interne et du sinus caverneux. Thesis, Paris
26. Dolenc V (1983) Direct neurological repair of intra cavernous vascular lesions. JNS 58: 824–884
27. Dolenc V (1986) Presentations int symp on CS. June 1986, Ljubljana, Yugoslavia
28. Dorrance GM, Loudenslager PE (1934) Physiologic considerations in treatment of pulsating exophthalmos. Ann J Ophthalmol 17: 1099–1111
29. Dott NMc (1969) Congress of neurosurgery. Montreal
30. Elschnig A (1893) Arch F Ophthalmol 39: 151–177. Quoted by Hamby WB [39]
31. Fujii K, Chambers SM, Rhoton (1979) Neurovascular relationship of the sphenoid sinus, a microsurgical study. JNS 50: 31–39
32. Galen C, quoted in: Margotta R, Limes P (eds) (1968) An illustrated history of medicine. Hamlen Publishing, Feltham, Middlesex, p 96

33. Gigli L (1898) Zur Technik der temporalen Schädelresektion mit einer Drahtsäge. Centralbl Chir 25: 245
34. Goshal NG (1986) Dural sinuses in the pig and their extra cranial venous connections. Am J Vet Res 47: 1165–1169
35. Goshal NG, Khamas WM (1985) Gross and histomorphological study on the tostral epidural rete mirable of the pig. Int J Anim Sci 55: 304–310
36. Goshal NG (1985) Thermo regulatory role of the cranial circulation in cerebral temperature control. Vlaam Diergeneeskungid Tijdschrift 54: 246–261
37. Goshal NG (1986–87) Personal communication
38. Graf CJ, Hamby WB (1966) Personal communication
39. Hamby WB (1966) Carotid cavernous fistula. ChC Thomas Publishers, Springfield, Illinois
40. Hamby WB, Gardner WJ (1933) Treatment of pulsations exophthalmos with report of two cases. Arch Surg 27: 676–685
41. Hamby WB (1963–1973) Personal communication
42. Hamby WB, Dohn DF (1964) Carotid cavernous fistula: report of 36 cases and discussion of their management. Clin Neurosurg 11: 150–170
43. Harrison CR, Hearn JB (1961) A new aspect of collateral circulation of internal carotid artery. JNS 18: 542–545
44. Hayes GJ (1985) Carotid cavernous fistulas: diagnosis and surgical management. Ann Surg 24: 839
45. Hollinshead WH (1954) Anatomy for surgeons, vol 1. Haeber Harper, New York, p 560
46. Holman E (1923) Physiology of an anteriovenous fistula. Arch Surg 7: 64–82
47. Horsley V (1887) Remarks on ten consecutive cases of operation on the brain and cranial cavity to illustrate the details and safety of the method employed. Br Med J, Apr 16: 862
48. Hoyt WF (1968) Personal communication
49. Hunter WM (1762) Further observations upon a certain species of aneurysm. Observ Enqui 2: 390–414
50. Isamat F, Salleras V, Miranda AM (1970) Artificial embolization of CCF with post operative patency of internal carotid artery. J Neurol Neurosurg Psychiatry 33: 674–678
51. Jaeger R (1949) Intracranial aneurysms. South Surg 15: 205–217
52. Jefferson G (1938) The vascular aneurysms of the internal carotid artery in the cavernous sinus. Br J Surg 26: 267–302
53. Johnson JH, Parkinson D (1974) Intracranial sympathetic pathways associated with the sixth nerve. J Neurosurg 40: 236–243
54. Jones RR, Weitzel H (1970) Bilateral carotid vertebro basilar rete mirable. JNS 33: 581–586
55. Kocher T, Richardson RG (ed) (1968) Surgery old and new frontiers. Ch Scribner's Sons, New York, p 126
56. Krayenbühl HD (1967) Unilateral exophthalmos. Clin Neurosurg 19: 289–301
57. Kubic S, Youmans JR (eds) (1982) Neurosurgical surgery, vol 5. Saunders, Toronto, p 3112

58. Laws E (1965) Personal communication
59. MacEwen W (1881) Tumor of the dura mater. Lancet 2: 581
60. McConnell EM (1953) The arterial blood supply of the human hypophysis cerebri. Anat Rec 15: 175–203
61. Mahoney GCG de, Schachter MH (1972) The myth of the rete mirable in man. Neuroradiology 4: 141–158
62. Malpighi M (1686) De pulmonibus in opuscula anatomia, Balogna 1680. Opera omnia. R Scott, London, 2 vols
63. Margotta R, Limes P (eds) (1968) An illustrated history of medicine. Hamlin Publishing, Feltham, Middlesex, p 96
64. Manti-Albanez (1971) A tale of tubes. Canada, 12: 133–141
65. Moniz E (1928) La radioanteriographie et la topographie cranio-encéphalique. J Radio Electrol 121: 1
66. Monro A (1746) The anatomy of the humor bones and nerves. Hamilton & Balfour, Edinburgh, p 363
67. Mont RR, in discussion of Dandy WE [24]
68. Mullan, quoted by Peterson E [101]
69. Nafziger H, in discussion of Dandy WE [24]
70. Nelaton H (1873) Carotid cavernous fistula. Lancet (Holmes lecture) 2: 142
71. Nishimato A, Takewchia S (1968) Abnormal network related to the internal carotid artery. JNS 29: 256–260
72. Obrador S (1974) Spontaneous CCF produced by rupture of aneurysm of meningo hypophyseal branch of internal carotid artery. JNS 40: 539–543
73. Paget DH (1948) The development of the cranial arteries in the human embryo. Contrib Embryol 32: 205–262
74. Paget DH (1961) Personal communication
75. Pare A, Keyres G (eds) (1968) The apologies and treatise containing the voyages made into diverse places with many of his writings upon surgery. Dover Publications, New York, p 19
76. Parkinson D, Ramsay RM (1963) Carotid cavernous fistula with pulsating exophthalmus: a fortuitous care. Can J Surg 6: 191–195
77. Parkinson D (1964) Collateral circulation of cavernous carotid artery: anatomy. Can J Surg 7: 251–268
78. Parkinson D (1965) A surgical approach to the cavernous portion of the carotid artery. Anatomical studies and case report. J Neurosurg 23: 474–483
79. Parkinson D, MacPherson RA, Childe AE, Middlecote LR, Morrow IM, MacEwan DW (1967) Routine simultaneous biplane stereoscopic angiography. J Can Assoc Radiol 18: 371–376
80. Parkinson D (1969) Transcavernous repair of carotid cavernous fistula. J Neurosurg 26: 420–424
81. Parkinson D (1972) Carotid cavernous fistula. In: Vinken PJ, Bruyn GW (eds) Handbook of clinical neurology, vol 12. North Holland, Amsterdam, pp 267–288
82. Parkinson D (1972) Anatomy of the cavernous sinus. In: Smith JL (ed) Neuroophthalmology , vol 6. CV Mosby Company, St. Louis, pp 73–101
83. Parkinson D (1973) Carotid cavernous fistula: direct repair with preservation of the carotid artery. J Neurosurg 38: 99–106

84. Parkinson D, Shields CB (1974) Persistent trigeminal artery: its relationship to the normal branches of the cavernous carotid. J Neurosurg 40: 245–248
85. Parkinson D (1974) Rete mirabile, the marvellous network. Can J Neurol Sci 1: 121–123
86. Parkinson D (1974) Carotid cavernous fistula: direct repair with preservation of the carotid artery. Surg 76: 882–889
87. Parkinson D (1975) Editorial communication. Carotid cavernous fistula. J Neurosurg 42: 1, 119
88. Parkinson D (1976) Carotid cavernous fistula, direct approach with repair of fistula and preservation of the artery. In: Morley TP (ed) Current controversies in neurosurgery. Saunders, Philadelphia, pp 237–249
89. Parkinson D, Legal J, Holloway AF, Walton RJ, LaFrance RT, MacEwan DW, Johnston J (1978) A new combined neurosurgical headholder and cassette changer for intraoperative serial angiography. J Neurosurg 48: 1038–1041
90. Parkinson D (1979) Anatomy of the cavernous sinus. In: Pia HW, Langmaid C, Zierski J (eds) Cerebral aneurysms. Springer Verlag, Berlin Heidelberg New York, pp 62–67
91. Parkinson D (1979) Intraoperative angiography. In: Pia HW, Langmaid C, Zierski J (eds) Cerebral aneurysms. Springer Verlag, Berlin Heidelberg New York, pp 181–184
92. Parkinson D (1979) Surgical approach to cavernous sinus aneurysms. In: Pia HW, Langmaid C, Zierski J (eds) Cerebral aneurysms. Springer Verlag, Berlin Heidelberg New York, pp 224–228
93. Parkinson D (1980) Venous anatomy of the cavernous sinus. In: Williams PL, Warwick R (eds) Gray's anatomy. Churchill Livingstone, Edinburgh, p 751
94. Parkinson D, West M (1982) Lesions of the cavernous plexus region. In: Youmans JR (ed) Neurological surgery, vol 5. Saunders, Philadelphia, pp 3004–3024
95. Parkinson D (1981) Surgical management of internal carotid artery aneurysms within the cavernous sinus. In: Schmidek HH, Sweet WH (eds) Operative neurosurgical techniques, vol 2. Grune & Stratton, New York, pp 819–829
96. Parkinson D, Wilkins RH, Rengachary SS (eds) (1985) Anatomy of the cavernous sinus in neurosurgery, vol 2. McGraw-Hill, New York, pp 1473–1483
97. Parkinson D (1957) Internal carotid insufficiency, a useful physical sign. CMAJ 76: 488–489
98. Parkinson D, Johnson J, Chaudhuri A (1978) Sympathetic connections of the fifth and sixth cranial nerves. Anat Rec 191: 221–226
99. Parkinson D, Bernard M (1979) Horner syndrome and others. Surg Neurol 11: 221–223
100. Pernkoph E (1963) Atlas of topographic and applied human anatomy, vol 1. Saunders, Philadelphia, pp 65, 73, 75
101. Peterson E (1970) Personal communication
102. Pool VL, Potts DC (1965) Aneurysms and anteriovenous anomolies of the brain. Harper and Row, New York

103. Power JH (1863) Anatomy of the arteries of the human body. JB Lippincott & Co, Philadelphia, p 130
104. Rhoton AL, Hardy DG, Chambers SM (1979) Micro surgical anatomy and dissection of the sphenoid bone, cavernous sinus and sella region. Surg Neurol 12: 63–104
105. Ridley H (1965) The anatomy of the brain. Smith and Walford, London, p 39
106. Sanders MD, Hoyt WF (1969) Hypoxic sequelae of CCF. Br J Ophthalmol 53: 82–97
107. Schnitzlein F, Muntagh R, Arrington JA, Parkinson D (1985) The sinus of the Dorsum sellae. Anat Rec 213: 587–589
108. Schnurer LB, Stattin S (1963) Vascular supply of intra cranial dura from internal carotid artery with special reference to its angiographic significance. Acta Radiol [Diagn] (Stockh) 1: 441–450
109. Schnurer LB (1965) Personal communication
110. Seftel DL, Kalson H, Gordon BS (1959) Ruptured intra cavernous carotid aneurysm with fatal epistasis. Arch Otolaryngol 70: 52–60
111. Seljeskog EL (1973) Carotid cavernous fistula. Minnesota Med: 929–950
112. Serbinenko F (1970) Personal communication, Moscow
113. Singleton AO (1939) Intracranial arterio venous aneurysms. Ann Surg 110: 525
114. Solasol A, Zidunc C, Slimanc-Taleb S et al (1966) The veins of the cavernous sinus in the four months old human fetus. CR Assoc Anat 149: 1009–1015
115. Spalteholz W (1935) Hand atlas of human anatomy, vol 2, 7th edn. JB Lippincott, Philadelphia, pp 415, 459
116. Speakman TJ (1964) Internal occlusion of a carotid cavernous fistula. J Neurosurg 21: 303–305
117. Sweet WH, Bennett HS (1948) Changes in internal carotid pressure during carotid and jugular occlusion and their clinical significance. JNS 5: 178–196
118. Thalamon J (1978) Volume neuroradiologic 14-2. Masson et cie Éditions, St. Germain Paris, p 333
119. Tandler J (1906) Zur Entwicklungsgeschichte der arteriellen Wundernetze. Anat Hefte 31: 235–265
120. Taptas JN (1949) La loge du sinus caverneux rev. Atoneuraophthalmol 21: 193–199
121. Taveras JM, Mount LA, Friednberg RM (1954) Arteriographic demonstration of external carotid anastomosis through the ophthalmalous anterior. Radiology 63: 525–530
122. Taylor CR (1969) The eland and the oryx. Scientific American 220: 88–95
123. Travers B (1811) A case of aneurysm of anastomosis in the orbit, by ligation of the common carotid artery. Med Clin Tr 2: 1–16
124. Twitchell A (1984) Gunshot wound of the face and neck. Ligation of the common carotid artery. N Engl J Med 1: 188–193
125. Umansky F, Nathan H (1982) The cavernous sinus with special reference to its lateral wall. JNS 56: 288–234
126. Uihlein A, Terry HR Jr, Payne WS, Kirklin JW (1962) Operations on intra cranial aneurysms with induced by hypothermia below 15 °C and total circulatory arrest. JNS 19: 237–239

127. Vesalius A, quoted in: Garrison FH (1966) History of median. Saunders, Philadelphia, p 219
128. Wallace S, Goldberg GI, Leeds ME, Mishlin MM (1967) The cavernous branches of the internal carotid artery. Am J Roentgenol Radium Ther Nuc Med 1: 34–46
129. Winslow JB (1734) Exposition anatomique de la structure du corps humain, vol 2. Prevast, London, p 31
130. Zeal AA, Rhoton AL (1978) Microsurgical anatomy of posterior cerebral artery. JNS 48: 534–551

Must we still call cavernous sinus the parasellar vascular and nervous crossroads? The necessity of a definite topographical description of the region

J. N. Taptas

Athens, Greece

The parasellar space known since Winslow (1732) as the cavernous sinus, although an important vascular and nervous crossroads, has for long been a matter of controversy. The fact that its description still differs from one book to another and that the same term is used to designate the space itself and one of its components, is confusing, particularly for the medical student.

The so-called cavernous sinus (CS) is not a trabeculated venous canal but a network of extradural veins that is part of the venous network of the base of the skull.

The venous pathways, the internal carotid artery, and the oculomotor cranial nerves

The venous pathway, the internal carotid artery (ICA) and the oculomotor cranial nerves cross the medial portion of the middle cerebral fossa in an extradural space formed on each side of the sella turcica by the diverging aspects of a dural fold which is the temporal segment of the tentorium cerebelli. In this space the venous pathway has only neighborhood relations with the carotid artery and the cranial nerves. The author presents a topographical description of the parasellar space, its dural walls, the vascular and nervous elements it contains and their relationship with the dura. A new terminology is proposed.

My personal struggle with this region started more than 40 years ago when as a young medical student in Paris, I could not understand the cavernous sinus described in the French anatomy textbooks as a trabeculated venous canal, bearing a close resemblance to the corpus cavernosum of the penis, through which the internal carotid artery and the abducens nerve traveled freely. After dissections of fresh specimens of adults and newly born and premature infants, I reached the conclusion that the parasellar venous pathway and its relationship with the carotid artery and the cranial nerves were very different from the classical description, but also that it was impossible by dissection alone to understand and conceptualize the anatomy of this particular region as well as that of the cranial dura in general. Indeed the adherence of the dura propria (internal layer of the pericerebral dura) to the intracranial periosteum (external layer of the dura) allows the inspection and description only of the interior aspect of the dura and this was probably the cause of many misinterpretations.

In my opinion the only way to understand the morphology of the cranial dura propria was to consider it as a continuous fibrous sheath formed and shaped around the brain, its vessels and nerves, during embryonic development. It is evident that the morphology of the cranial dura and that of the cranial bones, both originating from the initial ectomeninx, as well as the disposition of the cerebral vessels and cranial nerves, are the direct consequence of the development of the brain. One of the consequences of the embryonic development of man's frontal and temporal lobes is the formation of the anterior and middle cerebral fossae with the forward displacement of the eye and the orbit. Another consequence in regard to the morphology of the dura is the formation around the brain of dural folds involving the dura propria. The falx cerebri and the tentorium cerebelli, described as dural septae or dural expansions, are dural folds formed between the cerebral hemispheres, the hemispheres and the cerebellum. Every dural fold (Fig. 1) has two aspects, a free border and a peripheral border or convex margin. The two aspects of each fold closely adhere except when there are vessels or nerves between them.

In anatomy textbooks it is said that the extremity of the free border of the tentorium cerebelli attached to each anterior clinoid process, crosses above the peripheral border attached to the posterior clinoid process, forming a triangular field at the side of the diaphragma sellae (Fig. 2). This field is described as the roof of the cavernous sinus, the posterior and lateral walls of the sinus being formed by dural expansions.

In reality there is no such crossing of the two borders of the tentorium cerebelli. The extremity of the peripheral border is not attached to the posterior clinoid process. The two borders of the tentorium, free and peripheral, both cross over the apex of the petrous bone and the medial portion of the middle fossa on each side of the sella turcica (Figs. 3 and 4), the anterior attachment of the tentorium to the anterior clinoid process being at a higher level.

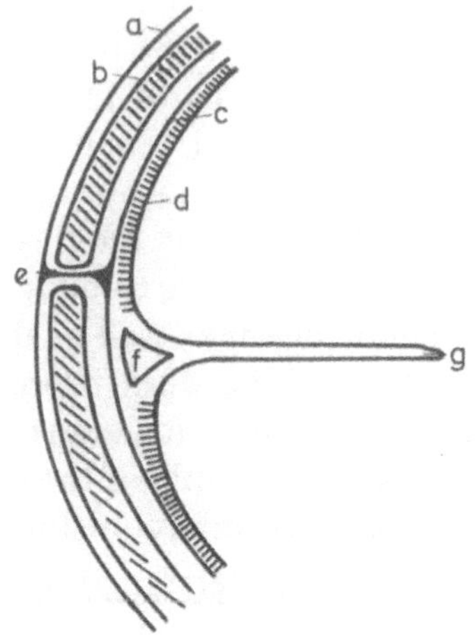

Fig. 1. Dural fold. Extracranial periosteum (*a*), cranial bone (*b*), intracranial periosteum or external layer of the dura (*c*), dura propria or internal layer of the cerebral dura (*d*), suture (*e*), venous sinus along the convex margin or peripheral border (*f*), free border (*g*)

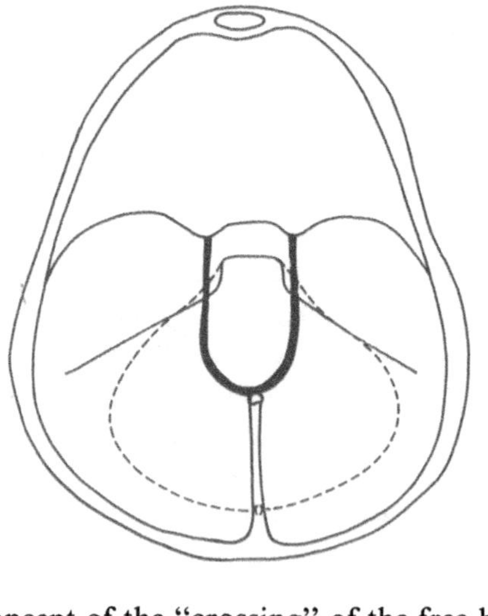

Fig. 2. The classical concept of the "crossing" of the free border of the tentorium over the peripheral border. Free border (black line), peripheral border (dotted line)

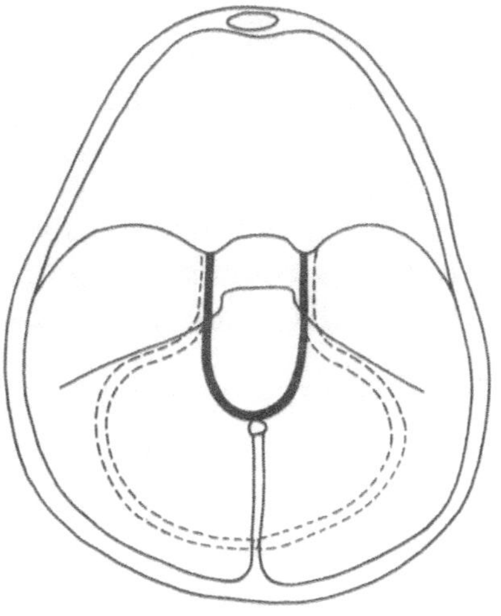

Fig. 3. Personal conception of the crossing of the medial portion of the middle cerebral fossa by the temporal segment of the tentorium cerebelli. Free border (black line), peripheral border (dotted line)

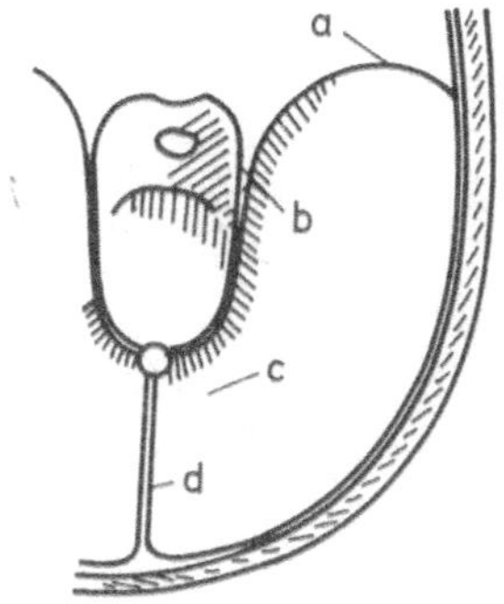

Fig. 4. Schematic view of the parasellar dural fold. Dural and cranial fold between the frontal and temporal lobes (*a*), the parasellar fold forming the space of the so-called cavernous sinus (*b*), tentorium cerebelli (*c*), section of the falx cerebri (*d*)

In the parasellar region, because of the existence of vascular and nervous elements, the two aspects of the tentorial dural fold diverge and form an extradural space (Fig. 6) which in 1949 [23] I called the "space of the cavernous sinus" to distinguish the space itself from part of its contents (the venous pathway). The superomedial aspect of this space is in continuity with the dura forming the diaphragma sellae while its lateral aspect is in continuity with the temporal dura propria along a line extending from the superior orbital fissure anteriorly to the apex of the petrous bone posteriorly. The osseous boundaries of this grossly triangular space are the lateral wall of the body of the sphenoid bone and the apex of petrous bone with their periosteum (Fig. 6). That this space is formed by the diverging aspects of the tentorium has been confirmed by the cross sections carried out by Parkinson and West [29]. Included in this interperiosteodural space are a venous pathway (the so-called cavernous sinus), the internal carotid artery, the oculomotor cranial nerves and in a lesser way the two first divisions of the trigeminal nerve.

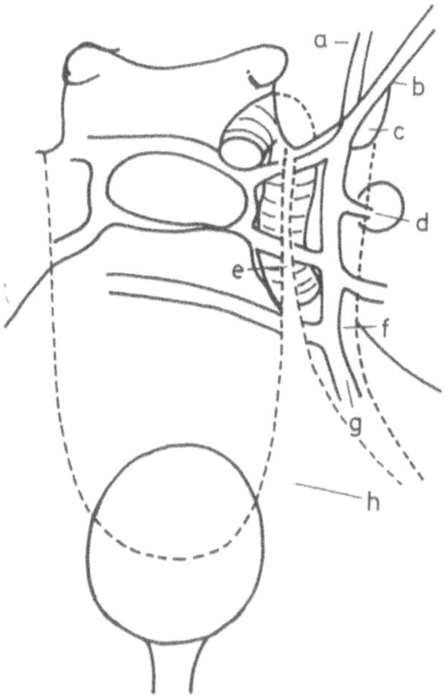

Fig. 5. The parasellar venous pathway and the ICA (schematic). The superior ophthalmic vein (*a*), the sphenoparietal sinus (*b*), the superior orbital fissure (*c*), the foramen rotundum (*d*), the free border of the tentorium cerebelli (*e*), the peripheral border (*f*), the superior petrosal sinus (*g*), the tentorium cerebelli (*h*)

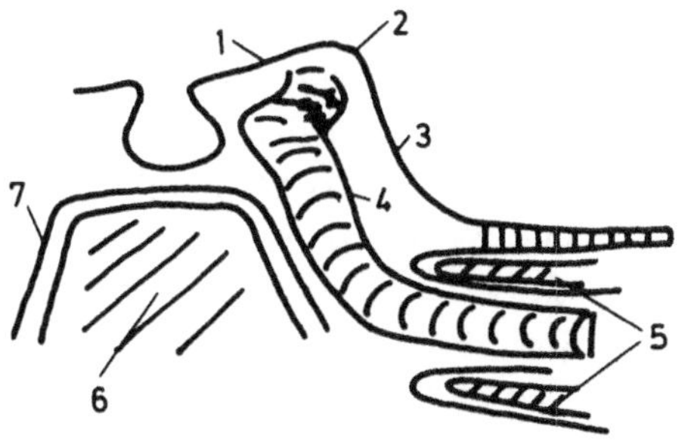

Fig. 6. The walls of the parasellar space. Superomedial aspect of the dural fold in continuity with the diaphragma sellae and the intrasellar dura around the hypophysis (*1*), the free border of the fold (*2*), the lateral aspect of the fold in continuity with the temporal dura which adheres to the intracranial periosteum (*3*), the internal carotid artery (*4*), the apex of the petrous bone with its periosteum (*5*), the sphenoid bone (*6*), the intracranial periosteum (*7*)

The venous pathway

It is not a trabeculated canal but a network of small caliber veins mainly draining the venous blood of the orbit towards the petrosal sinuses. After crossing the superior orbital fissure the ophthalmic vein, or veins, continue their course along the medial portion of the middle fossa, without change of character, and this anteroposterior canal takes a plexiform pattern by the adjunction and coalescence of other veins, like the sphenoparietal sinus and the bridging intercavernous sinuses when they exist (Fig. 5). This venous plexus communicates with the extracranial veins of the pterygoid fossa by connecting veins through the foramen rotundum, ovale and lacerum and is part of the rich venous plexus of the base of the skull. In the venous phase of carotid angiography the parasellar veins are quite clear, while phlebography gives a misleading image due to the coalescence and superposition of the different venous components.

The internal carotid artery

ICA emerges from its petrous segment over the foramen lacerum and bends upwards included in the parasellar space without piercing a floor which does not exist (Fig. 6). The artery ascends along the body of the sphenoid bone marking a groove on the bone, then makes a right angle and passes horizontally forwards to the anterior clinoid process. Along the bone the artery is in contact with the intracranial periosteum while in its horizontal portion the artery may bulge into the pituitary fossa and be in contact with the intrasellar dura surrounding the hypophysis. Along the medial side of the anterior clinoid process the artery makes another acute angle to continue its course upwards intradurally.

In its parasellar course the ICA has only neighborhood relations with the veins forming the venous network which incompletely surround the artery. This parasellar segment of the ICA is improperly called "intracavernous" and ought to be called "the parasellar extradural segment" of the carotid. From the artery arise small dural branches which with their divisions probably created the impression of trabeculation of the space. The ophthalmic artery may also have its origin in the parasellar space. The curves of the carotid siphon are the consequence of the formation of the anterior and middle fossae and not a system protecting the brain, on the contrary the curves of the artery may be a cause of ischemia of the brain, particularly in sclerotic individuals, each plicature of the artery narrowing its caliber.

As stated by Parkinson [29] except for the small branches of the ICA, the sympathetic fibers, the thin-walled veins and some fat there are no other structures in the parasellar space. We may add that a tortuous, elongated carotid may partly obliterate the space without impairing the venous drainage through the middle fossa thanks to the numerous intra- and extracranial venous connections. The existence of fat in the parasellar space is important as it proves that this space is in direct communication with the orbit. To become intradural the ICA does not pierce, traverse or perforate the dura, as is usually stated. During embryonic development the brain, it vessels and the cranial nerves are all enclosed by the original ectomeninx from which derives the dura propria, a thin fibrous formation, and the artery from extracranial becomes intracranial in its laterosellar segment, but still extradural, then intradural, without piercing or the bone or the dura. The involvement of the ICA by the dura propria corresponds to the base of the anterior clinoid process; here because of the adhesion of the dura propria to the intracranial periosteum, the artery is "fixed" to the bone, whereas in its extradural and intradural segments the ICA has some mobility. In its intradural segment the carotid has a thin fibrous (dural) sheath and a leptomeningeal sheath which when distended by cerebrospinal fluid forms a cisterna as described by Yaşargil et al. (1976) [27].

The cranial nerves in the middle cerebral fossa

As a consequence of the formation of the frontal and temporal lobes of man, the oculomotor cranial nerves III, IV and VI to reach the orbital fissure and the orbit must pass through the middle fossa included in the parasellar extradural space. To enter this space the nerves do not "pierce" the dura, the dura propria forms a sheath around each nerve and in the middle fossa the nerves have two sheaths, a leptomeningeal or epineurium and a dural or perineurium. (In the posterior fossa the leptomeningeal sheath around each cranial nerve when distended by CSF forms a cisterna [27]). In the middle fossa nerve VI is generally between the ICA and the lateral dural wall of the space. Nerves III and IV are very close to the temporal wall and the contact of the sheaths of these nerves with the dura explains why in 1927 Hovelacque [10] described the lateral wall as "multilayered". The ophthalmic and to a lesser extent the maxillary division of the trigeminal nerve, with their sheaths, are also against the temporal dural wall of the space. In addition to the cranial nerves, the sympathetic fibers cross the area, first on the surface of the ICA, to join nerve VI, then the first division of the trigeminal nerve.

Discussion

Since my first publication in 1949 numerous authors have studied the so-called cavernous sinus. Some defended the classical conception of an unbroken trabeculated canal [1, 8], others and mainly Parkinson [17, 18, 29], Kaplan [11], Papadakis [16], demonstrated by dissection and corrosion casts that the parasellar venous pathway is indeed a plexiform network of veins. Parkinson certainly made a major contribution to the understanding of the region and showed that the ICA can be approached through a triangular field of the dural lateral wall [17], thus opening up a new chapter in the surgery of the laterosellar carotid. Some of the authors who studied the parasellar space were not aware of may previous reports describing the parasellar venous pathway as a plexus, while I myself in 1949 as well as in 1982, when I reviewed the controversy about the region, was not aware that according to Poirier and Charpy (1901) [19] the concept of a venous plexiform canal had been published in 1884 by Langer [12] and in 1888 by Rudinger.

In 1901 in their textbook of anatomy Poirier and Charpy stated that in the newly born the cavernous sinus is not a cavernous formation but a venous network with two levels, a deep medial and a lateral superficial, but that in the adult it takes on its classical appearance by the coalescence and fenestration of its initial venous components. This concept of a plexus becoming in the adult a trabeculated canal was adopted in 1956 by Duroux et al. [5]. In 1970 Solassol [22] also described a parasellar venous plexus in 4-month-old fetuses. According to Duroux, Eisler [6] too in 1930 had described the cavernous sinus as a plexus.

I tried to find these older descriptions of the CS by Austrian and German authors and in general to compare the German anatomy texts with the

English and French ones. It was not always easy as the references were often incomplete and some publications nearly a century old. I did not find Rudinger's article but I found Langer's publication, not in 1884 but another in 1902 [13]. This Viennese author, after mentioning that the CS results from the junction of the superior ophthalmic vein with the sphenoparietal sinus, wrote that "with a more precise observation the CS presents a dense network of veins of different caliber" connected with those of the other side as well as with the extracranial veins of the base of the skull. But although Langer considered the CS as a plexus of veins, in their textbook of anatomy in 1901 [19] and 1908 [20] Poirier and Charpy reproduce schematic coronal sections of the CS by Langer showing a large venous cavity through which passes the ICA! I also found Eisler's publication in 1930 [6]; contrary to Duroux's quotation the CS is described as a trabeculated canal which Eisler compares to the corpus cavernosum. Yet in the same volume of the German handbook of ophthalmology, another author, Löhlein [4], reproduces a figure of the intracranial venous drainage of the orbit clearly showing the CS as a plexiform formation. In Hafferl's Topographical Anatomy (1953) [9] as well as in Sobota's Atlas (1964) the CS is presented as a trabeculated space with the carotid in its middle. On the contrary in Benninghoff's Anatomy in the 1950 edition [2] the CS is described as a cavernous tissue ressembling a bundle of veins (Venengeflechte) and in the 1971 edition [3] as a multilocated venous plexus.

I have not the possibility of finding the description of the CS in the anatomy textbooks of other countries but in recent English and French literature the uncertainty about the venous parasellar pathway persists. Thus, in Gray's Anatomy, 36th edition, 1980 [7], it is said that the CS is so named because it presents a spongy structure but that according to Parkinson it is a plexus of veins and that Pernkopf also depicted it as a plexus. According to Cunningham's Anatomy (1981) [4] the cavity of the sinus is divided by fibrous stands so as to give the appearance of cavernous tissue. In the last edition (1985) of Rouvière and Delmas' Human Anatomy [21] the description and drawing of the CS are the same as in 1927, similar to those of Testut in 1889 [26]. In Youman's Neurological Surgery (1982) in one chapter [28] it is said that the CS is a continuous trabeculated structure but that Taptas and Parkinson dispute this conception, in another chapter [29] that the ICA passes in the interior of the sinus which is subdivided into several canals by numerous septae and in another chapter [30] that the venous parasellar pathway is a plexiform canal. Most descriptions of the dural walls of the parasellar space are inaccurate and nowhere is the involvement by the dura of the ICA and the cranial nerves taken into consideration.

It is difficult to understand why for so long, and particularly in the Anglo-French literature, the concept prevailed of a large trabeculated sinus through which passes the ICA: perhaps because this anatomic pattern of the artery surrounded by venous blood allowed an easy explanation of the pathogenesis of the pulsating exophthalmos supposed to be the consequence of a traumatic or spontaneous rupture or fissuration of the carotid into the sinus. This pathogeny of the pulsating exophthalmos had first been presented by Nelaton in 1856 [15] in Paris and was admitted by all in the middle of our century when I started disputing the classical concept of the CS as well as that of the rupture of the carotid into the sinus [23, 24, 25]. Precise angiography has, since then, clearly demonstrated the possibility of numerous arteriovenous connections between dural branches of the internal carotid artery and/or branches of the external carotid artery and the parasellar veins resulting in pulsating exophthalmos, traumatic or spontaneous.

In my opinion a definitive topographical description of the parasellar space known as the cavernous sinus is necessary including its dural walls, the vascular and nervous elements which cross it and their precise relationship with the dura. A new terminology must be adopted distinguishing the space itself from its contents in the same way Meckel's Cave is distinguished from the Gasserian ganglion it contains. This description must be made available to editors of medical textbooks and to professors of medical schools so that centuries old misinterpretations are progressively forgotten.

References

1. Bedford MA (1966) The "cavernous" sinus. Br J Ophthalmol 50: 41–46
2. Benninghoff A (1950) Lehrbuch der Anatomie des Menschen. Urban und Schwarzenberg, München Berlin, p 205
3. Benninghoff A (1971) Lehrbuch der Anatomie des Menschen. Urban und Schwarzenberg, München Berlin, pp 481–482
4. Romanes GJ (1981) Cunninghman's textbook of anatomy. Oxford University Press, Oxford, p 953
5. Duroux PE, Bouchet A, Bossy J et al (1956) Contribution à l'étude du sinus caverneux. CR Ass Anat 90: 486–490
6. Eisler P (1930) Die Anatomie des menschlichen Auges. Kurzes Handbuch der Ophthalmologie. Springer, Berlin, pp 335–336
7. Gray H (1980) Anatomy of the human body, 36th edn. Churchill Livingstone, Edinburgh, p 746
8. Harris FS, Rhoton AL Jr (1976) Anatomy of the cavernous sinus. A microsurgical study. J Neurosurg 15: 169–180
9. Hafferl A (1953) Lehrbuch der topographischen Anatomie. Springer, Wien, p 2930

10. Hovelacque A (1927) Anatomie des nerfs craniens et rachidiens. Doin et Cie, Paris, p 61
11. Kaplan HA, Browder J, Krieger AJ (1976) Intracavernous connections of the cavernous sinuses. J Neurosurg 45: 166–168
12. Langer C (1884) Der Sinus cavernosus. CR Acad Sci Vienne. In: Duroux et al [5]
13. Langer C (1902) Lehrbuch der systematischen Anatomie. Braumüller, Wien Leipzig, pp 672–673
14. Löhlein W (1930) Erkrankungen der Lider. Kurzes Handbuch der Ophthalmologie. Springer, Berlin, p 268
15. Nelaton (1856) In: Thesis of Henri: Considérations sur les anévrysmes artério-veineux. Paris
16. Papadakis N, Lukl ND (1976) The cavernous sinus. Presented at the 44th ann meet of the am assoc of neurological surgeons. San Francisco, California
17. Parkinson D (1972) Anatomy of the cavernous sinus. In: Smith JL (ed) Neuro-ophthalmology, vol 6. Mosby Co, St. Louis, pp 73–101
18. Parkinson D (1973) Carotid-cavernous fistula: direct repair with preservation of the carotid artery. J Neurosurg 38: 106
19. Poirier P, Charpy A (1901) Traité d'anatomie humaine. Masson, Paris, pp 968, 973, 978, 981
20. Poirier P, Charpy A, Cunéo B (1908) Abregé d'anatomie. Masson, Paris, pp 723, 926
21. Rouvière H, Delmas A (1985) Anatomie humaine, 12e edn. Masson, Paris
22. Solassol A, Zidane C, Sliman TS et al (1970) The veins of the cavernous sinus in 4 months old foetuses. CR Ass Anat 149: 1009–1015
23. Taptas JN (1949) La loge du sinus caverneux, sa constitution et les rapports des éléments vasculaires et nerveux qui la traversent. Sem Hop Paris 25: 1719–1722
24. Taptas JN (1960) Loge du sinus caverneux et sinus caverneux. Rapports méningés des nerfs craniens et de l'artère carotide interne dans leur traversée de la fosse cérébrale moyenne. Sem Hop Paris 36: 1853–1860
25. Taptas JN (1982) The so-called cavernous sinus: a review of the controversy and its implications for neurosurgeons. Neurosurgery 11: 712–717
26. Testut L (1889) Anatomie générale, vol 2. Doin et Cie, Paris, p 212
27. Yaşargil MG, Kasdaglis K, Jain KK et al (1976) Anatomical observations of the subarachnoid cisterns of the brain during surgery. J Neurosurg 44: 298–302
28. Landolt AM, Wilson CB (1982) Tumors of the sella and parasellar area in adult. In: Youmans JR (ed) Neurological surgery, vol 5. Saunders, Philadelphia, pp 3111–3112
29. Parkinson D, West M (1982) Lesions of the cavernous plexus region. In: Youmans JR (ed) Neurological surgery, vol 5. Saunders, Philadelphia, pp 3004–3023
30. Day AL, Rhoton Jr AL (1982) Aneurysms and arterio-veneous fistulas of the intracavernous carotid artery and its branches. In: Youmans JR (ed) Neurological surgery, vol 3. Saunders, Philadelphia, pp 1764–1768

Anatomy

Gross anatomy of the cavernous region

H. A. Conesa[1], E. A. Zadorecki[2] and M. C. Lozano[3]

[1] Department of Anatomy, School of Medicine, University of Buenos Aires
[2] Neurosurgery Division and Emergency Department, and
[3] Neurosurgery Divison, Hospital General de Agudos "Ignacio Pirovano",
Buenos Aires, Argentina

The surgical disciplines understandably resort to the biostructural sciences as their fundamental basis for the determination of technical and tactical aspects. Nevertheless, faced with the technological breakthroughs which now support surgical practice, pure science is often relegated to the background and its value in research and explanation is not fully appreciated.

Anatomy is clear example of the aforementioned. Its passing from merely descriptive to topographic was a great step toward its application. The other anatomies, *i.e.*, radiological, correlative, projective, functional, clinical and surgical, focus on specific aspects from distinct angles.

These isolated concepts are now insufficient and only an integrated viewpoint will provide the surgeon with a clear, precise and useful anatomy.

The transcription of classical textbook knowledge is the best example of what applied anatomy is not.

Most textbooks on general anatomy or neuroanatomy include the cavernous sinus as an element to be described in the chapter on dural venous sinuses. It is considered to be found in a dural unfolding as an irregular space located at the sides of the sphenoidal bone, outside the sella turcica. The internal carotid artery is regarded as one of its main elements and some definitions state that it is a true mass of intercommunicating cavernous canals which enclose the internal carotid artery related to the cranial nerves and V/1. Other authors include part of the path of the V/2 and V/3.

The cavernous sinus is commonly illustrated as a coronal section diagram with the pituitary gland as a reference point. It shows a quadrilateral space with the cranial nerves in close relationship to the external wall and one of them within it in relation to the internal carotid artery.

Classical considerations of the cavernous sinus connections describe a bilateral communication made through the basilar plexus and the coronary sinus. The cavernous sinus is supplied by the two ophthalmic veins (superior and inferior) and the spheno-parietal sinus and drains into the superior and inferior petrous sinuses.

Textbooks which dwell more on the application of anatomy point out that both cavernous sinuses intercommunicate by means of conduits which course in front of and behind the pituitary gland and the basilar plexus. The latter, which extends along the clivus up to the foramen magnum links it to the venous plexus of the vertebral canal.

Surgical approaches with minimal craniotomies of deep zones and sectors which were until recently unreachable require another kind of appreciation. Microscopy, experimental and functional studies are forerunners supporting new techniques.

It is more difficult for gross anatomy to adapt itself to these constantly evolving sciences. Even so, practice on the dissection table can provide many answers, especially to beginners in neurosurgery.

The cavernous region is a deep bilateral osteomeningeal compartment, belonging to the anterior basal region, parasellar and subquiasmatic, which presents two areas of controversy. One regarding the venous tissue arrangement and its sinusal function, the other concerning its meningeal disposition. Since this chapter refers to the general anatomy of the region and is based on formalized cadaverous material (featured in all the illustrations), considerations on connective tissue and venous vascular pattern are not included herein.

The pure morphological considerations of the meningeal layers will preclude diverse interpretations as to the composition of the dura mater and the intradural/extradural internal carotid artery controversy.

The meningeal components which relate the Gasserian ganglion and the pituitary gland to the cavernous region are referred to the peculiarities of both tentorial circumferences. The dura mater layers separate at the apical level of the temporal petrous portion, forming a compartment with partitions which lodge the Gasserian ganglion and its branches, the pituitary gland, the internal carotid artery, oculomotor nerves and the venous sinuses.

The lesser circumference (free border) of the tentorium proceeds forward from the vertex of the petrous portion up to its definite insertion in the vertex of the anterior clinoid process and in the external facet (posterior) of the lesser sphenoidal wing behind the optic canal. The lesser circumference passes outside the posterior clinoid process in that stretch—slightly superior—forming the free border of the tentorium. It then emits a basal

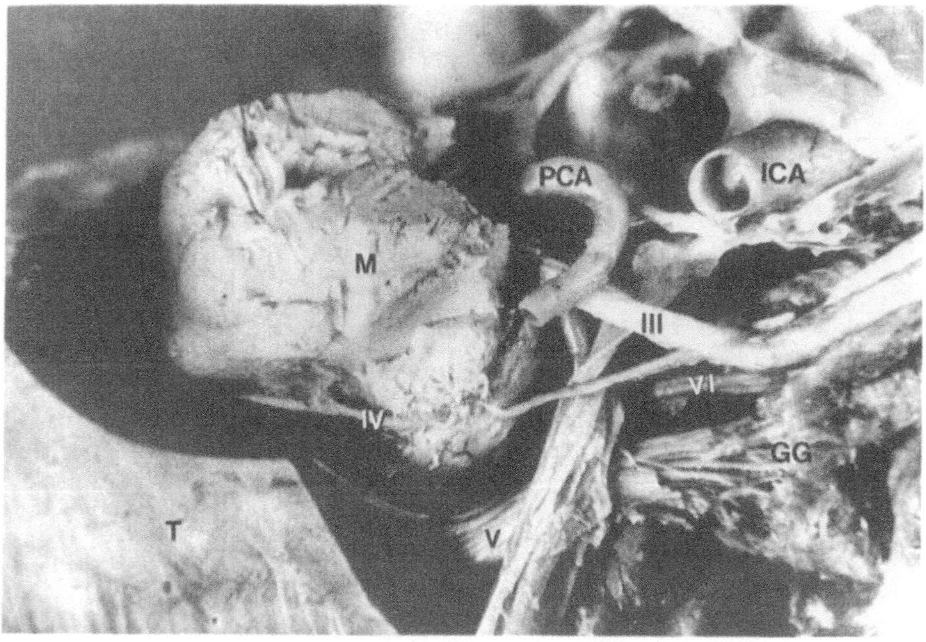

Fig. 1. Dissection of basal and cavernous regions. Superolateral view. Midbrain (*M*), posterior cerebral artery (*PCA*), internal carotid artery (*ICA*), cranial nerves (*III, IV, V, VI*), Gasserian ganglion (*GG*), tentorium (*T*)

expansion which inserts itself longitudinally on the sphenoidal floor of the medial cranial fossa. This insertion takes place between the petrous portion at the level of the foramen lacerum medium and the lateral ridge of the orbital fissure, constituting the external wall of the cavernous compartment. The continuity of this partition wall with the rest of the skull base lining goes towards the back with the petrous portions, and sidewards and forwards with the horizontal and vertical portions of the sphenoidal bone.

The greater circumference (peripheral border) of the tentorium inserts into the superior edge of the petrous portion up to the posterior clinoid process (free angle of the clivus). It then expands towards the base, constituting the posterior sector of the cavernous region contour. It continues with the basal lining of the clivus, where it forms the posteroinferior sector of the cavernous region contour, which allows the passage of the internal carotid artery and oculomotor nerves. This stretch is not continuous because there are three notches which become osteomeningeal rings: one, on the superior edge of the petrous portion (for the passage of both trigeminal roots) and the other two, of the clivus, for the passage of the medial oculomotor nerves (IIIrd and VIth nerves).

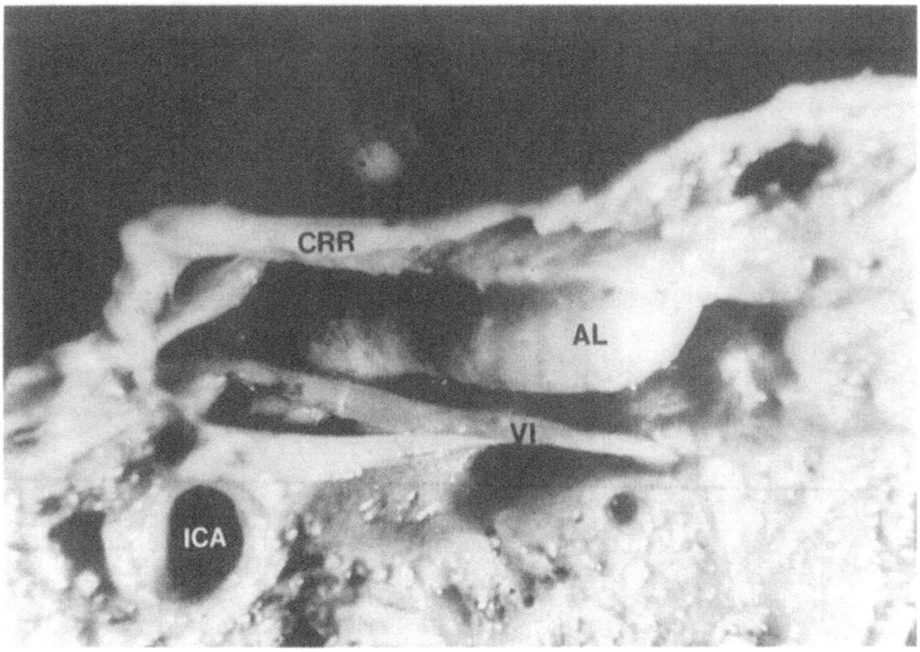

Fig. 2. Sagittal section (right). Lateral view. The section plane cuts the external wall of the cavernous region, permitting a view of the compartment space. Internal carotid artery (*ICA*), cavernous region's roof (*CRR*), anterior loop of ICA (*AL*), cranial nerve (*VI*)

Another expansion of the greater circumference takes place as it crosses the lesser circumference. It goes towards the back and covers the space between both circumferences. It corresponds to the roof of the region.

There are crossed meningeal bands between the heterolateral homolog clinoid process. A protuberance called the medial clinoid process is found between the homolateral processes. The internal carotid artery courses between the medial and the anterior clinoid process. The venous communication between the cavernous sinus and the coronary sinus takes place between the medial and the posterior clinoid processes. Thick meningeal fibroconjunctive tracts or even ring-like calcific bands may be found between these processes.

Figure 3 presents as points of reference for the section tha anatomical formation of the middle ear outside and behind, and the pneumatization of the sphenoidal sinus inside and in front. Cranioencephalic landmarks are the temporal lobe, orbital portion of the frontal lobe and the basal projection of the Sylvian fissure. The cavernous region extends within and inferior to these, between the aforementioned section landmarks and the osseous structures of the middle endocranial fossa.

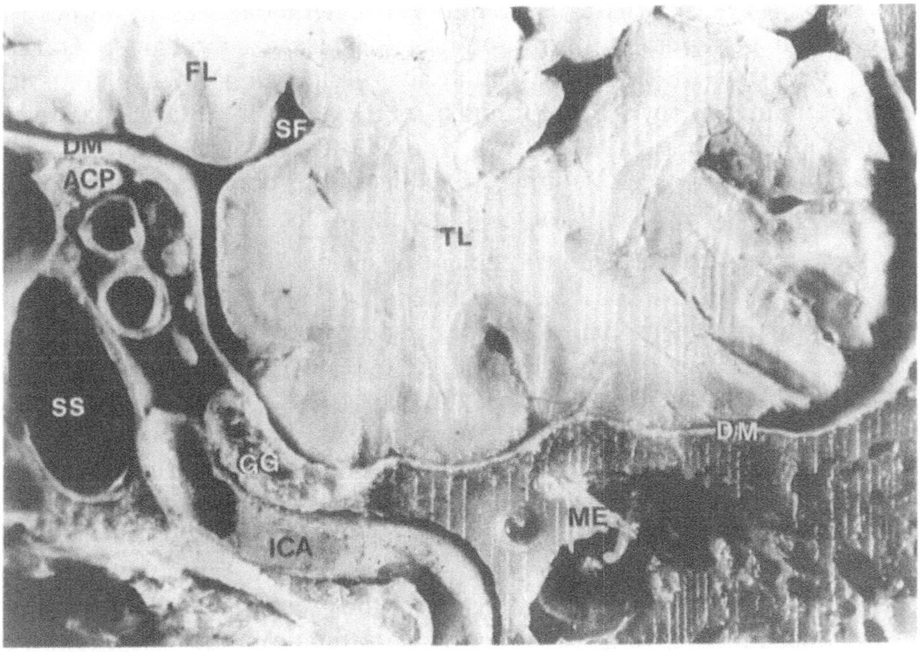

Fig. 3. Cranioencephalic coronal section with 30° anteroposterior obliquity. Posterior view. ICA entrance and its anterior loop are visualized. Frontal lobe (*FL*), temporal lobe (*TL*), Sylvian fissure (*SF*), dura mater (*DM*), anterior clinoid process (*ACP*), sphenoid sinus (*SS*), Gasserian ganglion (*GG*), internal carotid artery (*ICA*), middle ear (*ME*)

The dural layer separating the petrous portion from the temporal lobe at the height of the middle ear section is clearly differentiated. As previously described, this meningeal layer continues towards the Gasserian ganglion and from there the sagittal partition wall, which extends to the anterior clinoid process, is well noted. The external wall of the cavernous region is this sagittal partition wall which separates it from the temporomedial portion. This oblique sectioning permits us to follow this external wall and observe how the meninx unfolds to form the upper limit of this cavernous region, at the lower level of the frontal and temporal lobes.

The basal osteoligamentary structures, which enclose the carotideal conduit up to the foramen lacerum medium, are observed beneath the petrous portion of the internal carotid artery where it relates to the greater superficial petrous nerve. It is here where the artery penetrates into the cavernous region and approaches the lateral facet of the sphenoidal bone. This osseous differentiation is located between the sella and the origin of the greater sphenoidal wing. Here the internal carotid artery leaves an impression which is called the cavernous canal. It is siphon-shaped in all its extension from the tip of the petrous portion to the anterior clinoid process.

The oblique sectioning of the anterior sphenoidal section allows the observation of its sinus (corresponding to a large subsellar sphenoidal sinus). Three overlapping planes of the cavernous region's medial limits can be differentiated. They are, beginning from the outer: the internal periosteal lamina, the thin parietal bone wall, and the mucous sinus. The anterior clinoid ligament process complex completes the contour of the region continuing between the superior and medial walls.

Both ends of the cavernous segment of the carotid are observed in this slice. The petrous portion is seen at the back, and its relation to the optic nerve is observed in front. Its course remains above the section plane.

The petrous part of the internal carotid artery presents the classic "S" inflection. Its external bend is lodged in a bony compartment formed by the base of the petrous portion underneath the artery and its anterointernal edge over it. It goes through the skull along with tiny sympathetic branches which originate in the superior cervical ganglion (carotideal nerve). Branches for the vidian and third nerves arise from this carotideal plexus. The base of the petrous portion continues above the sphenoid bone coinciding with the shift of the direction of the internal carotid artery up to its entrance in the cavernous region. It is in that situation where it can be observed sliced in bevel (Figs. 3 and 4). A kidney-shaped mass is depicted outside and in front of this section: it is the plexiform portion of the Gasserian ganglion. Note the close relationship by contiguity of these two structures, which represent the posterior sector of the cavernous region floor.

After a short course where it enters the cavernous region, the internal carotid artery becomes horizontal towards the front and upwards. The V/1 arises from the Gasserian ganglion in the same direction and position. The structures observed (with greater detail in Fig. 4) are, starting at the bottom: the VIth nerve, the IVth nerve in close relationship to the wall and the IIIrd nerve. The inflection of the anterior carotid genu (C 3) is observed towards the interior with two section images. The lower corresponds to the horizontal portion and the upper to the cavernous part previous to the arising to the chiasmatic cistern in inferolateral relationship to the internal carotid artery. An ophthalmic vein is observed above the IIIrd nerve. A section of the optic nerve approaches the carotideal exit in the anterior upper inner angle.

Figure 5 presents as reference to the cavernous region the sellar medial relationship. It is a specimen with scarce sphenoidal pneumatization and with a pituitary gland which might correspond to the anatomical basis of an empty sella.

Figure 5 complements Fig. 4. It is observed from the back: the constitution of the foramen ovale and the free border of the tentorium crossing above the petrous portion to form the external wall of the

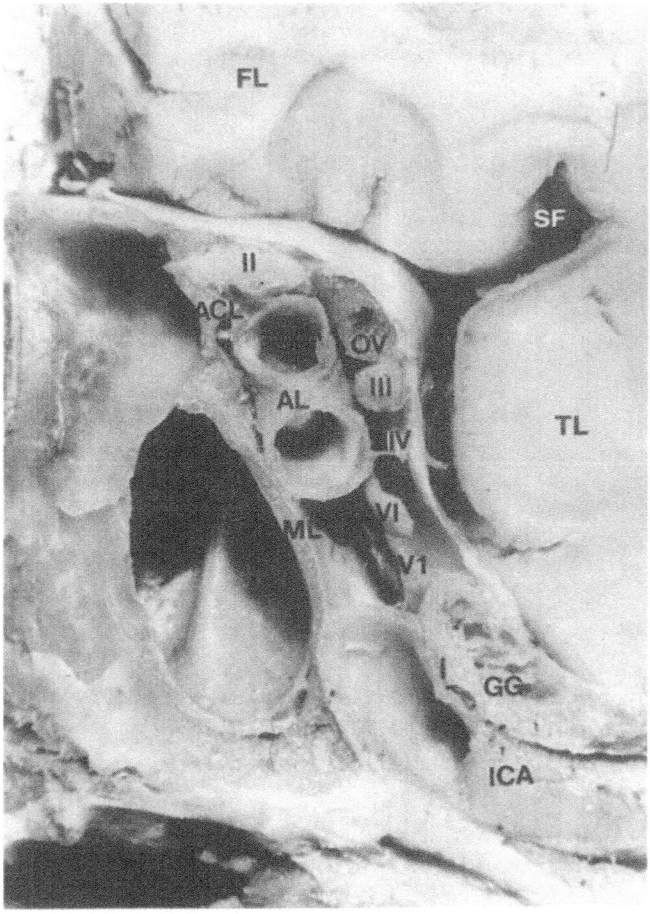

Fig. 4. Detail of cavernous area of Fig. 3. Anterior loop of ICA (*AL*), frontal lobe (*FL*), Sylvian fissure (*SF*), anterior clinoid ligament (*ACL*), ophthalmic vein (*OV*), temporal lobe (*TL*), medial limit of the cavernous region (*ML*), Gasserian ganglion (*GG*), internal carotid artery (*ICA*), cranial nerves (*II, III, IV, V/1, VI*)

cavernous region. It demonstrates the dural meningeal continuity with the basal covering of the horizontal and anterior portions of the middle cranial fossa. As it does, not have intradural elements the two layers face and touch each other.

The sellar meningeal lining between the gland and the osseous floor is clearly defined. This layer is a continuation of the dura mater from the base where it unfolds at its insertion into the dorsum sellae. The internal layer lines the sella floor, while the external layer jumps from the dorsum of sella up to optic canal, forming the so-called diaphragm of sella. The latter is

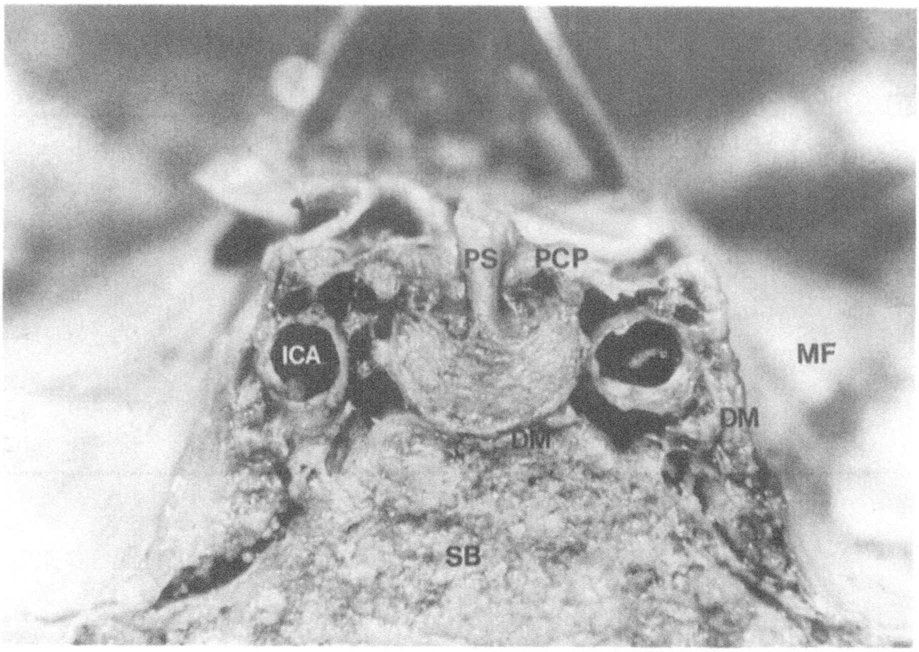

Fig. 5. Midhypophyseal coronal section shows the anterior loop of ICA. Anterior view. Internal carotid artery (*ICA*), pituitary stalk (*PS*), posterior clinoid process (*PCP*), sphenoid bone (*SB*), dura mater (*DM*), middle fossa (*MF*)

depicted vertically sectioned at the level of the pituitary stalk. The cavernous region is seen occupied mainly by the internal carotid artery in a high location—more parahypophysiary than parasellar. Lax tissue corresponding to venous vascular differentation is seen under the internal carotid artery (image of the so-called trabecular disposition of the cavernous sinus).

Figure 6 is a posterior view of a cavernous region section with the pituitary gland as a landmark. It is possible to differentiate and point out the carotideal ligament (Trolard) as a set of fibrous trabeculae that links the superior facet of the artery to the osteomeningeal sector of the region. The cavernous sinus anteromedial communicating holes are observed: the first under the pituitary gland, connecting the cavernous sinuses; the second hole over and in front of the gland, which has the same communicating function, known as the coronary sinus (Ridley), the third hole is located between the latter and the carotideal ligament. It corresponds to the unvalved outlet of one of the ophthalmic veins. The first two holes are elliptic in their sectioning because of the obliquity of the anatomical stretch. The terminal portion of the internal carotid artery is seen on the roof of the cavernous region. This anterior sector corresponds to the ventral boundary of the

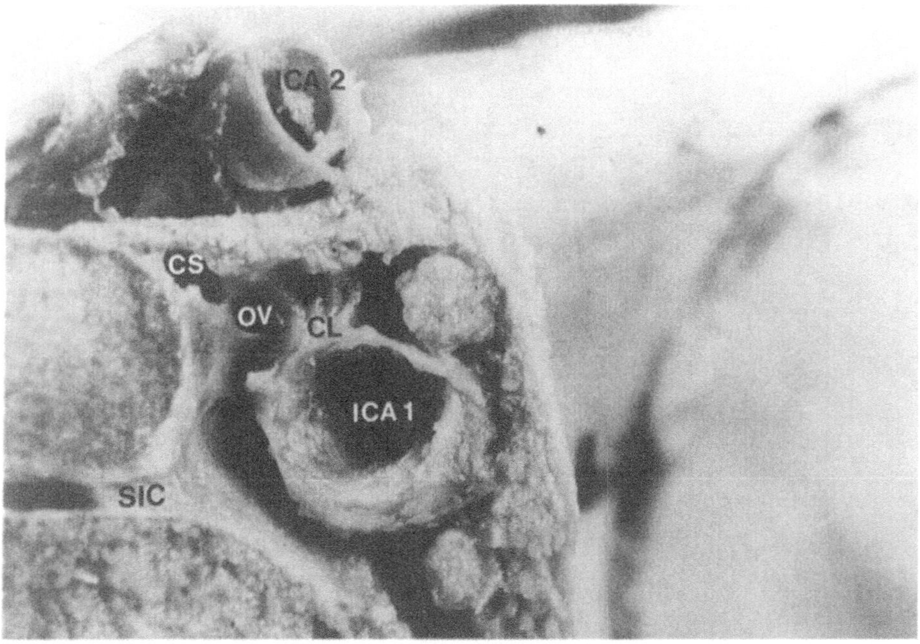

Fig. 6. Coronal hypophyseal section through the anterior part of the right cavernous region. Posterior view. Internal carotid artery (cavernous portion) (*ICA 1*), internal carotid artery (intradural portion) (*ICA 2*), carotideal ligament (*CL*), coronary sinus (*CS*), ophthalmic vein (*OV*), subsellar intercavernous communication (*SIC*)

cavernous region. A meningeal reflection in the sphenoidal bone (between the wings) is on one side, and on the other side continues with the orbital cavity through the superior orbital fissure, permitting the passage of the intracavernous nerves and the ophthalmic veins.

The cavernous branches of the internal carotid artery are not described here due to the thorough microanatomical description in other chapters.

The sellar and parasellar meningeal setting is demonstrated in Fig. 7. The entrances of the cranial nerves corresponding to the cavernous region are also shown. The nerves penetrate the narrow transdural zone which goes from the Gasserian ganglion to the posterior clinoid process. They approach the first portion of the carotid siphon. This zone, corresponding to the petrous vertex, was described by Jacod as a crossroads or "the petro-sphenoidal vascular nervous set". The external layer that covers the Gasserian ganglion was dissected at the right from the osteomeningeal trigeminal ring up to the individualization of its branches. This ganglion does not lean on the internal lamina but is suspended from the dura by connective bundles that are known in classical anatomy as Pricentau's

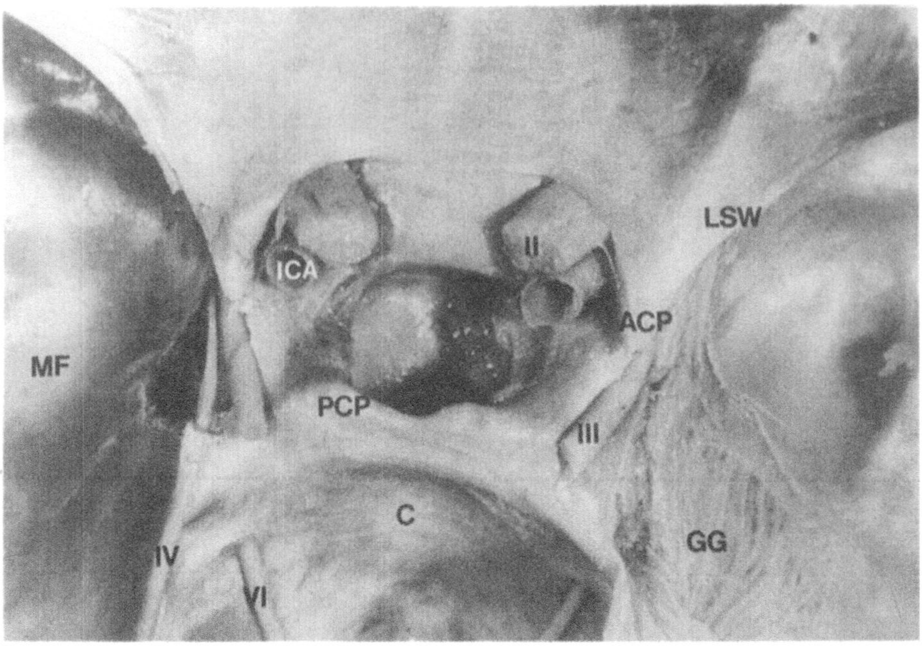

Fig. 7. Meningeal base. Superior view. The dura mater overlying the Gasserian ganglion is resected. Internal carotid artery (*ICA*), cranial nerves (*II, III, IV, VI*), lesser sphenoidal wing (*LSW*), anterior clinoid process (*ACP*), posterior clinoid process (*PCP*), Gasserian ganglion (*GG*), middle fossa (*MF*)

ligamentary system. This feature makes it difficult to dissect the Gasserian ganglion. It is necessary to uncover the plexii and separate them carefully from the vertical meningeal tracts, which must be cut as a last step.

Figure 8 represents a case of intracavernous carotideal loop. The lateral wall was resectioned in its posterior two thirds of the region, from a pregasserian plane. The resection continues horizontally along the ophthalmic branch up to the anterior third of the region perpendicularly with respect to the anterior clinoid process. The roof of the region is cut obliquely from the latter to the middle of the sellar region. The cranial nerves and the ophthalmic trigeminal branch can be seen in their relation to the carotideal inflections. From this perspective the anatomical intrasinal elements are clearly identified. They are respected by Parkinson and Dolenc's surgical approaches.

In 1986, in Ljubljana, the authors presented a self-instruction model based on planimetric patterns for sectioning and techniques for dissection. The result is a rapidly obtainable model (45 minutes) of multiple utility for the recognition and differentiation of the cranial nerves in general and the three-dimensional relationship of the cavernous region in particular.

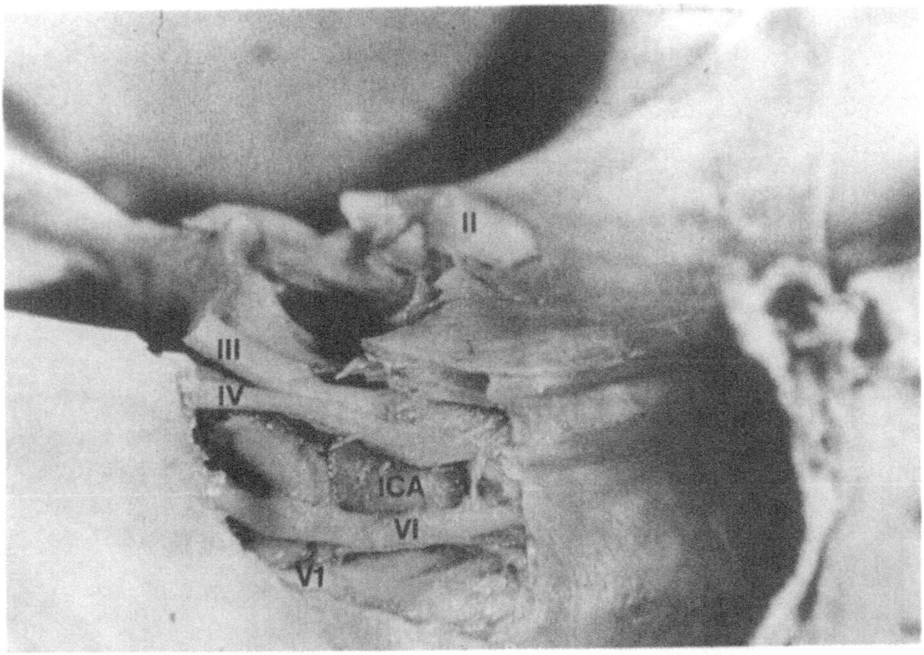

Fig. 8. Lateral view. Right. Dura mater overlying the cranial nerves is resected. Internal carotid artery (*ICA*), cranial nerves (*II, III, IV, V/1, VI*)

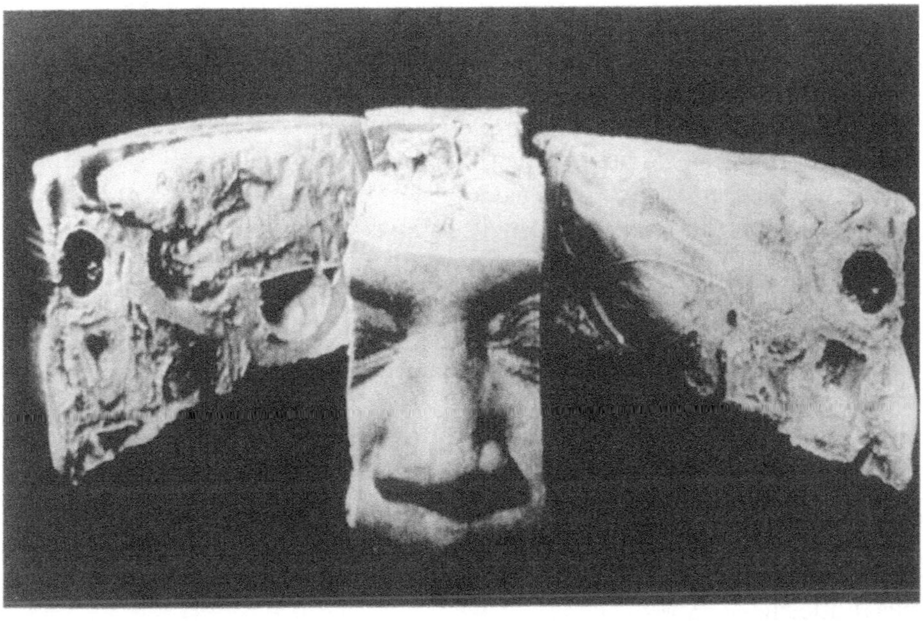

Fig. 9. Central block and lateral segments of the model depicting the sectional planes

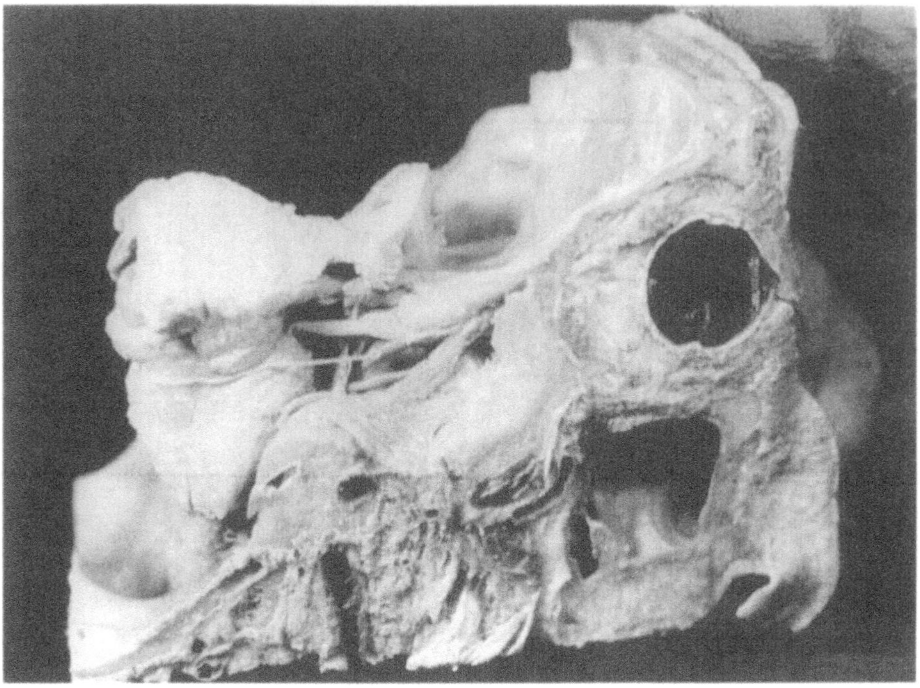

Fig. 10. Central block. Lateral view

1. A formalized or frozen human head is sectioned at the level of the 4th cervical vertebra. It must be completely shaved.

2. Sectioning is carried out with a "butcher's saw".

2.1. Axial sections.

2.1.1. Superior axial section: it follows the plane which passes one finger's breadth above the supraciliary arches.

2.1.2. Inferior axial section: it follows the tangential plane to the superior dental arc.

2.2. Sagittal sections: two symmetrical cuts that pass through the orbital midline.

2.3 Coronal section (posterior): midcerebellum.

3. Over the central block, the dissection is continued in stages.

3.1. The frontal lobe is resected preserving the olfactory nerves.

3.2. The temporal lobe is resected up to the lateral half of the cavernous region, completing it vertically up to the top of the piece, sectioning the basal nucleii.

3.3. The cerebellum is resected using the cerebellar penduncles as references.

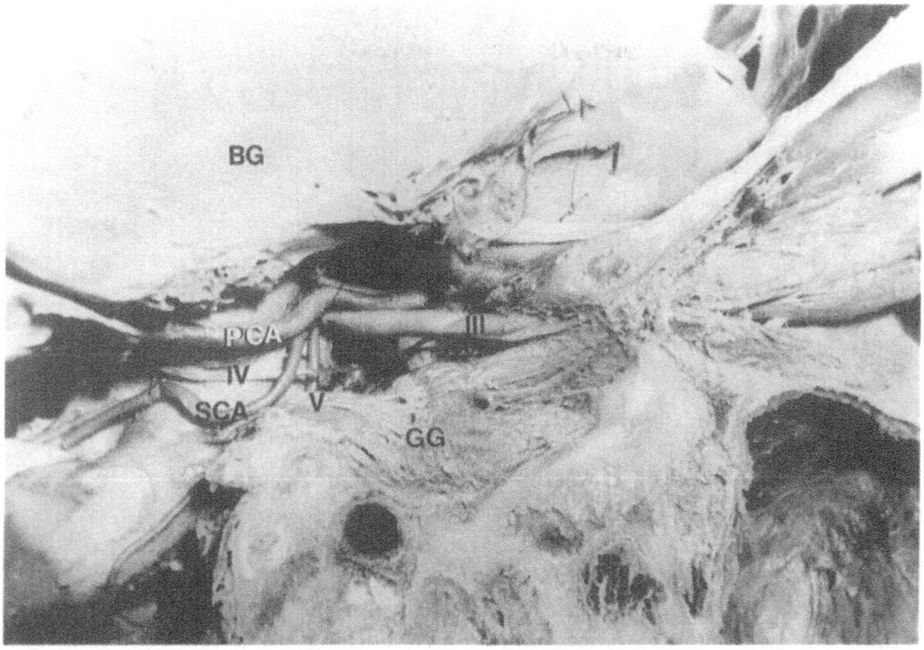

Fig. 11. Central block. Parasellar detail. Right. Basal ganglia (*BG*), posterior cerebral artery (*PCA*), superior cerebellar artery (*SCA*), Gasserian ganglion (*GG*), cranial nerves (*III, IV, V*)

3.4. The dura mater is totally resected from the medial fossa compartments.

3.5. The pia mater and the arachnoidal reticulum are dissected and resected.

The result is an anatomical model which presents all the cranial nerves from their apparent origins to their apparent emergences, preserving the topography and relationships. The cavernous region is the center of the model, the vascular nervous crossroads being the parasellar relationship of greatest importance. The lateral segments of the sections may be used for simulating surgical approaches in the previously dissected central block. This allows a clear view of the operating field according to the different surgical tactics.

The cavernous sinus. An anatomical study of its lateral wall

F. UMANSKY[1] and H. NATHAN[2]

[1] Department of Neurosurgery, Hadassah University Hospital, Jerusalem
[2] Department of Anatomy and Anthropology, Sackler School of Medicine, Tel Aviv University, Tel Aviv, Israel

The cavernous sinus has been and remains an anatomical enigma. Although Galen described with considerable accuracy the sinuses or dura-matral canals as collectors of the meningeal veins, Vesalius asserted that the sinuses received arteries as well as veins and that a pulsation was transmitted from the former. Probably the earliest description of the cavernous sinus was by Ridley (1695) [12] who placed the internal carotid artery (ICA) against the lateral wall. He also suggested the term "circular sinus" a name still sometimes applied. It was Winslow (1732) [23] who compared the interior of the sinus to that of the corpus cavernosum of the penis and applied the term "cavernous" which has been used ever since. After these first discriptions of the cavernous sinus, numerous anatomical studies have emphasized the importance of this paired venous canal. It is generally accepted that the sinuses are located between the two layers of the dura mater: the periosteal (endosteal) layer forming the floor and most of the medial wall of the cavernous sinus, and the dural layer forming its roof, lateral wall, and the upper part of the medial wall (Fig. 1 a). Different opinions are still found in the literature regarding the lateral wall and its relationship to the structures passing through the sinus (Fig. 1).

In most classical textbooks [3, 13, 16, 20] nerves III, IV, and V/1, V/2 are described as being embedded in the lateral wall of the sinus, while the internal carotid artery (ICA) with its sympathetic plexus and sixth nerve are located in the cavity of the sinus.

Other textbooks [9, 10, 14] describe the lateral wall as being split into superficial and deep layers (Fig. 1 b). The deep layer, according to these descriptions, forms a kind of septum in the sinus cavity and divides it into two compartments: a deep broad main compartment medial to the septum, containing the ICA and the sixth nerve; and a narrow, more superficial one

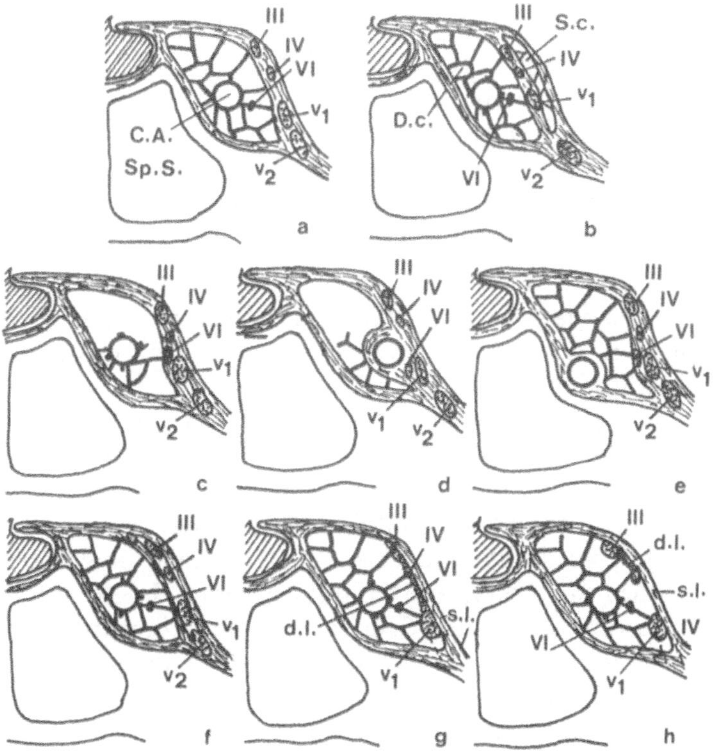

Fig. 1. Diagrams of the cavernous sinus as described by different authors, with special reference to the lateral wall of the sinus and the structures related to it. *Pit.* Pituitary gland; *Sp.S.* sphenoid sinus. **a** Classic textbooks. The lateral wall is formed by the dura mater in which nerves III, IV, and V 1 are embedded. The internal carotid artery (*C.A.*) and nerve VI pass through the cavity of the cavernous sinus. **b** French and Spanish authors. The septum divides the sinus into two compartments. The ICA and nerve VI pass through the deep compartment (*D.c*); nerves III, IV and V/1, V/2 are located within the septum. *S.c* Superficial compartment. **c** Anatomy similar to **a** except that nerve VI is included in the lateral wall. **d** Anatomy similar to **c**, except that the ICA is also included in the lateral wall. **e** Anatomy similar to **c** except that the ICA is included in the middle wall. **f** The lateral wall is split into two layers, with nerves III, IV, and V/1 passing between the layers. **g** Present observations. The lateral wall is composed of two layers: a superficial (*s.1.*) dural layer and deep layer (*d.1.*) formed by the sheaths of nerves III, IV and V/1 with a reticular membrane between these sheaths. **h** Anatomy similar to **g** except that the membrane of the deep layer is incomplete between nerve IV above and V/1 below (from Umansky F, Nathan H (1982) J Neurosurg 56: 228–234, with permission)

lying lateral to the septum. Nerves III, IV, and V/1, V/2 are described by these authors as running through the septum and not in the superficial layer.

Some authors [6, 11] recognized two "dural leaves" in the lateral wall of the sinus, and described the course and relationships of nerves III, IV, and V/1, running between them (Fig. 1 f). Others [4, 5, 15, 17], have described the III, IV and V/1, V/2 nerves as running in the lateral wall, between an endothelial or connective tissue lining and the dura mater. Furthermore, in some studies [2, 18, 21] the sixth nerve is considered as running in the lateral wall, together with the other nerves (Fig. 1 c).

In view of these varied concepts and contradictory descriptions it was decided to investigate the anatomy of the sinus with special regard to its lateral wall. For this purpose seventy cavernous sinuses were dissected in cadavers and in autopsy material [19].

Beginning the dissection at the posterosuperior angle of the lateral wall where the fourth nerve enters the sinus, and continuing the incision forward along the superior border of the wall, a layer of dura mater could be separated from a deeper layer containing nerves III, IV, and V/1 (Figs. 2, 3, 4, 5, and 6). Two additional incisions were made downward from the entrance of the fourth nerve and from the anterior clinoid process, in order to allow reflection of the superficial layer laterally toward the floor of the middle cranial fossa, enough to uncover nerve V/1 in its sheath. The lateral wall of the cavernous sinus was consistently found to be formed of two layers: a smooth superficial layer formed by the dura mater, and a deep layer containing nerves III, IV, and V/1 (Figs. 3 and 6). The two layers of the wall were only loosely attached to each other and could therefore be easily separated (Fig. 3). Only in its more anterior part, where nerves III, IV, and V/1 met, crossed, and branched before entering the superior orbital fissure, did the layers of the wall merge and become difficult to separate, resulting in a uniformly thick single wall. In no case was a separate superficial compartment of the sinus found between the layers. The deep layer was less defined than the superficial layer and was more irregular and variable in its texture and morphological characteristics. It was found to be formed by the sleeves or sheaths of dura mater accompanying the corresponding nerves from their points of penetration into the sinus walls, that is, nerve III through the roof close to the lateral wall in front of and slightly medial to nerve IV; nerve IV at the posterosuperior angle of the lateral wall, exactly where the free and attached borders of the tentorium cerebelli cross each other; and nerves V/1, V/2 through the posteroinferior angle of the lateral wall. The sheaths of these latter nerves are extensions forward of Meckel's cave where the trigeminal Gasserian ganglion is located. The sheaths around nerves III and V/1, V/2 were rather thick and constantly distinct, while that of nerve IV was thin and often inconspicuous. A membrane of a reticular texture extended between the sheaths of the nerves, thus complet-

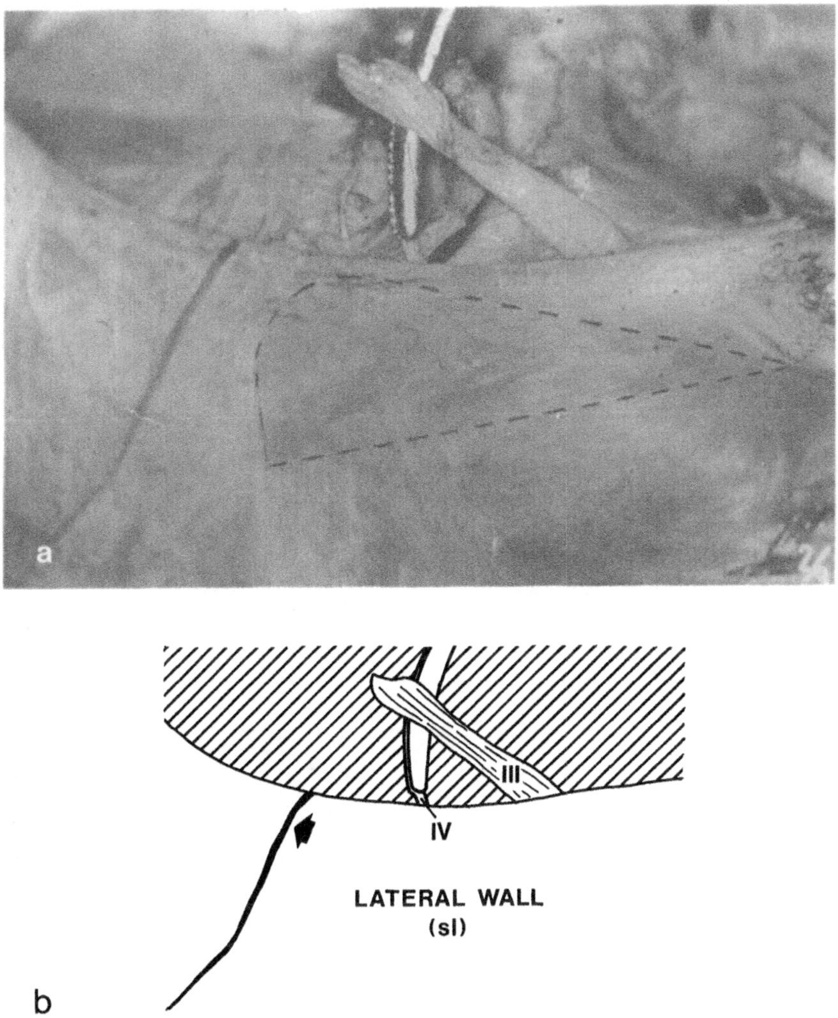

Fig. 2 a and **b.** Unopened right cavernous sinus as seen from the right. Nerve III enters the sinus through its roof; nerve IV, slightly raised by the forceps, is seen disappearing under the free border of the tentorium to enter the lateral wall where this border crosses the attached border of the tentorium. The triangular darker area (surrounded by broken line) of the lateral wall, corresponds to the area between nerves III and IV above, and nerve V/1 (not seen here) below, where the wall is thinner and formed only by the superficial dural layer (*sl*). In the diagram the arrow points to the incision made in the lateral wall to allow reflection of the outer layer

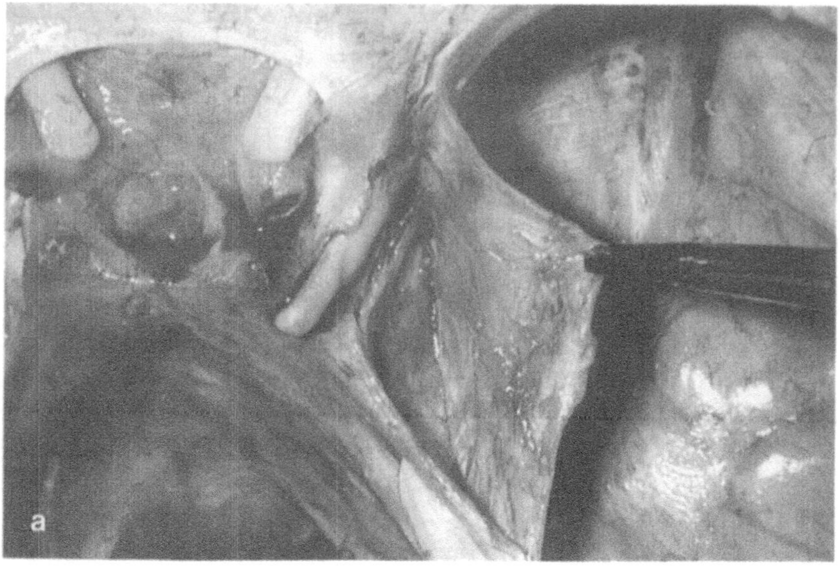

b

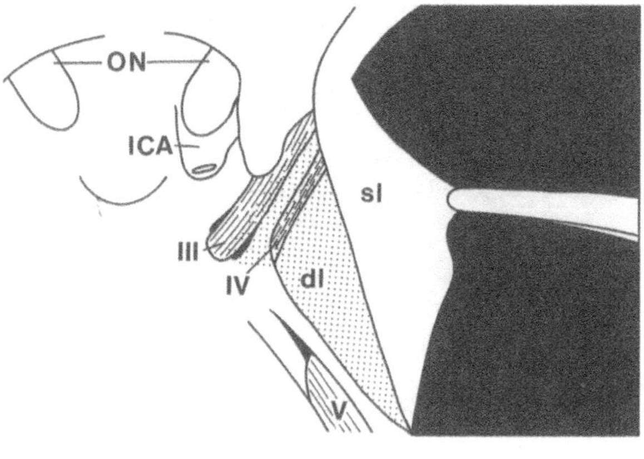

Fig. 3 a and **b.** Superior view of a right cavernous sinus. After separating the superficial layer (*sl*) from the deep layer (*dl*), nerves III, IV and V can be seen embedded in the deep layer. *ON* Optic nerve; *ICA* internal carotid artery

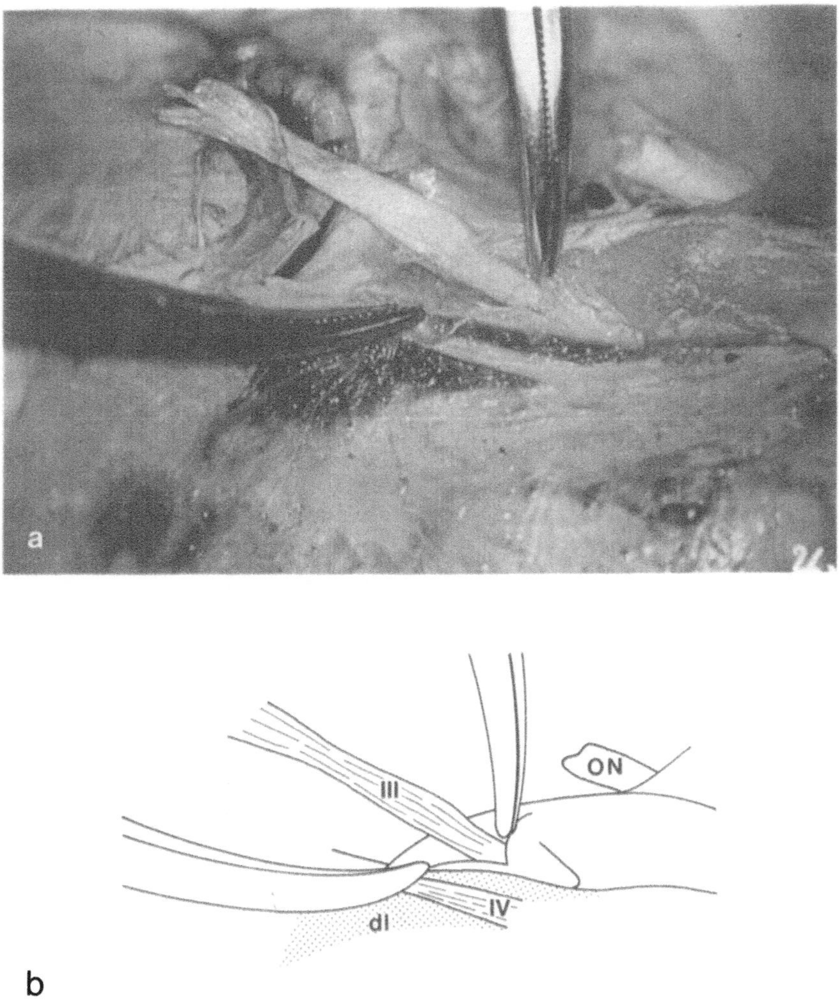

Fig. 4 a and **b.** Lateral view of a right cavernous sinus. The superficial dural layer of the lateral wall has been separated from the deeper layer (*dl*) and reflected downward. Nerves III and IV are clearly seen in their dural sheaths; the sheath of nerve III was opened, and lifted by the forceps to expose the nerve. Note the window, through which the dark contents (blood) of the cavernous sinus are seen. Nerve IV crosses the window and divides it into an upper narrow space and a lower broader one. The window corresponds with the shaded triangular area of the wall seen in Fig. 2a (marked by broken line). *ON* Optic nerve

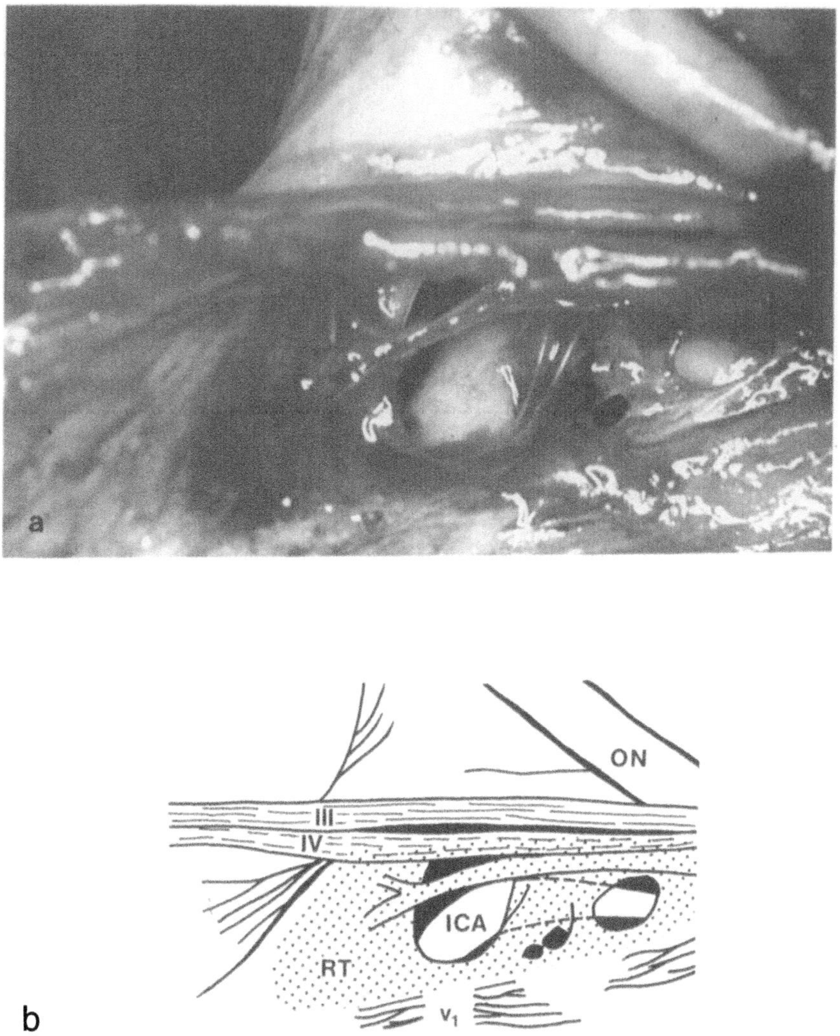

Fig. 5 a and **b.** Lateral view of a right cavernous sinus in an autopsy specimen. An incomplete reticular membrane (*RT*) which forms part of the deep layer of the lateral wall extends between nerve IV and nerve V/1. There is a window triangular in shape through which the cavity of the sinus and the ICA can be seen. *ON* Optic nerve

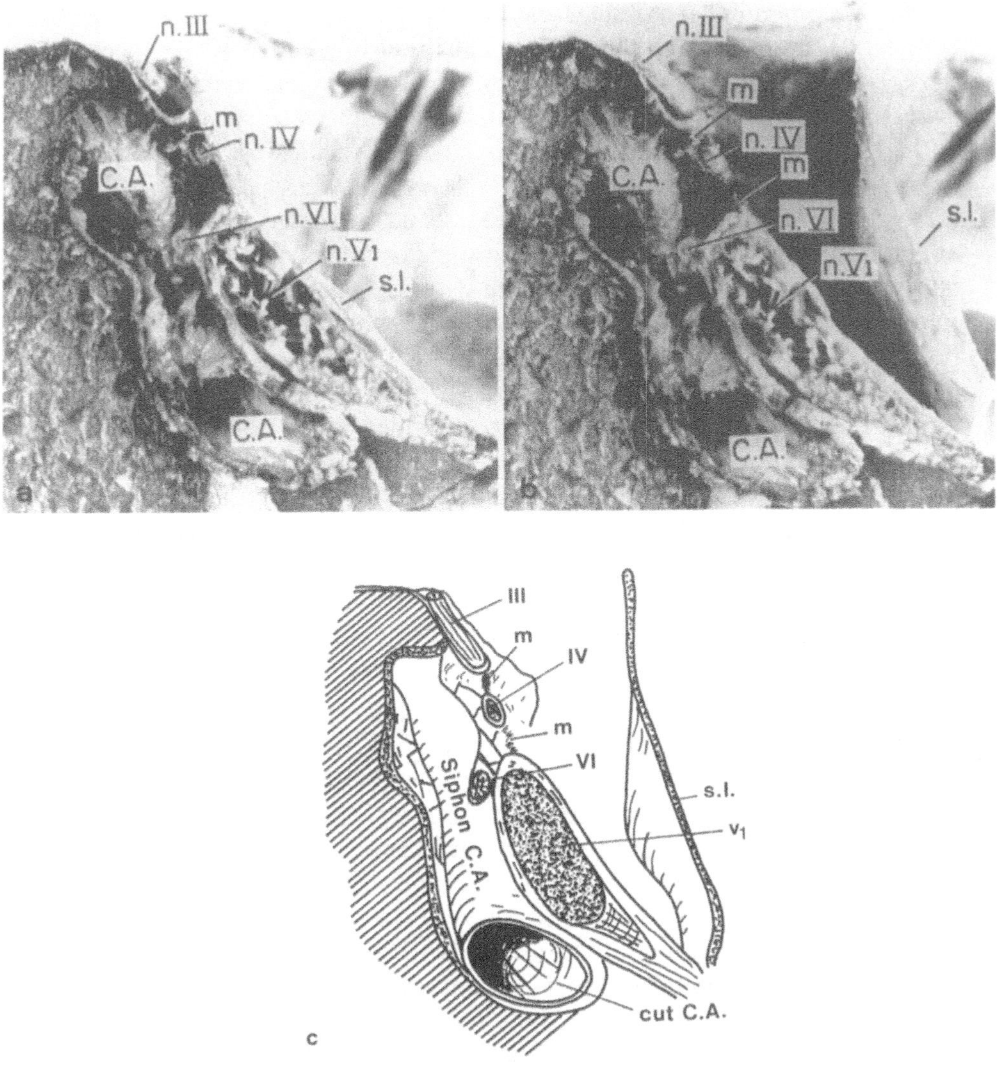

Fig. 6. Frontal (coronal) section of the right cavernous sinus at the site of entrance of nerve III, as seen from behind. **a** The superficial layer (*s.l.*) is attached in place to the deep layer. **b** The superficial layer (*s.l.*) of the lateral wall has been incised and separated from the deep layer. The latter is clearly seen to be formed by the sheaths of nerves III, IV, and V/1 connected by an irregular reticular membrane (*m*). Note that this membrane is incomplete between nerves III and V/1. Here the contents of the sinus come in contact with the superficial layer. Nerve V/1 is seen in its sheath, split into a number of small fascicles. The internal carotid artery (*C.A.*) is cut in its inferior portion, while its "siphon" can be seen within the cavity of the sinus, surrounded by trabeculae. Nerve VI passes between the artery and nerve V/1. **c** Artist's drawing of the anatomical features shown in **b** [from Umansky F, Nathan H (1982) J Neurosurg 56: 228–234 with permission]

ing the deep layer (Fig. 6). This membrane seemed to be composed of the connective tissue forming the trabeculae of the sinus cavity. In 42 specimens (60%), it was found as a thin but definitely complete membrane. In 28 (40%), it was incomplete, and often missing in the space between nerves III and V/1. In these cases (Figs. 4 and 5), a kind of window between these two nerves appeared when the superficial layer was dissected and reflected; through this window, the cavity of the sinus was revealed with its trabeculae and blood remnants. When these were cleared away, the ICA and sixth nerve could be seen in the cavity. The window was generally triangular in shape with its base situated posteriorly, corresponding to the posterior border of the wall. The superior border of the triangle corresponded to nerve III with its meningeal sheath, and the inferior border to nerve V/1 with its sheath. The apex of the triangle corresponded to the point where the two nerves met and decussated in the anterior part of the sinus wall. Nerve IV generally ran parallel with and close and inferior to nerve III at the superior limit of the window. When nerve IV was at a distance from III (Fig. 4), it crossed the window anteroposteriorly dividing it into a narrow superior and a broader inferior part. In the area of the window, the lateral wall of the sinus was much thinner than at the level of nerves III and V, since it was formed here only by the superficial layer.

Parkinson [8] defined a triangular space between nerve III and IV above and V/1 and VI below, which corresponds with the area we have described here where the lateral wall is much thinner because the deep layer is incomplete or missing. He described his surgical approach through this triangle in order to reach the ICA and some branches in the cavernous sinus.

Regarding the relationship of the ICA and sixth nerve in the sinus, most authors describe both these structures as passing through the cavity. However, other opinions differ. Thus, Bedford [1] considers the ICA and sixth nerve as being in the cavity of the sinus in only 8% of cases studied. In the great majority, he considers them to be outside the lumen of the sinus, forming its lateral boundary (Fig. 1 d). McGrath [7] states that the relationship of the ICA to the medial and lateral walls of the sinus is variable. Even in the same individual it may change at different levels. Indeed, we also very frequently found the ICA displaced towards the medial or the lateral wall of the sinus, with nerve VI in these latter cases being pushed against the lateral wall at the level of V/1. We interpret these changes in many cases as a displacement of the ICA due to the enlargement, elongation, and tortuousity of the vessel as a result of arteriosclerosis, and not as a normal basic anatomical relationship. It should be kept in mind that most dissected cadavers are of elderly people affected by this condition. In the fetuses studied by Bedford [1], the ICA was found "clearly in the sinus". Weizenhoffer [22] describes the ICA as running in the medial wall of the sinus (Fig. 1 e), and Rhoton et al. [11], state that the ICA may protrude through the medial wall of the cavernous sinus and indent the pituitary gland or produce a prominence of the wall into the sphenoid sinus. We have very often observed similar changes during our dissection. From our study it appears that the structure of the lateral wall of the cavernous sinus does not conform either to descriptions that include a septum dividing the cavity into two compartments, or to other descriptions of a single dural layer of the wall with nerves embedded in it.

For the neurosurgeon approaching the cavernous sinus through its lateral wall the presence of two layers lossely attached to each other and easy to separate has practical implications. In most cases (60% in our study) the outer layer can be dissected free allowing a better view of nerves III, IV and V/1 which are included in the deep layer of the wall. In other cases (40% in our study) an incomplete deep layer will result in bleeding from the sinus when performing the dissection. Sometimes and due to its transparency a thinner wall can be suspected by its darker color (Fig. 2).

Detailed and more precise anatomical investigations of the sinus and of the structures related to it may still contribute to a better understanding of the hemodynamics of the sinus as well as being helpful for correct interpretation of the pictures obtained either by arteriography or phlebography, or by the more sophisticated modern computerized tomography and magnetic resonance imaging technique.

References

1. Bedford MA (1966) The "cavernous sinus". Br J Ophthalmol 50: 41–46
2. Bonnet P (1955) La loge caverneuse et les syndromes de la loge caverneuse. Arch Ophthalmol (Paris) 15: 357–372
3. Christensen JB, Telford IR (1978) Synopsis of gross anatomy, with clinical correlations, 3rd edn. Harper and Row, New York, p 275
4. Crafts RD (1979) A textbook of human anatomy, 2nd edn. Wiley, New York, pp 503–505
5. Gardner E, Gray DJ, O'Rahilly R (1975) Anatomy. A regional study of human structure, 4th edn. Saunders, Philadelphia, p 609
6. Harris FS, Rhoton AL Jr (1976) Anatomy of the cavernous sinus. A microsurgical study. J Neurosurg 45: 169–180
7. McGrath P (1977) The cavernous sinus: an anatomical survey. Aust NZ J Surg 47: 601–613
8. Parkinson D (1965) A surgical approach to the cavernous portion of the carotid artery. Anatomical studies and case report. J Neurosurg 23: 474–483
9. Paturet G (1964) Traité d'anatomie humaine, vol 4, système nerveux. Masson, Paris, pp 721–722
10. Quiroz-Gutierrez F (1965) Tratado de anatomia humana, vol 2. Editorial Porrua, Mexico City, pp 146–389

11. Rhoton AL Jr, Hardy DG, Chambers SM (1979) Microsurgical anatomy and dissection of the sphenoid bone, cavernous sinus and sellar region. Surg Neurol 12: 63–104
12. Ridley H (1695) The anatomy of the brain. Smith and Walford, London, p 39
13. Romanes GJ (ed) (1981) Cunningham's textbook of anatomy, 12th edn. Oxford University Press, London, p 953
14. Rouviere H (1970) Anatomie humaine. Descriptive et topographique, 10me edn. Masson, Paris, p 678
15. Snell RS (1981) Clinical anatomy for students, 2nd edn. Little, Brown and Co, Boston
16. Testut L, Latarjet A (1974) Tratado de anatomia humana, vol 2, angiologia-sistema nervioso central. Salvat Editores, Barcelona, p 441
17. Thompson JS (1977) Core textbook of anatomy. JB Lippincott, Philadelphia, pp 204–206
18. Thorek P (1951) Anatomy in surgery. JB Lippincott, Philadelphia, p 58
19. Umansky F, Nathan H (1982) The lateral wall of the cavernous sinus with special reference to the nerves related to it. J Neurosurg 56: 228–234
20. Warwick R, Williams PL (eds) (1973) Gray's anatomy, 35th edn. Longman, Edinburgh, p 695
21. Weinberger LM, Adler FH, Grant FC (1940) Primary pituitary adenoma and the syndrome of the cavernous sinus. A clinical and anatomic study. Arch Ophthalmol 24: 1196–1236
22. Weizenhoffer A (1932) Contralateral cavernous sinus thrombosis. NY State J Med 32: 139–142
23. Winslow JB (1732) Exposition anatomique de la structure du corps humain, vol 2. Prevost, London, p 31

The blood supply of the cranial nerves in the lateral wall of the cavernous sinus

E. Knosp[1], G. Müller[2], and A. Perneczky[1]

[1] Department of Neurosurgery and [2] Institute of Anatomy, University of Vienna, Vienna, Austria

Cranial nerves III, IV, V, and VI are embedded in the deep layer of the lateral wall of the cavernous sinus, and are supplied by arteries which approach the nerves from medially. The arteries arise from two main stems of the internal carotid artery (ICA): the meningohypophyseal trunk (TMH), and the inferior lateral trunk (ILT). The ILT points towards the lateral wall of the cavernous sinus, where it supplies the cranial nerves which converge to the superior orbital fissure. The TMH points dorsally and supplies cranial nerve VI within Dorello's canal, the Gasserian ganglion, and the dural entrance area around cranial nerve IV. Branches and anastomoses from and to the middle meningeal and ophthalmic artery system, as well as from and to the internal maxillary artery system, may in part replace the arterial supply pattern of the TMH and the ILT. In the sella and clivus area there exist anastomoses with the contralateral intracavernous branches of the ICA. Many of the anastomotic vessels observed in this study can be explained as developmental remnants of ancestral arterial patterns of the skull base.

Introduction

Increasing neurosurgical interest in the cavernous sinus region, as reflected by this volume and recent literature, demands a more detailed and applied anatomical knowledge of the area. Gross anatomical descriptions lack the details necessary for the application of microneurosurgical techniques. The operation microscope brings blood vessels of small size, such as arteries that supply the cranial nerves, within the range of importance. The direct surgical approach to the cavernous sinus area, as well as the increasing use of embolization techniques, demand a better understanding of the arterial supply patterns to the cranial nerves.

The present study is exclusively confined to the arterial supply of the cranial nerves within the cavernous sinus region, and does not deal with the problems associated with the parasellar venous pathway. Therefore the term "cavernous sinus" will be used in this paper, although the anatomical concept of the area calls for revision (Knosp et al., this volume).

Material and methods

The arterial system of the head was injected with colored latex and dissection was carried out on total skull bases as well as on isolated blocks of the sella area. For better distinction and in an attempt to simulate the *in vivo* flow conditions the external and the internal carotid systems were injected with latex of different colors. For this purpose the carotid bifurcation was exposed and the external and internal carotid arteries were injected separately. After injection of the external carotid artery system was completed, a standard fronto-temporal craniotomy was performed. Filling of the internal carotid system was continued after clipping the supraclinoid ICA distal to the ophthalmic artery's origin. This was done in order to provide a better perfusion of the intracavernous arterial branches. All investigations were performed under magnification and photographs were taken with a Leitz M 8 stereoscope.

Results

The lateral wall of the cavernous sinus consists of two layers of dura, which can be separated by careful dissection. The dura of the middle cranial fossa was incised parallel to the lateral wall of the cavernous sinus from the lesser sphenoidal wing to the petrosal ridge. The superficial layer of the dura was easily removed from the middle cranial fossa as well as from the lateral cavernous sinus wall.

This dissection exposed cranial nerves III to VI and their relationship to each other along their course from the dural entrance to the superior orbital fissure. The nerves are embedded in the deeper layer of the lateral wall. This second layer contains less collagen fibers and is not always continuous. Especially in the dorsal part of the cavernous sinus wall, in the area between IV and V/1, this layer is thin or even missing. This area corresponds to Parkinson's triangle. Cranial nerves III–VI are embedded in the medial dural sheath and are supplied by vessels which come from the ICA. Thus the resection or lifting of the superficial dural layer will not compromise the blood supply of these nerves.

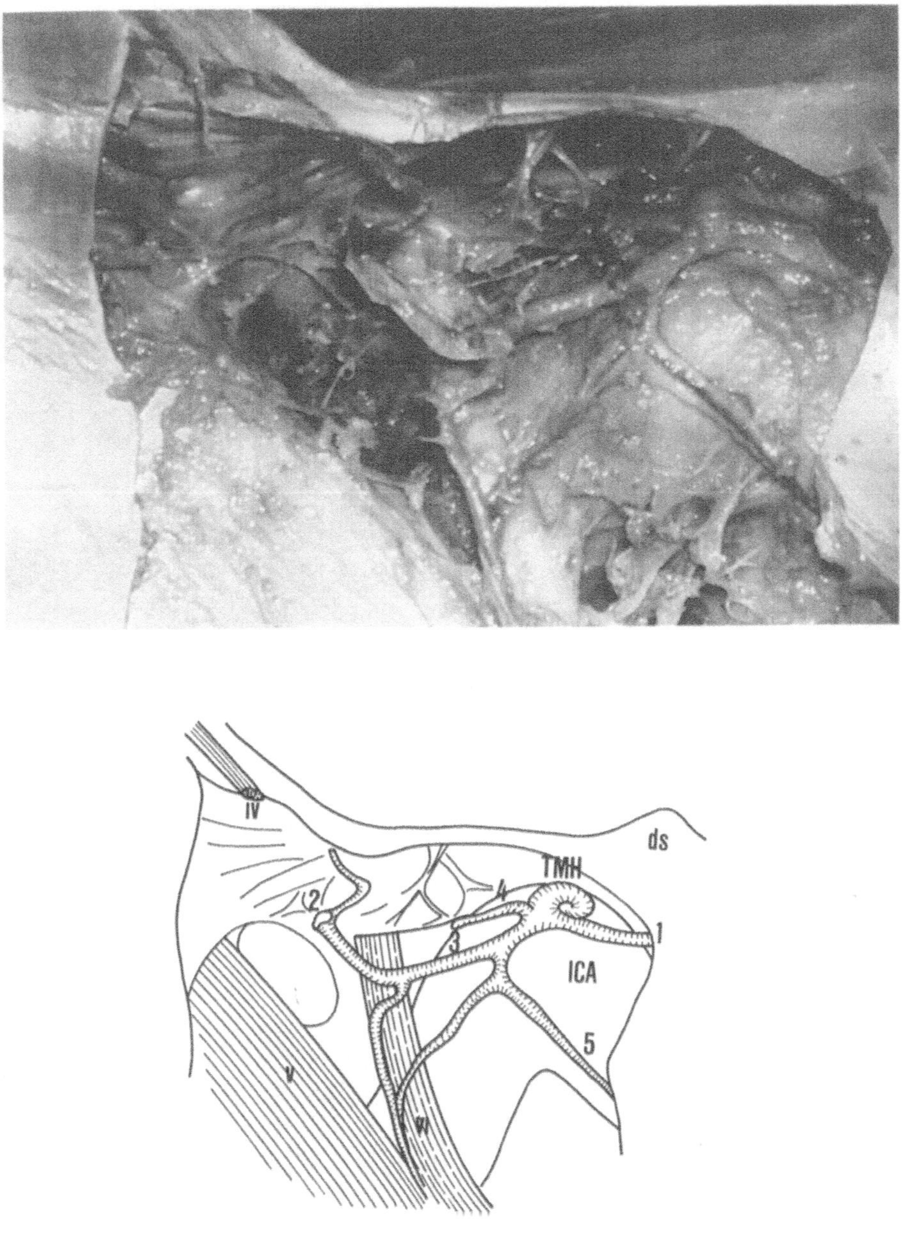

Fig. 1. Right cavernous sinus after partial removal of the lateral wall, anterolateral view. Meningohypophyseal trunk (*TMH*), inferior hypophyseal artery (*1*), tentorial artery (*2*), lateral clival artery (*3*), medial clival artery (*4*), anastomotic branch with the inferior lateral trunk (*5*). The trochlear nerve (*IV*) is cut at its dural porus. The abducent nerve (*VI*) is supplied by the lateral clival artery. Trigeminal nerve (*V*), dorsum sellae (*ds*), internal carotid artery (*ICA*)

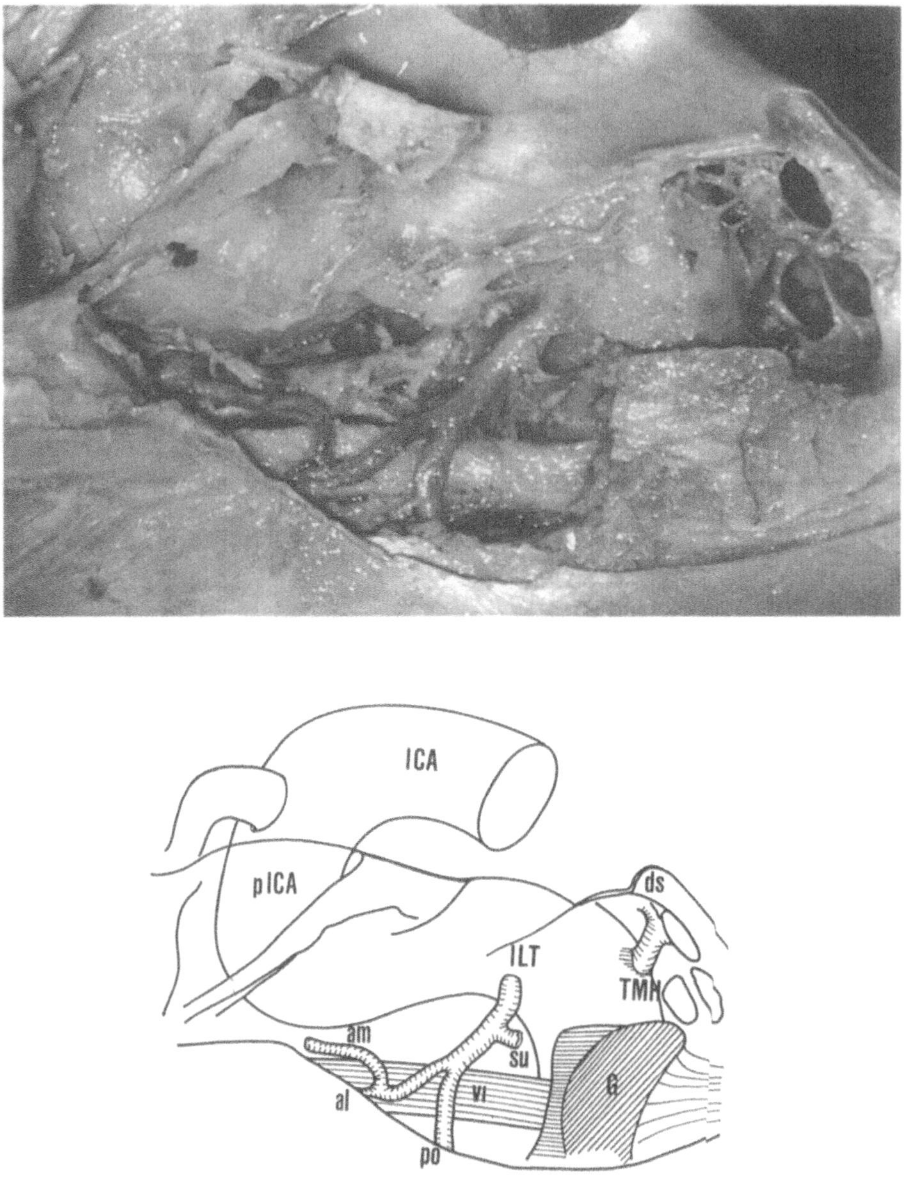

Fig. 2. Cavernous sinus of the left side after removal of the anterior clinoid process and parts of the lateral wall. The oculomotor nerve, the trochlear nerve, and the ophthalmic and maxillary division of the trigeminal nerve have also been resected. Note the origin of the inferior lateral trunk (*ILT*), in the C4 segment of ICA, just above the abducent nerve (*VI*). The anterior medial branch (*am*) and the superior branch (*su*) were removed together with the nerves. Anterolateral branch (*al*), posterior branch (*po*). Gasserian ganglion (*G*), meningohypophyseal trunk (*TMH*), dorsum sellae (*ds*), paraclinoid carotid artery (*pICA*)

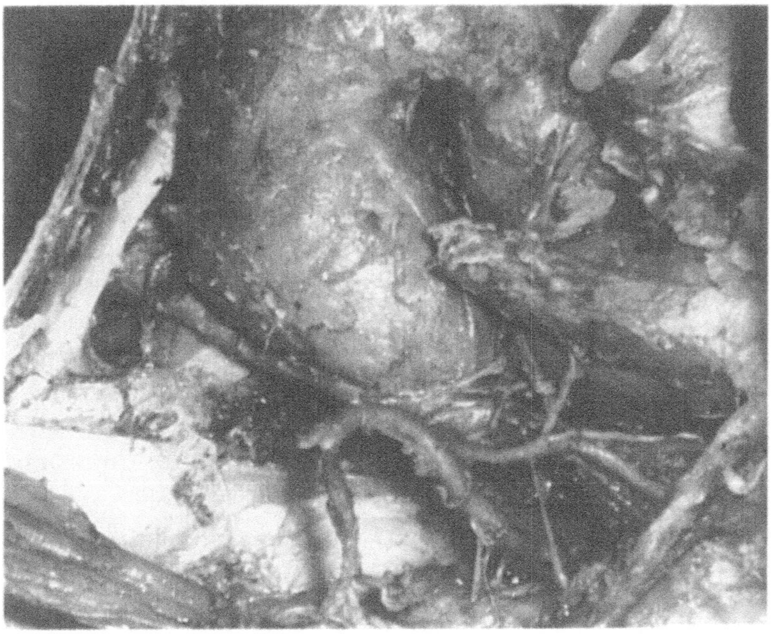

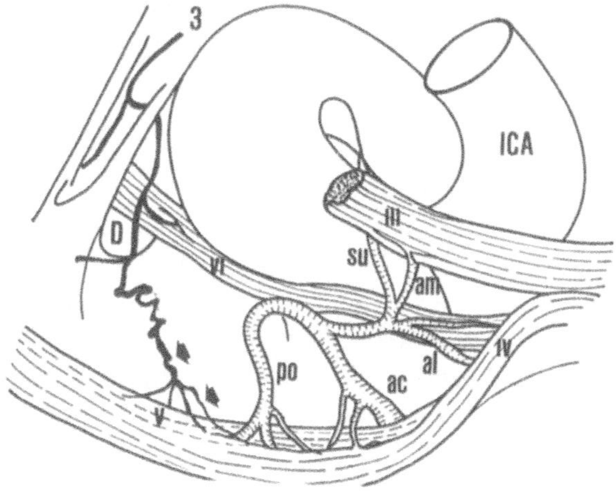

Fig. 3. Right cavernous sinus seen from above. Type of accessory meningeal artery supply of the structures of the lateral sinus wall, in the absence of ILT. The trochlear nerve (*IV*) and trigeminal nerve (V) are displaced laterally to demonstrate the accessory meningeal artery (*ac*) and its branches: anteromedial branch (*am*), anterolateral branch (*al*), posterior branch (*po*), superior branch (*su*). Note connection to the TMHs lateral clival artery (*3*) in the area of the Gasserian ganglion (🡅). Dorello's canal (*D*) with the abducent nerve (*VI*); the oculomotor nerve (*III*) is partially resected. Very tortuous cavernous carotid artery (*ICA*)

The intracavernous ICA gives rise to two main branches: the meningohypophyseal trunk (tr. carotico cavernosus posterior) and the inferior lateral trunk (tr. carotico cavernosus lateralis). The TMH originates from the apogee of the posterior intracavernous siphon loop (Fig. 1) and the ILTs origin is from the horizontal part of the ICA (C 4 segment). The ILT has a characteristic relationship to nerve VI, which passes just below its stem and was found to be in contact with the ICA. This situation was seen in all specimens except in those where no ILT was present (Fig. 3).

The capsular arteries (McConnell) which arise from the medial aspect of the ICA do not take part in the blood supply of the cranial nerves.

The TMH was always found to be present, whereas the ILT was replaced by the accessory meningeal artery in one case. In addition to this, various anastomoses may be present: to the ascending pharyngeal artery, to the middle meningeal-ophthalmic artery system and to the contralateral branches of the ICA. They can partly replace each other.

Cranial nerves III to VI converge to the superior orbital fissure: cranial nerves III and IV, descending from the tentorial margin, nerve V/1 in an almost horizontal way and nerve VI ascending from the clivus. The ILTs origin from the ICA corresponds to the center of the lateral cavernous sinus wall (depending on the tortuosity of the intracavernous segment). Thus the branches of the ILT reach the cranial nerves along the shortest route. Along the transcranial passage of the cranial nerves we always found anastomoses to the middle meningeal-ophthalmic artery system and to the internal maxillary artery, which are the main vessels that take over the blood supply of the nerves in the orbit and the face.

The ILT typically divides into four branches:

— the antero-medial branch of the ILT runs to the superior orbital fissure, supplying nerves III, IV, V/1 and VI. This branch gives rise to anastomotic vessels, through the superior orbital fissure, to the deep recurrent ophthalmic artery within Zinn's tendon ring (Fig. 4);

— the antero-lateral branch of the ILT accompanies nerve V/2 through the foramen rotundum and has anastomoses with branches of the internal maxillary artery;

— the posterior branch passes together with V/3 through the foramen ovale and has anastomoses with the internal maxillary artery and/or with the petrosal branch of the middle meningeal artery. This anastomosis is the cavernous branch of the middle meningeal artery (Fig. 7). In our series of preparations this branch was always found to pass between the motor and sensory root of V/3, on the medial aspect of the foramen ovale;

— the superior branch of the ILT runs adjacent to nerve IV to its dural entrance. On its way the artery supplies nerve IV (Figs. 5 and 6). In the region of the plica petroclinoidea posterior the area of supply of the superior branch overlaps with the territory of the TMHs tentorial branch. Anas-

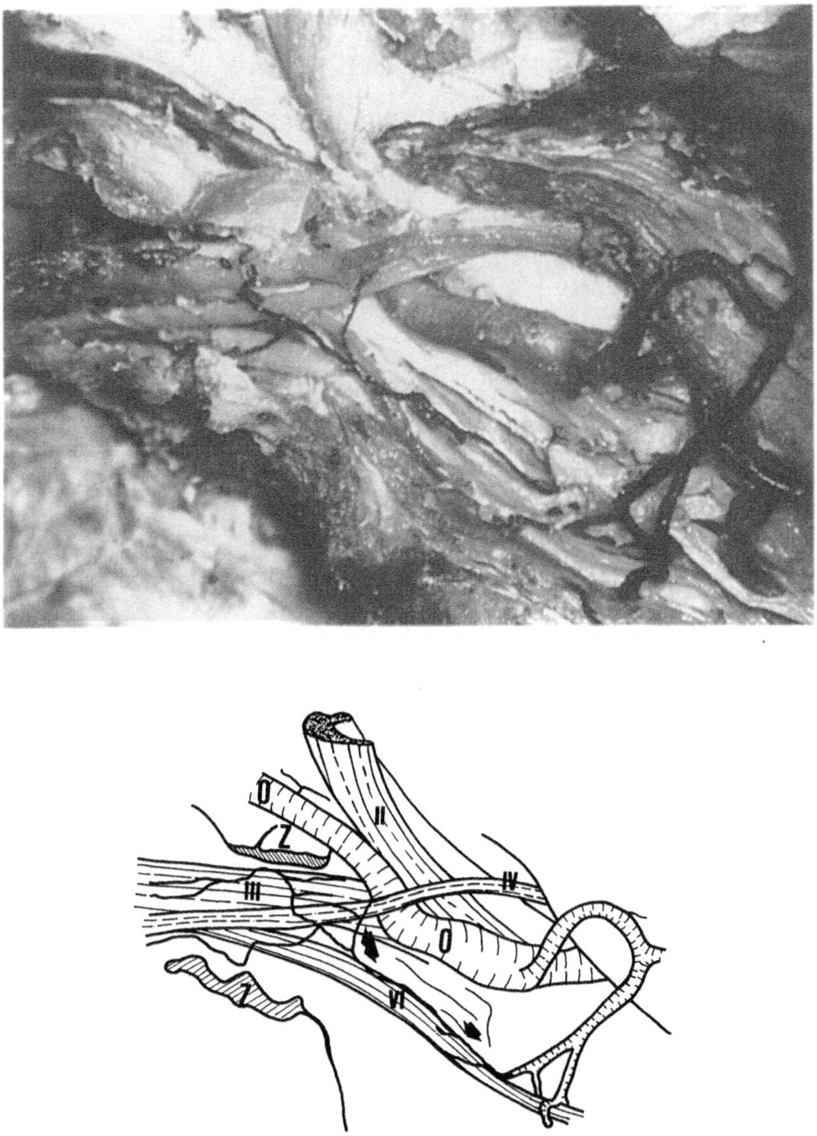

Fig. 4. Superior orbital fissure of the right side, after transection of Zinn's tendom ring (*Z*) and opening of the optic canal: the deep recurrent ophthalmic artery (⬆) runs with nerve VI (*VI*) to the superior orbital fissure. Anastomotic vessels with the anteromedial branch of ILT (⬆⬆). Elevated optic nerve (*II*), ophthalmic artery (*O*), oculomotor nerve (*III*), trochlear nerve (*IV*)

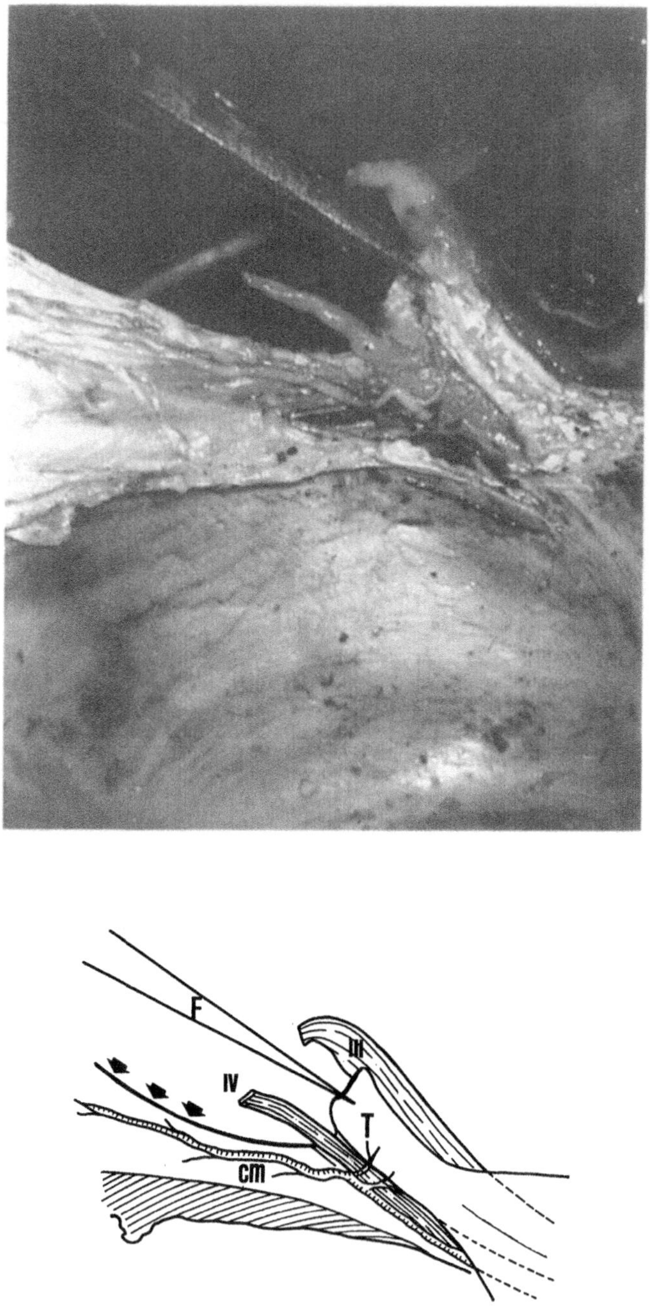

Fig. 5. Dural entrance area of the right trochlear nerve (*IV*) (same specimen as in Fig. 6). The central meningeal artery (*cm*) supplies exclusively the trochlear nerve from the orbit to the plica petroclinoidea posterior. Oculomotor nerve (*III*), forceps (*F*) holding a part of the tentorium (*T*), free margin of tentorium (🡅)

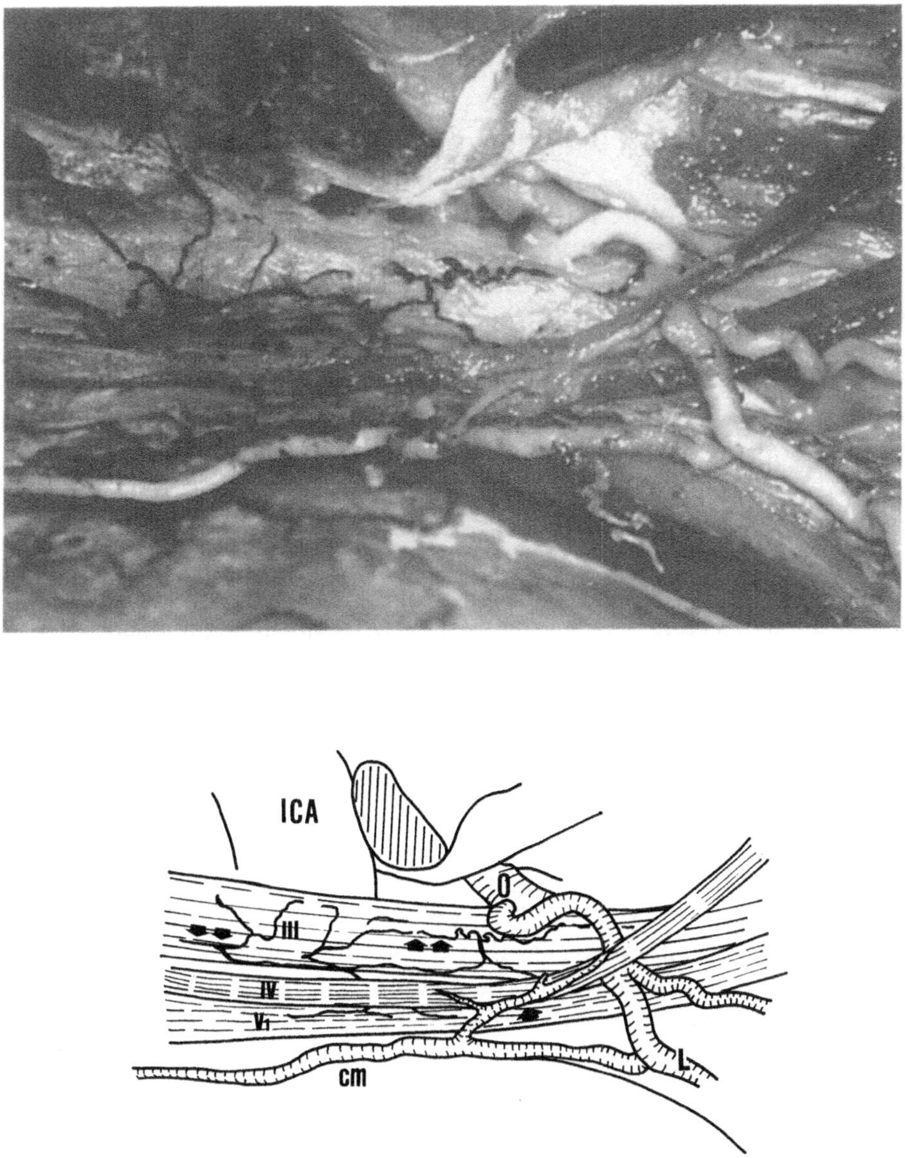

Fig. 6. Right superior orbital fissure. Example of central meningeal artery (*cm*) origin from the lacrimal artery (*L*). The trochlear nerve (*IV*) is exclusively supplied by this artery (⬆) (see also Fig. 5). The oculomotor nerve (*III*) and the ophthalmic branch of the trigeminal nerve (*VI*) are supplied by the ILT (dark color) (⬆⬆). Paraclinoid carotid artery (*ICA*), ophthalmic artery (*O*)

tomoses may be found in this area or the vessels may replace each other.

The TMH originates from the ICA at the top of the posterior siphon knee (Fig. 1). But, in contrast to the ILT, its origin points dorsally. After a very short common stem the TMH divides into its branches which run medial, lateral and dorsal to the ICA;

— the tentorial branch runs to the roof of the cavernous sinus as well as to the dural porus of nerve IV and supplies parts of the tentorium. It may replace the superior branch of the ILT or may form anastomoses with it;

— the inferior hypophyseal artery, which is the main branch of the TMH, turns medially and supplies the capsular and posterior part of the pituitary. In the sella area there exist anastomoses with the corresponding contralateral artery as well as with the superior hypophyseal arteries;

— the clival branch divides into the medial clival artery and the lateral clival artery. The medial clival artery runs to the dorsum sellae, forming an anastomotic ring, and supplies the superior clival dura. The lateral clival artery supplies the dura around the entrance area of nerve VI and nerve VI within Dorello's canal. Along the inferior petrosal sinus an anastomosis to the posterior meningeal artery was always found. Sometimes one of these vessels may originate separately.

Discussion

An intimate correlation between the structure of the sinus wall itself, the course of the cranial nerves within the wall, and their blood supply can be observed. Our findings [21, 22] support the concept of Umansky and Nathan [24], who demonstrated that the cranial nerves are situated in the deeper layer of the lateral wall of the cavernous sinus and that this layer may be missing in the area of Parkinson's triangle.

With his new anatomical and surgical concept Parkinson [18, 19, 20] pioneered intracavernous surgery more than twenty years ago. For operations within the cavernous sinus he suggests making the dural incision in the space between the trochlear nerve and the first division of the trigeminal nerve. In contrast to Harris and Rhoton [14] we could not always find a triangular space between nerve IV and nerve V/1. When the dura is opened between IV and V/1, one is able to approach the intracavernous ICA in the region of the TMH and its branches. Parkinson [19, 20], and Harris and Rhoton [14, 23] found this artery in 100% of their specimens, which is in contrast to Lasjaunias's [13] or Lang and Schäfer's [6] findings. Its very early branching and the initial course within the arterial adventitia of the ICA might be one reason for the different results [25]. In some cases the lateral clival branch (a. carotico cavernosa posterior [6]) has its own

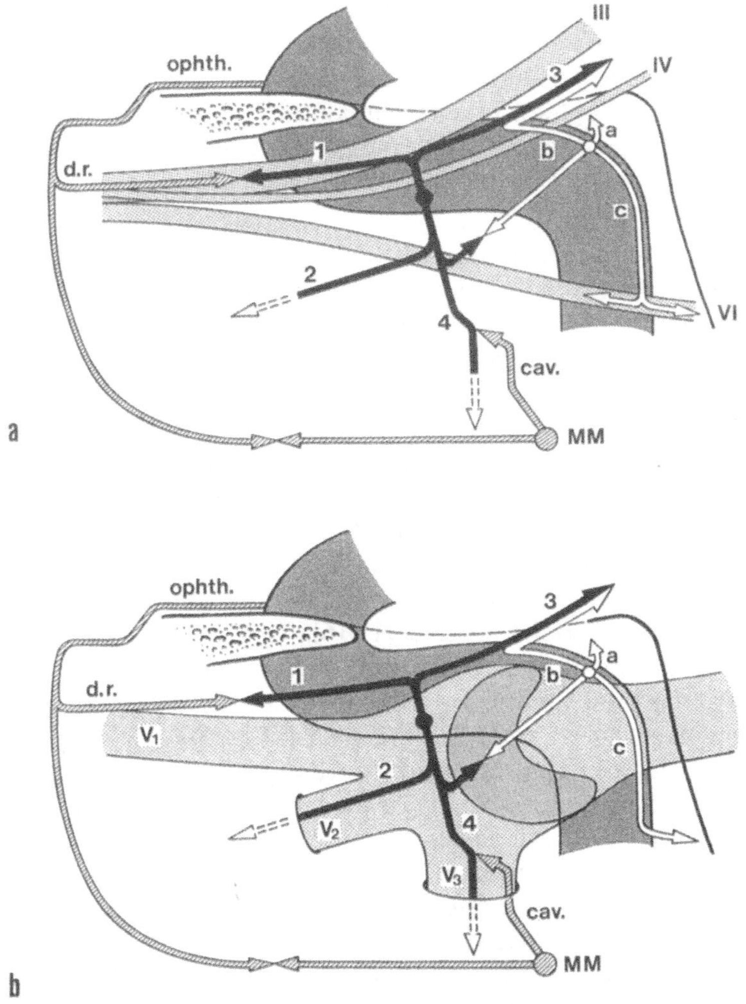

Fig. 7. Diagram of the blood supply of the extraocular motor nerves (**a**) and the trigeminal nerve (**b**): Oculomotor nerve (*III*), trochlear nerve (*IV*), abducent nerve (*VI*), trigeminal nerve (V/1, V/2, V/3). ILT: with its anteromedial (*1*), anterolateral (*2*), superior (*3*) and posterior branch (*4*). TMH: with its inferior hypophyseal artery (*a*), tentorial artery (*b*), and the clival artery (*c*). Note anastomotic branches in the area of the Gasserian ganglion, which arise from the ILT, the TMH, and the MM. *MM* Middle meningeal artery with its cavernous branch (cav.). *Ophth* Ophthalmic artery; *dr* Deep recurrent ophthalmic artery. ▬ ILT, ▭ TMH, ▨ MM-Ophth

origin from the C 5 segment of the ICA and is then regarded as the remnant of the primitive trigeminal artery [13].

In contrast to the constant presence of the TMH (tr. carotico cavernosus posterior [6]) the ILT (tr. carotico cavernosus lateralis [6]) is less frequent. Parkinson [19, 20], Lasjaunias [10, 11, 13], Harris and Rhoton [14], and Lang and Schäfer [6] found the ILT in about 80% of their cases. When the ILT is not present the accessory meningeal artery, passing through the foramen ovale, takes over its territory (Fig. 3).

This anastomosis is the largest and most important of the ILT. The connection between the anteromedial branch of the ILT and the deep recurrent ophthalmic artery, through the superior orbital fissure, is considered to be the remnant of a dorsal primitive ophthalmic artery [12, 13] (Fig. 4). This would explain the existence of an intracavernous origin of the ophthalmic artery in about 8% [14]. The connection of the posterior branch of the ILT with the cavernous branch of the middle meningeal artery is the remnant of the former stapedial artery [2, 13, 17]. The superior branch of the ILT runs along nerve IV to its dural entrance, and supplies the nerve and the medial part of the tentorium. This branch is also called the central meningeal artery [6, 7, 9], or artery of the free margin of the tentorium [13], or artery of Bernasconi-Cassinari [1, 16]. This artery may also originate from the middle meningeal artery itself or from the ophthalmic artery near the superior orbital fissure. In these cases it runs along nerve IV to the tentorium, exclusively supplying this nerve (Fig. 5).

With respect to the pattern of arterial supply of the cranial nerves found in this study, the surgical opening of the lateral wall of the cavernous sinus between nerve IV and V/1, as described by Parkinson [18, 19, 20] and others [3, 4, 21, 22] seems to be optimal. However we, and others [8], were not able to find a triangular space between nerve IV and V in all specimens. If the dural opening is performed caudal and parallel to nerve IV, preserving its accompanying artery, theoretically only the anastomoses between the TMH and ILT have to be sacrificed.

Injury of the accessory meningeal artery in the oval foramen, during puncture of the Gasserian ganglion for thermocoagulation [26] may eventually result in development of ophthalmoplegia, if the ILT is not present.

The increasing application of embolization techniques in the skull base area requires a more detailed knowledge of the blood supply of the cranial nerves to avoid cranial nerve palsies. Because of the anastomoses between the external carotid system and the ICA, which are described in this study, it becomes evident that embolization within the external carotid artery system not only carries the risk of cranial nerve palsies, but a potential risk of blindness and severe cerebral complications [3] as well.

This work was in part supported by a grant from Anton-Dreher-Gedächtnisschenkung (24/83).

References

1. Bernasconi V, Cassinari V (1956) Un segno carotidografico tipico di meningioma del tentorio. Chirurgia 11: 586–588
2. De la Torre E, Netsky MG (1960) Study of persistant primitive maxillary artery in human fetus. Am J Anat 106: 185–195
3. Debrun G, Lacour P, Viñuela F et al (1981) Treatment of 54 carotid cavernous fistulas. J Neurosurg 55: 678
4. Dolenc V (1983) Direct microsurgical repair of intracavernous vascular lesions. J Neurosurg 58: 824
5. Derome P (1984) 2nd "Skull-base Study Group" meeting. (Oral presentation) Mainz
6. Lang J, Schäfer K (1976) Über Ursprung und Versorgungsgebiete der intracavernösen Strecke der A. Carotis interna. Gegenbaurs Morphol Jahrb 122: 182–202
7. Lang J (1981) Klinische Anatomie des Kopfes. Springer, Berlin Heidelberg New York, p 200
8. Lang J, Reiter U (1984) Über den Verlauf der Hirnnerven in der Seitenwand des Sinus cavernosus. Neurochirurgia (Stuttg) 27: 93–97
9. Lanz T, Wachsmuth W [Lang J, Wachsmuth W (Hrsg)] (1979) Praktische Anatomie, Bd 1, Teil 1. Springer, Berlin Heidelberg New York, pp 63–90
10. Lasjaunias P, Merland J, Theron J, Moret J (1977) Dural vascularization of the middle cranial fossa. J Neuroradiol 4: 361
11. Lasjaunias P, Moret J, Mink J (1977) The anatomy of the inferior lateral trunk of the internal carotid artery. Neuroradiology 13: 215
12. Lasjaunias P, Brismar J, Moret J, Theron J (1978) Recurrent cavernous branches of the ophthalmic artery. Acta Radiol 194: 553
13. Lasjaunias P (1981) Craniofacial and upper cervical arteries. Williams and Wilkins, Baltimore, pp13–78
14. Harris FS, Rhoton AL Jr (1976) Anatomy of the cavernous sinus. J Neurosurg 45: 169
15. McConnell EM (1953) The arterial blood supply of the human hypophysis cerebri. Anat Rec 115: 175
16. Krayenbühl H, Yaşargil M, Huber P (1979) Zerebrale Angiographie für Klinik und Praxis. Thieme, Stuttgart, pp 68–71
17. Padget DH (1948) The development of cranial arteries in the human embryo. Contrib Embryol 32: 205
18. Parkinson D (1973) Carotid cavernous fistula: direct repair with preservation of the carotid artery. J Neurosurg 38: 99
19. Parkinson D (1964) Collateral circulation of the cavernous carotid artery: anatomy. Can J Surg 7: 251
20. Parkinson D (1965) A surgical approach to the cavernous portion of the carotid artery: Anatomical studies and case report. J Neurosurg 23: 474

21. Perneczky A, Knosp E, Vorkapic P, Czech TH (1985) Direct surgical approach to infraclinoidal aneurysms. Acta Neurochir (Wien) 76: 36
22. Perneczky A, Knosp E (1986) The intracavernous connective tissue cover of internal carotid artery: anatomy and surgery. In: Scheunemann H (ed) 2nd "Skullbase Study Group". W de Gruyter, Berlin, pp 171–175
23. Rhoton AL, Hardy DG, Chambers SM (1979) Microsurgical anatomy and dissection of the sphenoid bone cavernous sinus and sella area. Surg Neurol 12: 63
24. Umansky F, Nathan H (1982) The lateral wall of the cavernous sinus with special reference to the nerves related to it. J Neurosurgery 56: 228
25. Schnürer LB, Stattin S (1963) Vascular supply of the intracranial dura from the internal carotid artery with special reference to its arteriographic significance. Acta Radiol [Diagn] (Stockh) 1: 441–450
26. Siegfried J (1981) Percutaneous controlled thermocoagulation of Gasserian ganglion in trigeminal neuralgia: experience with 1000 cases. In: Samii M, Jannetta P (eds) The cranial nerves. Springer, Berlin Heidelberg New York, pp 323–331
27. Yaşargil G, Mortara RW, Curcic M (1980) Meningiomas of the basal posterior cranial fossa. In: Krayenbühl H et al (eds) Adavances and technical standards in neurosurgery, vol 7. Springer, Wien New York, pp 3–115
28. Yaşargil G (1984) Microneurosurgery, vol 1. Thieme, Stuttgart New York, pp 54–60
29. Xuerub GB, Prichard ML, Daniel PM (1954) The arterial supply and venous drainage of the human hypophysis cerebri. QJ Exp Physiol 39: 199–217

Microsurgical anatomy of collateral branches of the intracavernous internal carotid artery

G. Brassier[1], P. Lasjaunias[2], Y. Guegan[1], and J. Pecker[1]

[1] Department of Neurosurgery, Hospital Pontchaillou, Rennes, and
[2] Department of Neuroradiology, Hospital Bicetre, Le Kremlin-Bicetre, Paris, France

Since Winslow identified it in 1732, the cavernous sinus has given rise to numerous discussions about its description, its embryology, its dynamic, and even its own designation: cavernous sinus, cavernous area, parasellar region ...

The intracavernous collaterals of the internal carotid artery have been known since Luschka (1860) first described the postero-inferior hypophyseal artery. Then, Dandy [1], Schnurer and Stattin [34], McConnell [22], and more recently Parkinson [29, 30, 31, 32], Harris and Rhoton [4], and Rhoton [33] were interested in this field.

Our study took the following considerations into account:

to connect with the operation's (position, optical magnification, brain's consistency),

to explain the numerous anatomical descriptions by the different embryological developments;

to compare our results to previous studies.

Methods

The anatomical parts were embalmed with liquid of Winckler and arterial vascular injections were carried out on both sides of the internal carotid, external carotid and vertebral artery with colored latex.

Finally, we kept only 40 anatomical parts, enabling us to study 80 cavernous sinuses.

Embryological considerations

They are founded on the works of Lasjaunias, Moret et al. [9, 13, 14, 15, 25]. The human embryo has four vessels in this area.

The dorsal ophthalmic artery

At the embryo-stage of 4–8 mm, two arteries work towards supplying the orbit:

the ventral ophthalmic artery which arises from the anterior cerebral artery;

the dorsal ophthalmic artery, which arises from the carotid siphon (C 4) anterior to the trigeminal and the primitive maxillary artery. It supplies the eye ball and the optic nerve after entering the orbit through the superior orbital fissure. This artery, which usually regresses, may however more or less persist. Also its proximal remnant appears to be the inferior lateral trunk (ILT, whose the anterior medial branch anastomoses with the ophthalmic artery in the orbit) of the internal carotid siphon, while its distal remnant is the deep recurrent ophthalmic artery.

The stapedial artery

It arises from the internal carotid artery in the middle ear, runs through the crus of the stapes and enters the skull through a small foramen on the upper face of the petrous pyramid.

In the temporal fossa, it divides into the supraorbital artery (future middle meningeal) which remains in the skull, and the maxillomandibular artery (future maxillary artery) which leaves the cranial cavity through the foramen spinosum.

Usually (Fig. 1) the stapedial system regresses in the area of the stapes, while simultaneously its maxillo-mandibular branch is annexed by the external carotid and becomes the internal maxillary artery. Finally, the whole stapedial system arises from the external carotid artery. Its carotid remnant (proximal part) is the caroticotympanic artery.

The supraorbital artery (middle meningeal artery) divides again at the endocranium level into three branches:

the first, meningeal for the vault;

the second, recurrent tentorial for the free edge of the tentorium;

the third, orbital, which penetrates through the superior orbital fissure and gives rise in the orbit to two branches: the lacrimal artery (lateral) and the nasociliary artery (medial).

At this stage, the ophthalmic artery annexes the orbital branch:

firstly, by contracting an anastomosis with the nasociliary artery around the optic nerve. This anastomosis will become the second portion of the

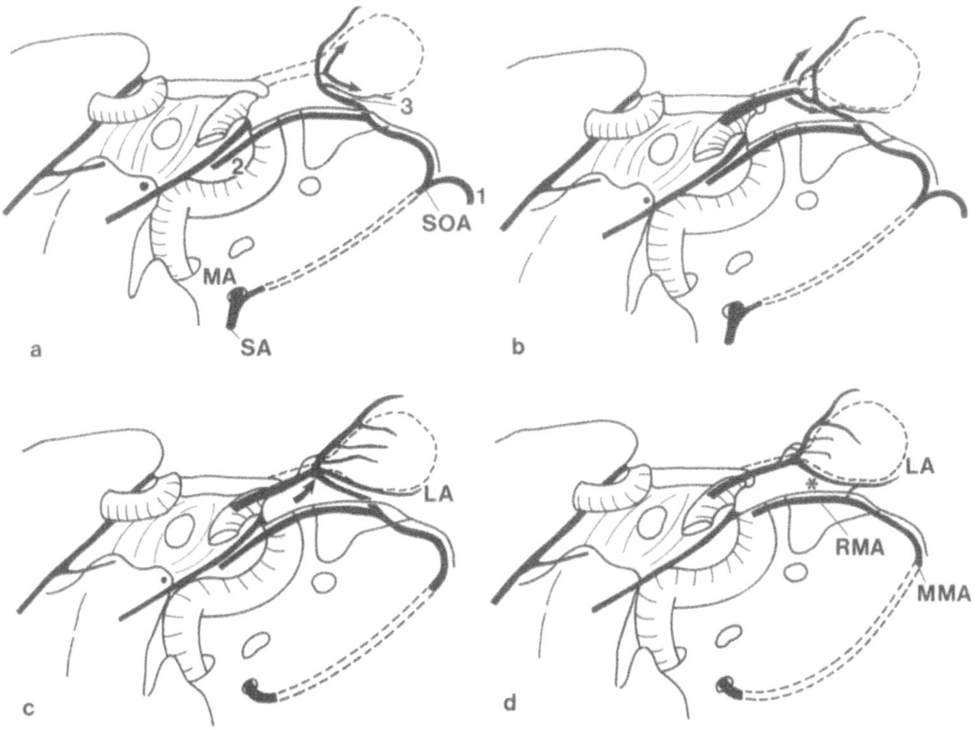

Fig. 1. Development of the orbital arterial system from the stapedial system: recurrent meningeal type (adapted from Lasjaunias). **a** The stapedial artery (*SA*) gives two branches: the maxillomandibular artery (*MA*) (exocranial), the supraorbital artery (*SOA*) (endocranial) which gives off three branches: meningeal (*1*), recurrent tentorial (*2*) and orbital (*3*). **b** Connection of the orbital branch (of the supraorbital artery) by the nasociliary branch of the ophthalmic artery. **c** From the stage 1 b follows an incomplete anastomotic circle, usually lateral, around the optic nerve, and corresponding to the path of the definitive ophthalmic artery. The stapedial artery is connected with the ventral pharyngeal artery (external carotid). *LA* Lacrimal artery. **d** Regression of the orbital branch at the level of the superior orbital fissure (*). The vestige of this branch corresponds to the anastomosis between lacrimal artery (*LA*) and middle meningeal artery (*MMA*): recurrent meningeal artery (*RMA*)

ophthalmic artery in the adult, while the remaining part of the nasociliary artery becomes the third extraconic portion of this same ophthalmic artery;

secondly, by regression of the orbital branch to the level of the superior orbital fissure. The remnant of this branch persists in the adult as an anastomosis through the superior orbital fissure between the lacrimal artery and the middle meningeal artery.

This evolution is the most frequent and individualizes a middle meningeal contribution to the orbit which is: the recurrent meningeal type.

A variation is possible in the development of the stapedial system (Fig. 2). Sometimes, the division of the orbital branch of the supraorbital artery into the lacrimal and nasociliary arteries is made in the temporal fossa.

The lacrimal artery penetrates the orbit through the greater wing of the sphenoidal bone by a canal called Hyrtl's canal. It is then named the meningolacrimal artery.

The nasociliary artery penetrates the orbit normally through the superior orbital fissure where it is annexed in its distal part by the primitive ophthalmic artery.

The proximal part regresses either partially or totally in the adult, and becomes an anastomosis between the trunk of the ophthalmic artery and the middle meningeal artery. It is called the meningoophthalmic artery. Another type of middle meningeal contribution to the orbital supply is thus individualized: the meningolacrimal type, which requires:

the presence of a Hyrtl's canal;

the absence of a lacrimal artery arising directly from the ophthalmic artery.

Three types of errors are possible in this evolution:

the regression takes place at the level of the trunk of the supraorbital artery. In this case, in the adult, the ophthalmic artery gives rise to the middle meningeal artery;

the regression takes place at the level of the ophthalmic artery. So it is the middle meningeal artery which gives rise to the ophthalmic artery;

absence of regression and of annexion of the orbital branch by the ophthalmic artery.

So the orbital supply depends on the internal carotid via the ophthalmic artery (globe and optic nerve) and on the middle meningeal artery (serving the aponevrotic, lacrimal glandular and annexial structures).

The trigeminal artery

This artery develops (Fig. 3) in the embryo at the 4 mm stage and disappears at the 7–12 mm stage. It may persist in the adult. Its frequency is estimated at 0.1–0.5%. It arises from the basilar artery between the anterosuperior and the anteroinferior cerebellar. It then runs medially to the trigeminal nerve. The trigeminal artery and the first division of the trigeminal nerve penetrate into the cavernous sinus, where the artery connects with the C 5 portion of the carotid siphon.

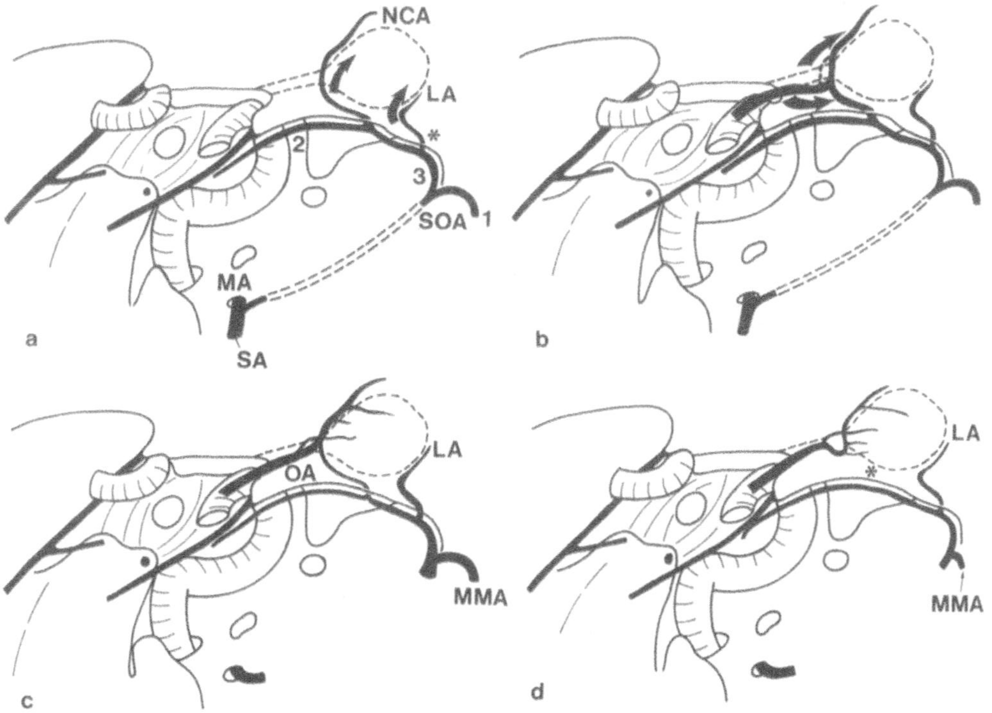

Fig. 2. Development of the orbital arterial system from the stapedial system: meningolacrimal type (adapted from Lasjaunias). **a** The stapedial artery (*SA*) divides into 2 branches: the maxillomandibular artery; the supraorbital artery, which gives off meningeal (*1*) and orbital (*3*) branches. The orbital branch divides in the temporal fossa into: lacrimal artery (*LA*), entering the orbit through Hyrtl's canal (*); nasociliary artery (*NCA*) which runs into the superior orbital fissure; recurrent tentorial artery (*2*). **b** Connection of the nasociliary artery by the primitive ophthalmic artery in its distal portion. **c** Incomplete regression of the proximal portion of the nasociliary artery: so an anastomosis exists between the ophthalmic artery (*OA*) and the middle meningeal artery (*MMA*). **d** Entire regression of the proximal portion of the nasociliary artery (*). The lacrimal artery (*LA*) depends only on the middle meningeal artery (*MMA*)

Three types of trigeminal arteries can be described:

type 1: the trigeminal artery supplies the two posterior cerebral arteries;

type 2: in which it supplies only one posterior cerebral artery, usually the contralateral, whereas the ipsilateral is supplied by the posterior communicating artery;

type 3: in which it supplies only the two anterosuperior cerebellar arteries.

If this trigeminal artery persists in its embryonic form, it gives off an arterial remnant to the area. Like the dorsal ophthalmic artery, this persistent vessel can take over the blood supply of number of structures, depending on what part regresses and what part persists, including the following:

a middle meningeal artery will arise from the basilar artery, if the basilar vestige of the trigeminal artery has taken over the endocranial branch of the stapedial artery;

a cerebellar artery will arise from the basilar artery, if the carotid remnant of the trigeminal artery has taken over part of the cerebellar territories which originally belonged to the basilar artery.

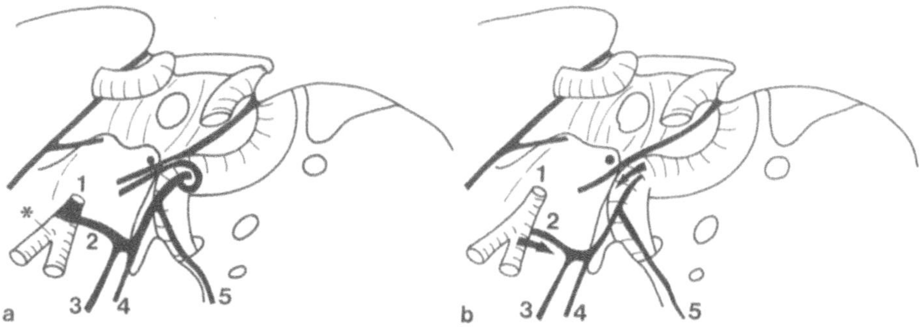

Fig. 3. Schematic drawing of the entire persistence of the trigeminal artery (adapted from Lasjaunias). **a** Aplasia of the basilar artery (*BA*) (*), basilar artery (*1*); trigeminal artery (*2*), cerebellar artery (*3*); lateral clival artery (*4*) (anastomosing with the jugular branch of the ascending pharyngeal artery); basal tentorial artery (*5*). **b** The basilar artery is persistent. There is a dual filling from the ICA and from the basilar artery

The primitive maxillary artery

This artery originates from the medial surface of the C 5 portion of the carotid siphon and supplies the posterior hypophysis where it anastomoses with its counterpart on the other side.

It may arise from a common trunk with the trigeminal artery and their common remnant is then a single artery which arises from C 5 and gives off all the meningeal, hypophyseal and neural branches of this region. So it is the meningohypophyseal trunk which Parkinson described. For us, this trunk is not always present and is a variant.

In addition to a branch supplying the hypophysis, the primitive maxillary artery also gives rise to a meningeal branch for the dorsum sellae (the medial artery of the clivus). This branch anastomoses with its counterpart on the other side and inferiorly with the clival branch of the hypoglossal branch of the ascending pharyngeal artery.

Certain variants may result from the persistance or unusual origin of the primitive maxillary artery:

the contralateral origin of the internal carotid artery by a transsellar anastomosis, supplying an internal carotid artery whose cervical portion has disappeared;

a supracarotid course of the posteroinferior hypophyseal artery, when all the embryonic branches arise from a common trunk.

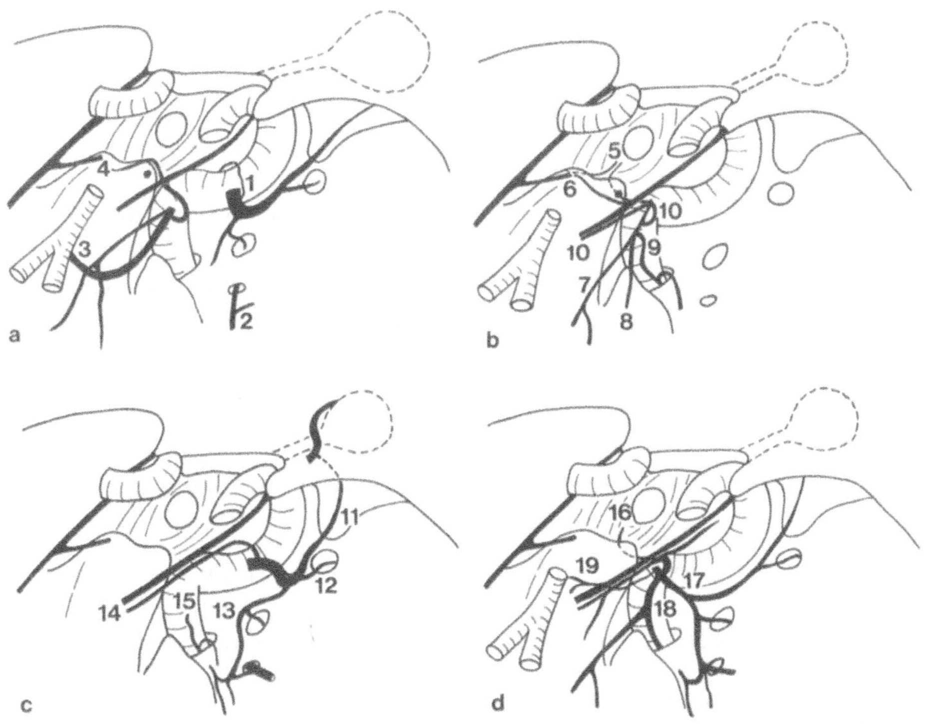

Fig. 4. Schematic drawing of the most frequent intracavernous arterial varieties (adapted from Lasjaunias). **a** Embryonic arrangement: dorsal ophthalmic artery (*1*); stapedial artery (*2*); trigeminal artery (*3*), primitive maxillary artery (*4*). **b** Branches of the C5 portion: hypophyseal branch (*5*); medial clival artery (*6*); medial branch of the lateral clival artery (*7*); lateral branch of the lateral clival artery (*8*); recurrent artery of the foramen lacerum (*9*); marginal tentorial artery (*10*). **c** Branches of the inferolateral trunk (C4): anteromedial branch (*11*); anterolateral branch (for the foramen rotundum) (*12*); posterior branch (*13*); superior branch (marginal tentorial artery) (*14*); carotid branch of the ascending pharyngeal artery (*15*). **d** Common trunk for all the embryonic vessels (variant): hypophyseal artery (*16*); inferolateral trunk (*17*); remnant of the trigeminal artery (*18*); medial clival artery (*19*)

Anatomical description and microsurgical study

Collateral branches of the C 5 portion of the carotid siphon

There are six possible arteries (Figs. 4, 5, 6).

The posteroinferior hypophyseal artery

This artery, present in about 90% of our specimens, may arise:

either independently from the posteromedial surface of the C 5 portion of the carotid siphon. Its origin lies between that of the recurrent artery of the foramen lacerum and that of the more or less complete posterosuperior trunk;

or from a common trunk (posterosuperior trunk).

The posteroinferior hypophyseal artery curves immediately, descending medially to supply the posterior hyophysis and anastomoses with its counterpart.

In one third of the cases, this artery branches off the medial artery of the clivus which runs towards the posterior clinoid process and then towards the dura of the clivus. At this level, the medial artery of the clivus passes into the transverse occipital plexus, where it supplies the meninges of this region and it anastomoses with the hypoglossal branch of the ascending pharyngeal artery.

The lateral artery of the clivus (dorsal meningeal artery for Parkinson and Rhoton)

Present in 82% of our cases, it arose:

independently from the lateral surface of C 5 (36%). Then it gives off two branches:

a medial branch which follows the superior edge of the lateral surface of the sixth nerve and always runs with it into Dorello's canal. This branch anastomoses with the jugular branch of the ascending pharyngeal artery;

another lateral branch which travels inside and beneath the trigeminal nerve, following the anterosuperior edge of the petrous bone. This branch supplies the fifth nerve and the ventral surface of the trigeminal ganglion. Finally it participates with the petrosal and petrosquamosal branches of the middle meningeal artery in a basal petrosal and tentorial arterial arcade, which supplies the basal edge of the tentorium cerebelli.

The origin of the lateral artery of the clivus lies above that of the recurrent artery of the foramen lacerum and beneath that of the posterosuperior trunk.

From a common posterosuperior trunk (40%), the meningohypophyseal trunk of Parkinson. After its origin, the artery immediately divides into medial and lateral branches.

From the recurrent artery of the foramen lacerum (3%). The artery thus observed fitted the medial branch and penetrated into Dorello's canal.

In this case, the lateral branch depends on the carotid branch of the ascending pharyngeal artery.

Beside it there usually exists a very important basal tentorial arcade in which the posterosuperior trunk participates.

In 21% of the cases, we observed a dual lateral artery of the clivus:

a medial which arose independently from the lateral surface of C 5 and then entered Dorello's canal;

another lateral, corresponding to the lateral branch and arising from the posterosuperior trunk.

The recurrent artery of the foramen lacerum

This small artery was found in 30% of cases. It may arise from:

for the most part the lateral surface of C 5, which means it is the first collateral of the carotid siphon, with which it remains in contact;

sometimes the posterosuperior trunk.

This artery penetrates into the foramen lacerum and then anastomoses with the carotid branch of the ascending pharyngeal artery.

It supplies the pericarotid autonomic nervous plexus and plays the role of vasa-vasorum.

The lateral artery of the trigeminal ganglion

This always present small branch arises for the most part from the superior part of the C 5 portion, courses laterally and above the trigeminal cistern and supplies the superficial part of the trigeminal ganglion and the adjacent duramater.

Sometimes this artery arises from either the lateral artery of the clivus or the cavernous basal branch of the middle meningeal artery.

The artery of the free margin of the tentorium cerebelli

This marginal tentorial artery, constantly present, may arise from the posterior trunk (45%). Other types of origin are possible (see later).

The basal tentorial artery

It usually divides into two branches. It arises from:

either the lateral branch of the lateral artery of the clivus;

or the posterosuperior trunk;

or independently and so corresponding to the cavernous branch of the middle meningeal artery.

Collateral branches of the C 4 portion of the carotid siphon

Capsular arteries

There are one, two or three arteries. These arteries arise from the medial surface of the C 4 portion of the carotid siphon. They run medially and anastomose on the midline with their counterparts, supplying the walls of the hypophyseal fossa, or at least the floor and lower part of the lateral wall.

One on each side may give off a branch which penetrates the bone vertically to descend into the sphenoidal sinus through which Rathke's pouch passed during embryonic development.

The inferolateral trunk

This artery is also called the lateral or inferior artery of the cavernous sinus. Its importance is usually underestimated.

The inferolateral trunk, present in 90% of our specimens, arises from the middle portion of the lateral surface of C 4. Occasionally is its origin more posterior, just after the first bend of the carotid siphon.

In its most frequent and complete form, it divides into four branches:

a superior or tentorial branch, which supplies the roof of the cavernous sinus, the third nerve (one or two branches), the fourth nerve (2 to 4 branches). This superior branch often takes part in the make-up of the marginal tentorial artery.

Rarely, the superior branch arises from a common trunk with:

an anteromedial branch, passing through the superior orbital fissure where it supplies the nerves as they enter the orbit and terminates as the deep recurrent ophthalmic artery. At the level of its origin, it is in contact with the superior margin of the sixth nerve;

an anterolateral branch which courses into the foramen rotundum. It seldom arises from a common trunk with the anteromedial branch, but on the other hand frequently with;

a posterior branch, which divides into an anterior ramus for the foramen ovale and a posterior ramus which passes under and supplies the trigeminal ganglion. This posterior ramus anastomoses with the middle meningeal artery at the level of the foramen spinosum.

The anterolateral and posterior branches, or their common trunk (when it exists), always pass at first between the lateral surface of the sixth nerve and the medial surface of the ophthalmic division of the fifth nerve that these arteries cross from the top downwards.

Sometimes, the inferolateral trunk gives off an anteroinferior branch, which does not pass through the superior orbital fissure but descends laterally in the duramater along the lesser wing of the sphenoid, to anastomosis with anterior rami of the middle meningeal artery.

The territories and anastomoses of these vessels are variable and numerous

Schematically, it should be understood that there exists a balance between the contribution of the maxillary artery through its transcranial branches and that of the internal carotid branches.

First case

The internal carotid branches are dominant. The C 4 segment gives off prominent inferolateral trunk which arches upwards over the sixth cranial nerve and gives rise to diverging branches of lesser caliber in the four territories of the inferolateral trunk. These branches anastomose with branches of the internal maxillary artery, which are smaller but present.

Second case

The transcranial branches of the internal maxillary artery are dominant. Therefore it is a branch of the accessory meningeal artery which enters this region via the foramen of Vesalius or via the foramen ovale to supply the whole area, giving four branches identical to those described in the inferolateral trunk. This variant is angiographically present in about 20% of cases. There is no anastomose with the cavernous internal carotid artery and no inferolateral trunk visible.

Intermediate forms

The region is supplied by two sources:

one via the accessory meningeal artery entering the skull through the foramen ovale, which supplies the anterolateral and posterior territories;

the other via the inferolateral trunk arising from the C 4 segment of the internal carotid artery, which supplies the superior and anteromedial territories.

In addition to the branches supplying the IIIrd, IVth, VIth, and Vth cranial nerves and their roots, the inferolateral trunk may also contribute through its posterior branch to the arterial supply of the intrapetrosal facial nerve.

The marginal tentorial artery
(or artery of the free edge of the tentorium cerebelli)

It is constantly present and supplies the anterosuperior third of the tentorium cerebelli. Its origin is variable. The different variants are located on an arterial arch which follows the posterior edge of the lesser wing of the sphenoid and the free margin of the tentorium. In our study, the following took part in its constitution:

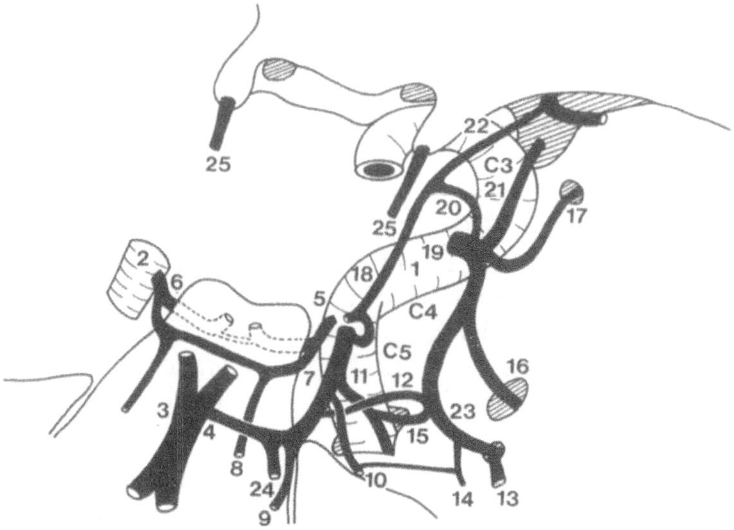

Fig. 5. Diagrammatic representation of the different anastomotic varieties in the parasellar area (adapted from Lasjaunias): right carotid siphon (*1*); left C 5 segment (*2*); basilar artery (*3*); trigeminal artery (*4*), right posterophypophyseal artery (*5*) and the left (*6*); medial clival artery (*7*); hypoglossal branch of the ascending pharyngeal artery (*8*); lateral clival artery or jugular branch of the ascending pharyngeal artery (*9*); basal tentorial artery (*10*); recurrent artery of the foramen lacerum (*11*); trigeminal meningeal anastomosis (*12*); middle meningeal artery (*13*); petrous branch of the middle meningeal artery (*14*); carotid branch of the ascending pharyngeal artery (*15*); cavernous branch of the accessory meningeal artery or artery of the foramen ovale (*16*); artery of the foramen rotundum (anterolateral branch of the ILT) (*17*); marginal tentorial artery (*18*); inferolateral trunk (ILT) (*19*); superior branch of the ILT (*20*); anteromedial branch of the ILT (*21*); recurrent meningeal artery (*22*); cavernous branch of the middle meningeal artery (*23*); cerebellar artery (*24*); free edge of the tentorium (*25*)

only the posterosuperior trunk in 20% of the cases;
posterosuperior trunk and inferolateral trunk (25%);
only the inferolateral trunk (43%),
the recurrent meningeal artery (12%) associated either for the most part with the inferolateral trunk or with the posterosuperior trunk.

However, the following arteries may participate in its constitution:
the middle meningeal artery;
the accessory meningeal artery;
the deep recurrent meningeal artery;
the lacrimal artery (meningolacrimal artery).

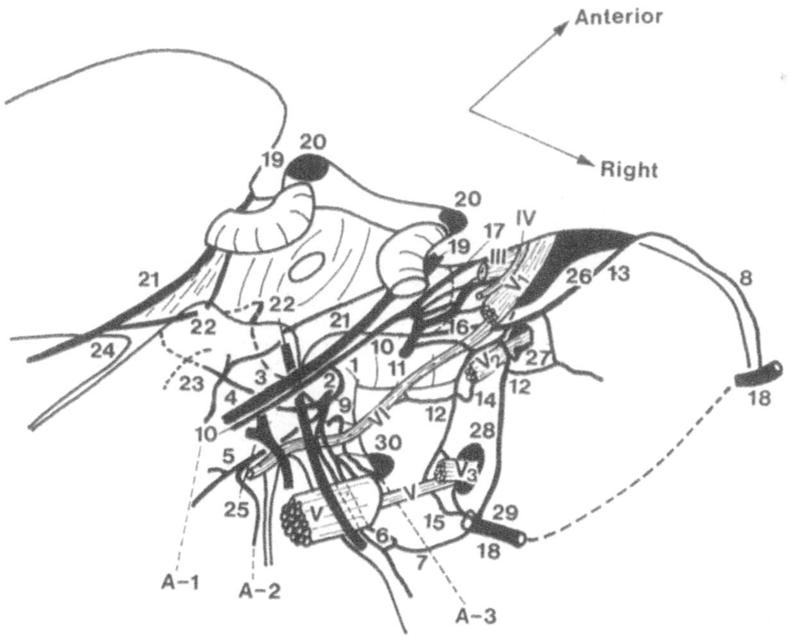

Fig. 6. Posterosuperior view and schematic representation of the collateral branches of the carotid siphon. *A-1* Anastomosis with the hypoglossal branch of the ascending pharyngeal artery. *A-2* Anastomosis with the jugular branch of the ascending pharyngeal artery. *A-3* Anastomosis with the carotid branch of the ascending pharyngeal artery. ICA (*1*); posterosuperior trunk (*2*); posteroinferior hypophyseal artery (*3*); medial clival artery (*4*); lateral clival artery (medial branch) (*5*); lateral clival artery (lateral branch) (*6*); basal tentorial branch of the petrous branch of the middle meningeal artery (MMA) (*7*); anterior branch of the middle meningeal artery (*8*); recurrent artery of the foramen lacerum (*9*); marginal tentorial artery (*10*); inferolateral trunk (*11*); posterior branch (*12*); anteroinferior branch (*13*); artery of the foramen rotundum (*14*); accessory meningeal artery (*15*); anteromedial branch (*16*); recurrent meningeal artery (*17*); middle meningeal artery (*18*); anterior clinoid process (*19*); optic canal (*20*); free edge of the tentorium (*21*); basal edge of the tentorium (*22*); clivus (*23*); petrous apex (*24*); petrous sphenoid ligament (*25*); superior orbital fissure (*26*); foramen rotundum (*27*); foramen ovale (*28*); foramen spinosum (*29*); foramen lacerum (*30*)

Hence, most often the marginal tentorial artery forms an arterial arcade along the free edge of the tentorium cerebelli, both destined for the meninges and also supplying the cranial nerves. So this artery is a "neuromeningeal artery".

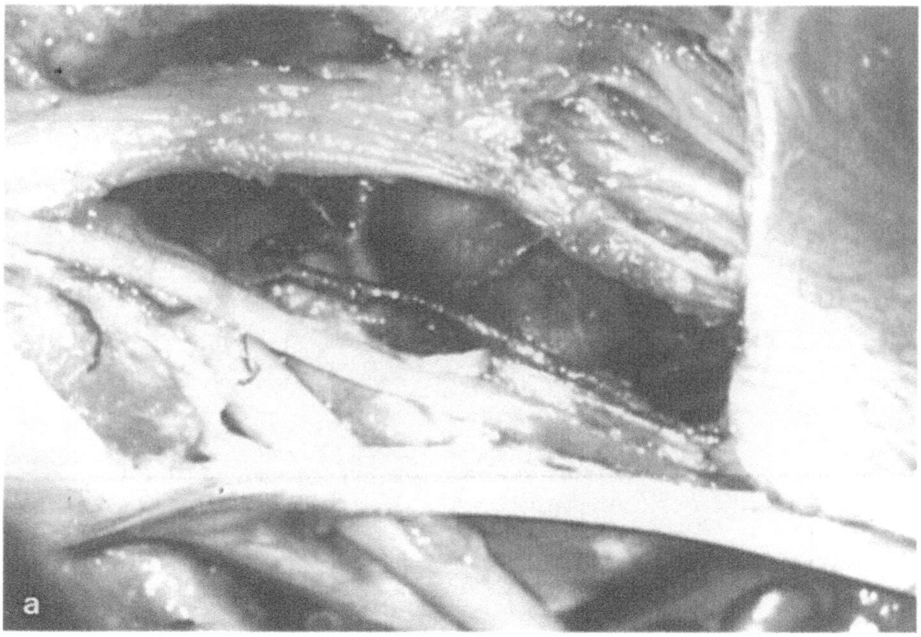

b

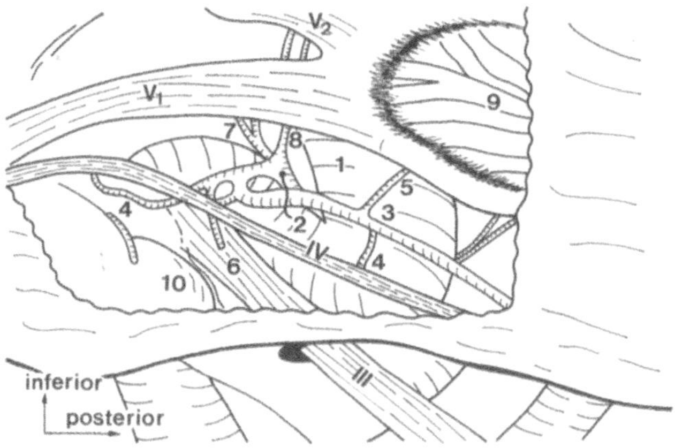

Fig. 7 a and **b.** Marginal tentorial artery which arises exclusively from the inferolateral trunk: ICA (*1*); inferolateral trunk (*2*); marginal tentorial artery (*3*); branch for the nerve IV (*4*); branch for the first division of the nerve V (*5*); branch for the nerve III (*6*); branch for the first division of the nerve V and for the nerve VI (*7*); artery of the foramen rotundum and ovale (*8*); area of the trigeminal ganglion (*9*); anterior clinoid process (*10*)

The basal edge of the tentorium cerebelli

It is supplied by two arcades, petrosal and occipital.

The petrosal arcade follows the superior petrosal sinus, courses laterally and receives:

the lateral branch of the lateral artery of the clivus;

the basal tentorial branch of the petrous ramus of the middle meningeal artery;

the basal tentorial branches of the petrosquamosal trunk of the middle meningeal artery.

The occipital arcade receives a contribution from two sources:

One, located supratentorially, is formed by terminal branches of the petrosquamosal trunk and descending branches of the occipital branch of the middle meningeal artery.

The other is infratentorial and formed by the superior branches of the artery of the cerebellar fossa laterally, the mastoid meningeal ramus of the occipital artery, a branch of the ascending pharyngeal artery, then of the vertebral artery posteriorly.

The territory apparently supplied by these basal arcades corresponds to the basal two thirds of the tentorium cerebelli. On the midline where the free margin crosses the confluence of the sinuses, and along the straight sinus, the left and right arteries anastomose, contributing in these instances to the supply of the inferior part of the falx cerebri.

Comparison with previous studies and discussion

Quite obviously, we have not made the same conclusions as the two most important microsurgical studies, which were carried out by Parkinson [29, 30, 31, 32] and then Rhoton [4, 33].

These authors describe three groups of collateral branches arising from the carotid siphon:

Firstly, the meningohypophyseal trunk. According to Rhoton, this artery is always present and its caliber is nearly the same as that of the ophthalmic artery.

The meningohypophyseal trunk divides almost immediately into three branches which are the tentorial artery (always present and arising from this common trunk), the dorsal meningeal artery and the inferior hypophyseal artery.

In 6% of Rhoton's specimens, the artery of the inferior cavernous sinus arises from the meningohypophyseal trunk. Parkinson finds a trifurcation of the meningohypophyseal trunk in 100% of his specimens and furthermore describes an arterial circle around the dorsum sellae. This arterial circle depends on both the left and right dorsal meningeal arteries and the left and right inferior hypophyseal arteries.

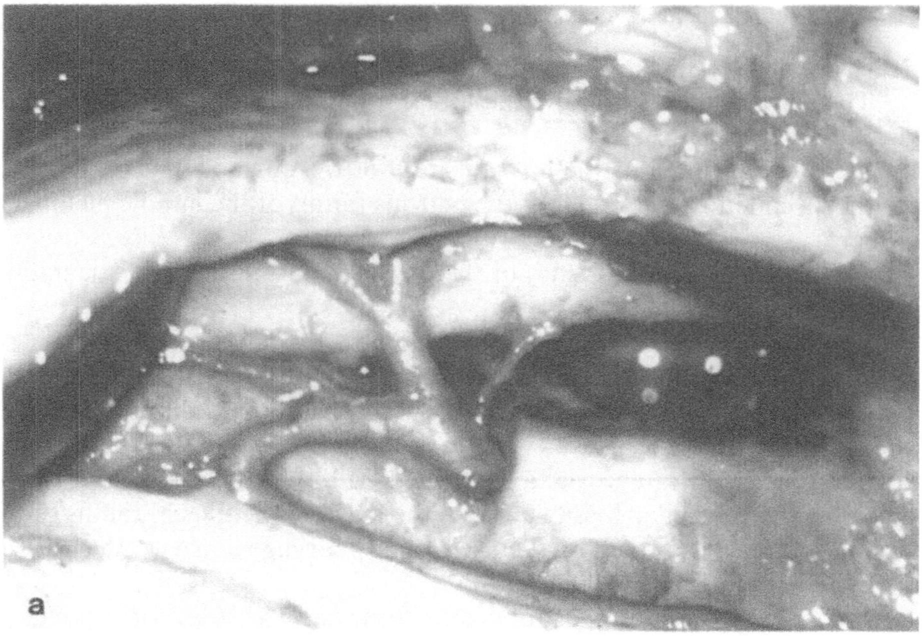

a

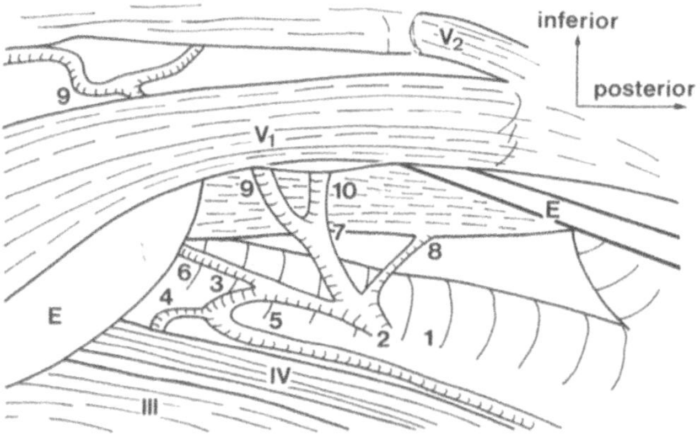

b

Fig. 8 a and **b.** Inferolateral trunk in its complete form: internal carotid artery (C 4) (*1*); inferolateral trunk (*2*); superior branch (*3*); branch for the nerve IV and the CS roof (*4*); marginal tentorial artery, running along the inferior edge of the nerve IV (*5*); anteromedial branch (*6*); common trunk giving (*9*) and (*10*), and passing between the nerve VI and the first division of the nerve V (*7*); branch for the nerve VI (*8*); anterolateral branch (*9*); posterior branch (*10*)

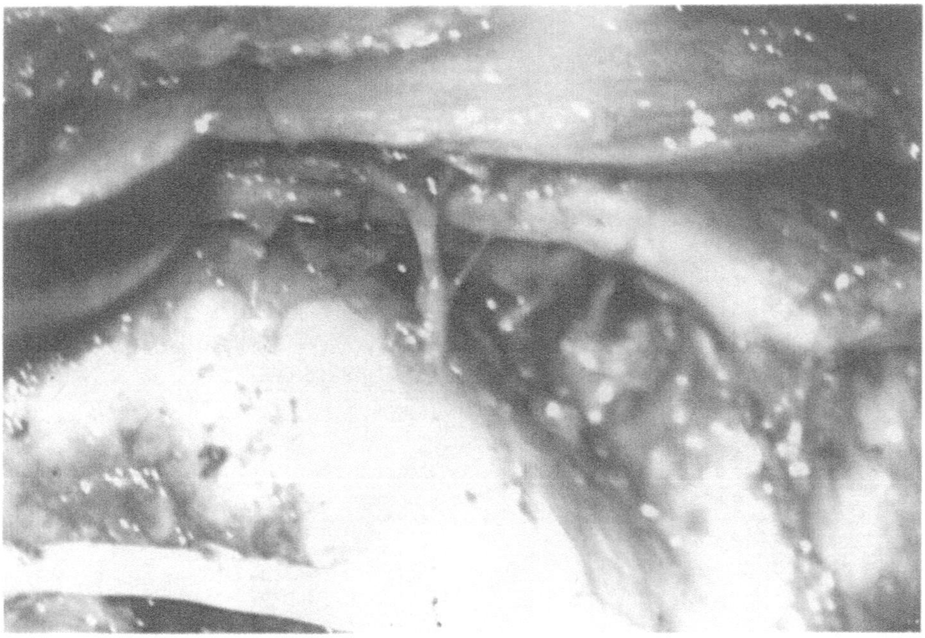

Fig. 9. Hypoplasic inferolateral trunk

The artery of the inferior cavernous sinus. It passes over the sixth nerve and downwards medial to the ophthalmic division of the fifth nerve, to supply the dura of the inferior wall of the cavernous sinus and the area of the foramina ovale and spinosum. It may anastomose with the middle meningeal artery at the foramen spinosum and gives off some branches to the Gasserian ganglion.

The McConnell's capsular arteries are present in 28% of Rhoton's specimens. These conclusions are about the same as ours.

Finally, Rhoton et al. found that the ophthalmic artery arose within the cavernous sinus in 8% of the cases.

As regards the possible persistent trigeminal artery, Parkinson and Shields [32] observe this artery in 0.5% of the cases. According to these authors, it courses laterally and posteriorly, passing immediately beneath the abducens nerve, then piercing the posterior dural wall of the cavernous sinus trough a separate foramen located 1 cm medial to the trigeminal root and 1 cm superolateral to Dorello's canal.

Our approach of the collateral branches of the carotid siphon was different from previous studies because we took into account:

observations through the superselective angiographies of the cranio-facial arteries [9], showing numerous variations and enabling a more dynamic approach than anatomical studies;

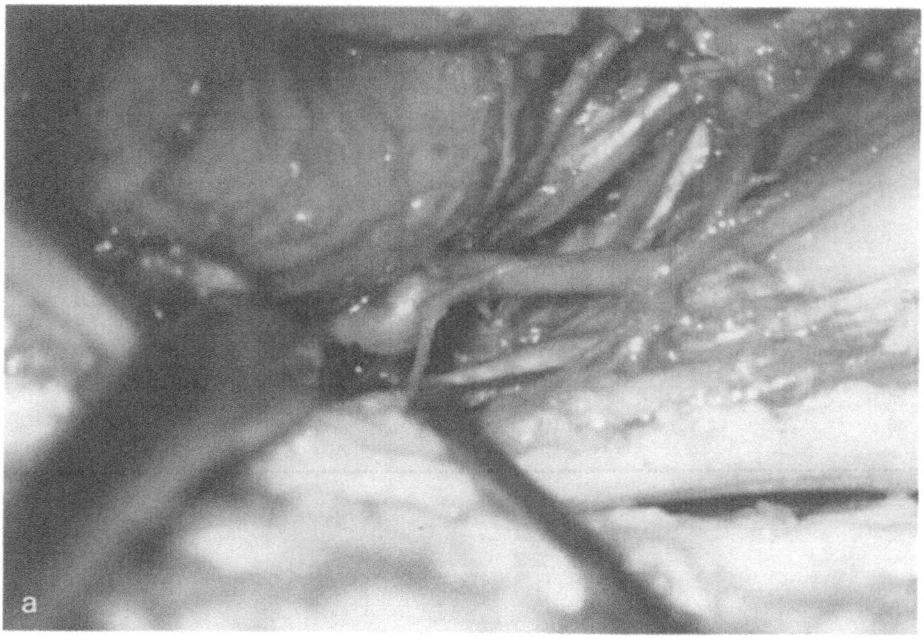

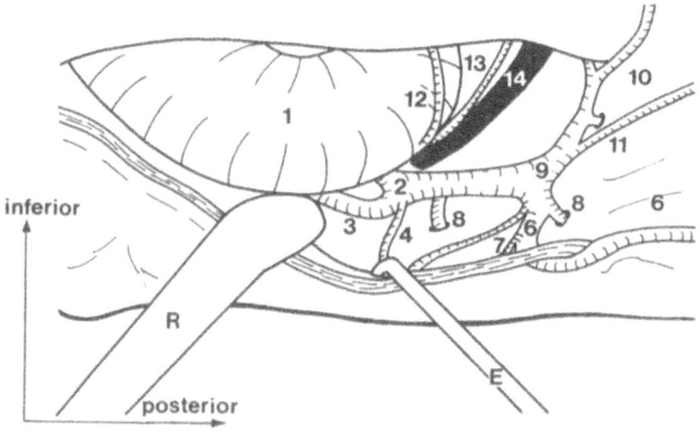

Fig. 10 a and **b.** Collateral branches of the C 5 segment: first bend of the carotid siphon (*1*); posterosuperior or meningohypophyseal trunk (*2*); posteroinferior hypophyseal artery (*3*); medial clival artery (*4*); common trunk giving (*9*) and (*6*) (*5*); marginal tentorial artery (arising here only from C 5) (*6*); branches for the nerve IV (*7*); rami for the dura (*8*); common trunk giving (*10*) and (*11*) (*9*); artery of the trigeminal ganglion (*10*); basal tentorial artery (*11*); recurrent artery of the foramen lacerum (*12*); lateral clival artery (*13*). (*12*) and (*13*) arise individually from C 5; petrous sphenoid ligament (*14*), *R* Retractor

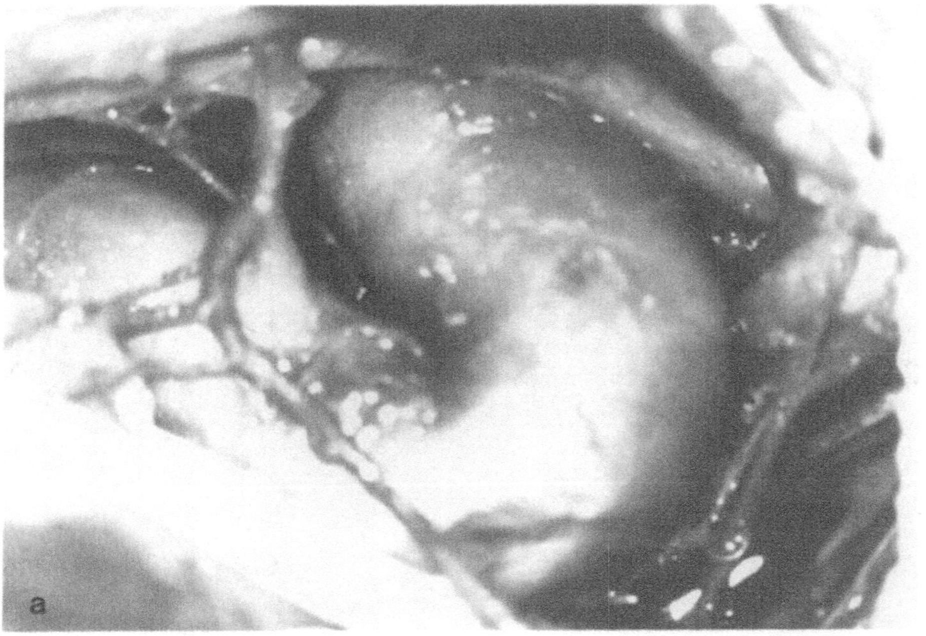

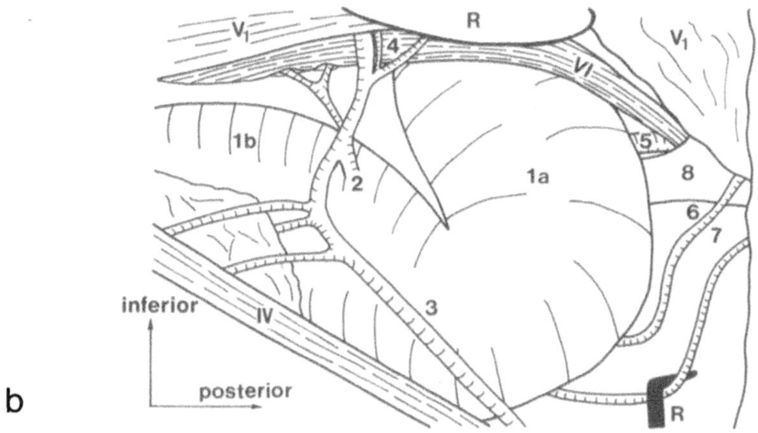

Fig. 11 a and **b.** Superior view of the content of the cavernous sinus. Here the marginal tentorial artery arises exclusively from the inferolateral trunk. There is no true posterosuperior trunk: carotid siphon (*1 a*: C 5) (*1 b*: C 4); origin of the inferolateral trunk (*2*); marginal tentorial artery (*3*); arteries of the foramen rotundum and ovale (*4*); lateral clival artery (*5*); artery of the Gasserian ganglion (*6*); basal tentorial artery (*7*); petrous sphenoid ligament (*8*), *R* Retractor

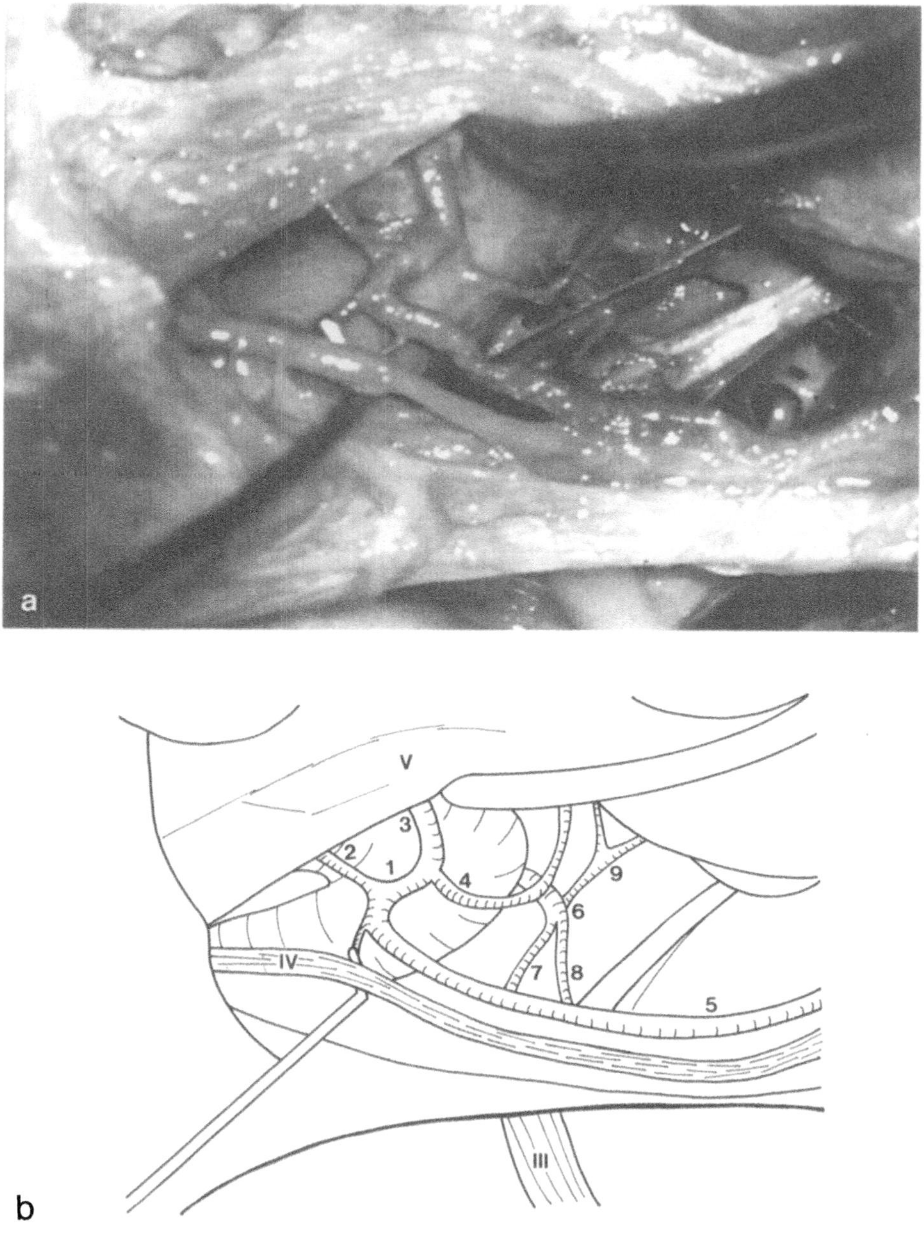

Fig. 12 a and **b.** Mixed formed with: an ILT notably giving rise to the marginal tentorial artery and a posterosuperior trunk, giving off three branches: ILT (*1*); anterolateral branch (*2*); posterior branch for the foramen ovale (*3*); posterior branch for the trigeminal ganglion (*4*); marginal tentorial artery (*5*); posterosuperior trunk (*6*); posteroinferior hypophyseal artery (*7*); medial clival artery (*8*); lateral clival artery (*9*)

the different possibilities of embryonic development, the possible hemodynamic balance between the internal carotid and external carotid respective systems, the right and left sides, the anterior, lateral or posterior areas;

so in fact there does not exist a so-called normal description contrasting with variations, which must be considered as abnormalities. On the other hand, we think it is not necessary to describe all the possibilities as a percentage, because any systematization is hazardous and the list of the anatomical variants is not completely established.

However, we would stress:

the respective importance of the branches arising from the C 4 segment (inferolateral trunk) and those arising from the C 5 segment (meningohypophyseal trunk or posterosuperior trunk),

a possible intracavernous origin of the ophthalmic artery and the role of the internal maxillary artery in supplying the orbit;

the importance of transosseous arterial anastomoses;

the role played by the internal maxillary artery, the ascending pharyngeal artery interconnected with the carotid siphon and thus which have areas dependent on them which are classically attributed to the internal carotid artery;

the anastomoses between both the carotid siphons by their respective C 5 segments;

the dual supply of the tentorium cerebelli in its anterior portion and the role of the marginal tentorial artery (classical artery of the free edge of the tentorium) both destined for meninges and also supplying cranial nerves.

Conclusion

As a result, two points should be emphasized:

firstly the presence in this area of a fundamental duality between internal carotid and external carotid arteries;

secondly, the importance of actively taking into consideration the branches of the carotid siphon, according to their own anastomoses and their respective areas of supply.

References

1. Dandy W, Goetsche E (1911) The blood supply of the pituitary body. Am J Anat 11: 137–150
2. Djindjian R, Hurth M, Bories J, Brunet P (1965) L'artère trigéminée primitive (aspects artériographiques et signification à propos de 12 cas). P Med 73: 2905

3. Dolenc V (1983) Direct microsurgical repair of intracavernous vascular lesions. J Neurosurg 58: 824–831
4. Harris FS, Rhoton AL (1976) Anatomy of the cavernous sinus. J Neurosurg 45: 169–180
5. Henderson WR (1966) A note on realtionship of the human maxillary nerve to the cavernous sinus and to an emissary sinus passing through the foramen ovale. J Anat 100: 905–908
6. Kuru Y (1967) Meningeal branches of the ophthalmic artery. Acta Radiol 6: 241–251
7. Lang J (1974) Eintritt und Verlauf der Hirnnerven (III, IV, VI) im Sinus cavernosus. Z Anat Entwickl Gesch 145: 87–89
8. Lang J (1981) Topographical anatomy of the cranial nerves. In: Samii M, Jannetta P (eds) The cranial nerves. Springer, Berlin Heidelberg New York, pp 6–15
9. Lasjaunias P (1981 and 1983) Cranio-facial and upper cervical arteries, 2 vols. Williams and Wilkins, Baltimore [Functional, clinical and angiographic aspects, vol 1, pp 13–99. Collateral circulation and angiographic protocols, vol 2, pp 115–128]
10. Lasjaunias P, Berenstein A, Moret J (1983) Signification de la vascularisation durale des lésions du système nerveux central. J Neuroradiol 10: 31–42
11. Lasjaunias P, Berges O, Doyon D (1979) Circulation collatérale de l'artère maxillaire interne. J Neuroradiol 6: 197–205
12. Lasjaunias P, Doyon D, Vignaud J et al (1975) Progress in the arteriographic study of cavernous sinus disease. In: Salamon G (ed) Advances in cerebral angiography. Springer, Berlin Heidelberg New York, pp 324–330
13. Lasjaunias P, Merland JJ, Theron J, Moret J (1977) Vascularisation méningée de la fosse cérébrale moyenne. Neuroradiology 4: 361–384
14. Lasjaunias P, Moret J (1976) The ascending pharyngeal artery: normal and pathological radioanatomy. Neuroradiology 11: 77–82
15. Lasjaunias P, Moret J, Mink J (1977) The anatomy of the inferolateral trunk (ILT) of the internal carotid artery. Neuroradiology 13: 215–220
16. Lasjaunias P, Picard L, Manelfe C, Moret J, Roland J (1981) Angiographic aspects of the arterial supply of the cranial nerves. In: Samii M, Jannetta P (eds) The cranial nerves. Springer, Berlin Heidelberg New York, pp 195–206
17. Lasjaunias P, Theron J (1976) Radiographic anatomy of the accessory meningeal artery. Radiology 21: 99–104
18. Lazorthes G, Gouaze A (1968) Voies anastomotiques de suppléance de la vascularisation artérielle de l'axe cérébro-médullaire. CR Assoc Anat 140: 5–79
19. Lazorthes G, Gouaze A, Salamon G (1976) Vascularisation et circulation de l'encéphale. Masson, Paris, pp 84–85, 220–235
20. Leclercq TA, Grisoli F (1983) Arterial blood supply of the normal human pituitary gland. An anatomical study. J Neurosurg 58: 678–681
21. Lie TA (1968) Congenital anomalies of teh carotid arteries. Excerpta Medica Foundation, Amsterdam, 1–13
22. McConnell EM (1953) The arterial blood supply of the human hypophysis cerebri. Anat Rec 115: 175–203

23. MacLennan JE, Rosenbaum AE, Haughton VM (1974) Internal carotid origins of the middle meningeal artery. Neuroradiology 7: 265–275
24. Merland JJ, Bories J, Djindjian R (1977) Vascularisation de la faux du cervau, de la faux et de la tente du cervelet. Neuroradiology 4: 175–202
25. Moret J, Lasjaunias P, Theron J, Merland JJ (1977) L'artère méningée moyenne. Son apport à la vascularisation de l'orbite. J Neuroradiol 4: 225–248
26. Mori K (1979) The cavernous sinus. Neurol Med Chir (Tokyo) 19: 757–769
27. Mori K (1982) A surgical approach to the carotid-cavernous fistulas: anatomical studies. No Shinkei Geka 10: 3
28. Padget DH (1948) The development of the cranial arteries in the human embryo. Contrib Embryol Carneg Instr 32: 205–262
29. Parkinson D (1965) A surgical approach to the cavernous portion of the carotid artery. Anatomical studies and case report. J Neurosurg 23: 474–483
30. Parkinson D (1973) Carotid cavernous fistula: direct repair with preservation of the carotid artery; technical note. J Neurosurg 38: 99–106
31. Parkinson D, Hunt Br, Zeal A (1978) Lateral sellar venous anatomy. Cavernous sinus. Anat Rec 190: 503
32. Parkinson D, Shields CB (1974) Persistent trigeminal artery: its relationship to the normal branches of the cavernous carotid. J Neurosurg 39: 244–248
33. Rhoton AL, Hardy DG, Chambers SM (1979) Microsurgical anatomy and dissection of the sphenoid bone, cavernous sinus and sellar region. Surg Neurol 12: 63–104
34. Schnurer LB, Stattin S (1963) Vascular supply of the intracranial dura from internal carotid artery with special references to its angiographic significance. Acta Radiol 1: 441–450
35. Stattin S (1961) Meningeal vessel of the internal carotid artery and their angiographic significance. Acta Radiol 55: 329

Anatomical remarks on the fetal cavernous sinus and on the veins of the middle cranial fossa

E. Knosp[1], G. Müller[2], and A. Perneczky[1]

[1] Department of Neurosurgery and [2] Institute of Anatomy, University of Vienna, Vienna, Austria

Introduction

Increasing surgical experience within the cavernous sinus region has generated increased interest in the region's anatomy. Despite many attempts to understand the morphological complexity of the cavernous sinus, its description and interpretation are still controversial. Two main views oppose each other: classic textbooks of anatomy, but also recent studies (e.g. Harris and Rhoton [11], Bedford [1]), interpret the cavernous sinus as an intradural venous canal, which is more or less trabeculated by fibrous strands. Several other workers of the present century, however, interpret the cavernous sinus as a network of extradural veins (e.g. Taptas [21, 22], Bonnet [3], Parkinson [15, 16, 17], a view which is not yet generally accepted. Other controversial problems of the area concern the relationship of the venous pathways with the structures that pass through the cavernous sinus area, like the internal carotid artery and the cranial nerves that run to the orbital cavity.

It is our view that these questions can only be solved by a developmental approach, which does not regard the cavernous sinus as an isolated adult structure, but as a result of the development of the entire venous arrangements at the skull base.

It will be argued in the present paper that, throughout the fetal period, the anatomical region named cavernous sinus in the adult consists of a network of distinct, individual, veins. Therefore the term "cavernous venous plexus" will be applied to this structure. In this terminology "cavernous" merely points to the anatomical region and provides a semantic link to the traditional name of the area, but does not indicate any cavernous condition of its morphology.

Method

Dissection of the parasellar area was carried out in 10 fetal skull bases. Six of these were formalin-fixed and two were fresh autopsy cases. According to their crown-rump length the age of the fetuses ranged from 17 to 40 weeks of gestation.

The skin of the heads was incised along the coronal suture, and the supratentorial calvaria and dura mater were removed while the tentorium was preserved. The midbrain, the optic nerves, the carotid arteries and the infundibulum were transsected and the cerebral hemispheres were removed. The anatomical preparation of both parasellar areas was carried out under a surgical microscope and included in every case the following steps: mapping of the veins in the middle cranial fossa (MCF); removal of the superficial dural layer of the MCF and of the lateral wall of the cavernous sinus region; study of the course and relationship of cranial nerves (CN) III, IV, and V; removal of these nerves and careful dissection of the veins, of the internal carotid artery (ICA) with its branches, and of CN VI.

Two fetal sella blocs were formalin-fixed, decalcified, sectioned in the coronal plane, and stained for connective tissue.

Results

Veins of the middle cranial fossa

Throughout all stages of development remnants of the tentorial sinus and of the prootic sinus could be seen. The middle cerebral veins drain into the tentorial sinus (Fig. 1), which runs from the lesser sphenoid wing along the bottom of the MCF towards the tentorium, usually without any connection to the cavernous plexus. The tentorial sinus either joins the superior petrosal sinus or directly joins the transverse sinus. In 3 cases, however, the middle cerebral veins unilaterally drained into the cavernous venous plexus. The location of this connection was found between CN III and CN IV. The middle cerebral veins were never seen to form a sphenoparietal sinus, which is commonly described as following the edge of the lesser sphenoid wing to join the cavernous sinus in its anterior portion.

Superior petrosal sinus

In all specimens the superior petrosal sinus could be observed. In 60% of these cases the sinus communicated with the veins of the cavernous plexus (Fig. 2). This connection usually is frail and always passes over CN V, but never underneath the nerve. Lateral to the entrance of the superior petrosal vein the diameter of the sinus always increases towards its junction with the

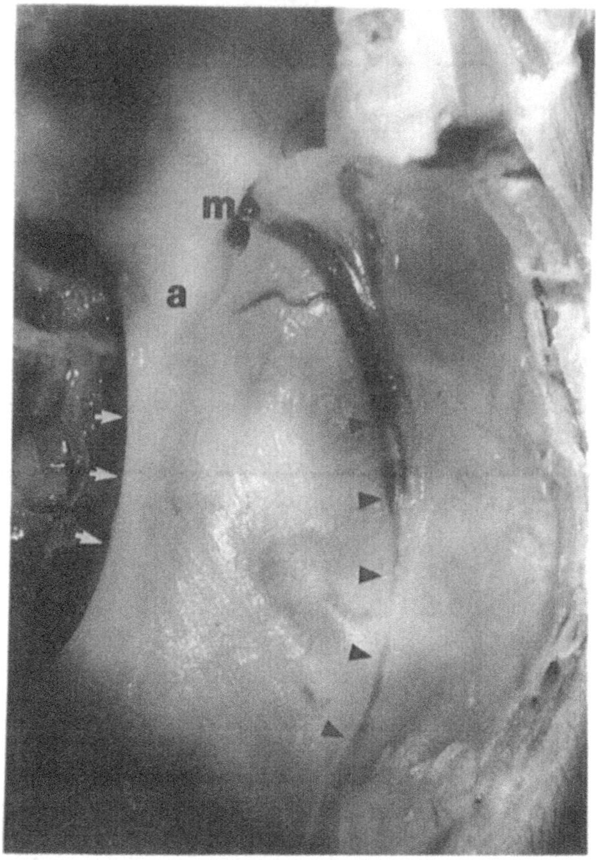

Fig. 1. Right middle cranial fossa (fetus of 18 cm CRL). The middle cerebral veins (*m*) drain into the tentorial sinus (black triangles) which joins the transverse sinus. In this case no connection to the cavernous venous plexus was present. Anterior clinoid process (*a*); tentorial rim (white arrows)

transverse sinus and thus mainly represents the drainage of this vein. In two of the skull bases the superior petrosal sinus appeared duplicated, because the superior petrosal vein ran parallel to the middle part of the sinus (Fig. 2).

Superior ophthalmic vein

This vein represents the main contribution to the cavernous venous plexus. The vein enters the MCF through the superior orbital fissure, lateral to the nerves, and follows the margin of the greater wing of the sphenoid. On its further course the vein passes between the first and second branch of the

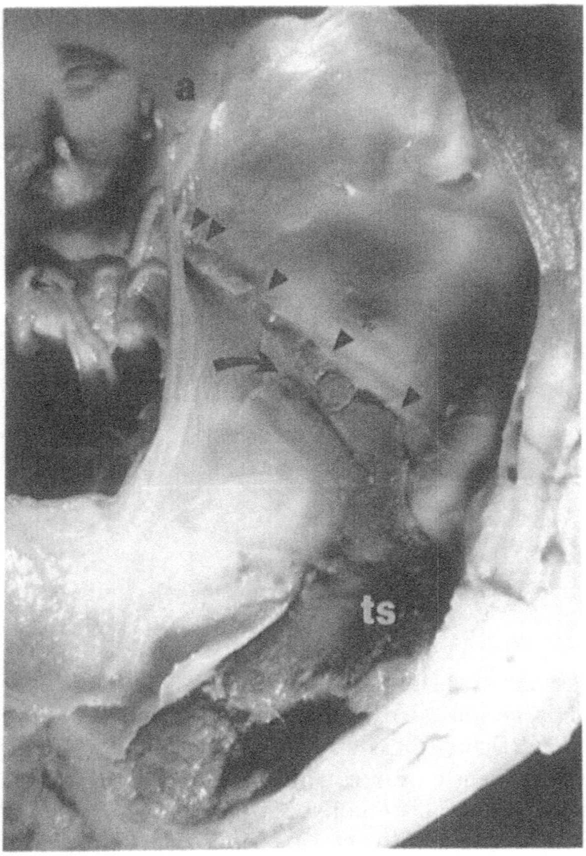

Fig. 2. Right middle cranial fossa (fetus of 14 cm CRL). The superior petrosal sinus (black triangles) has a significant communication with the cavernous venous plexus (pair of triangles). The anterior petrosal vein (arrow) parallels the superior petrosal sinus. Both venous structures join the transverse sinus (*ts*). Anterior clinoid process (*a*)

trigeminal nerve (Fig. 3). Medial to CN V/1 the superior ophthalmic vein divides into several branches and joints the cavernous plexus in its lower, anterior part.

Cavernous venous plexus

During the fetal period observed in our study, the parasellar venous pathway consists of individual vessels, which are clearly separated by abundant connective tissue (Fig. 4). The vessel walls consist only of an endothelial layer, without a muscular layer (Fig. 4). The venous vessels of

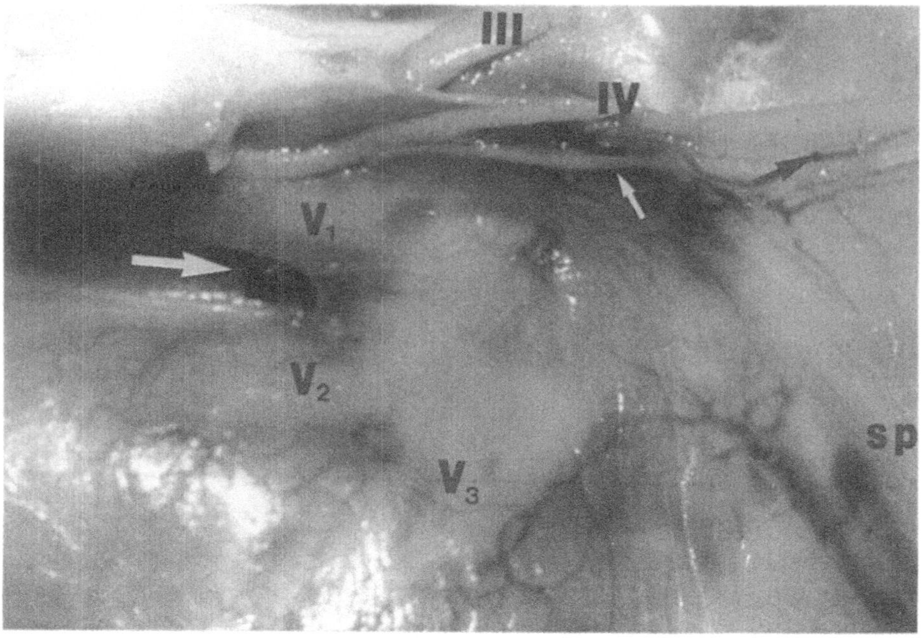

Fig. 3. Left parasellar area, lateral view (fetus of 18 cm CRL). The left superior ophthalmic vein (large white arrow) takes its regular course between V/1 and V/2. Oculomotor nerve (*III*); divisions of the trigeminal nerve (*V/1, V/2, V/3*). Trochlear nerve (*IV*) with a frequently occurring duplication (small white arrow). Tentorial branch (black arrow) of the meningohypophyseal trunk. No communication of the superior petrosal sinus (*sp*) with the cavernous venous plexus is present in this specimen

this area show several interconnections and thus appear as a plexiform network. The splitting of the superior ophthalmic vein marks the anterior beginning of the venous plexus. The main compartment of the plexus consists of a few large veins which run medial to the ICA (Fig. 5 a). A minor compartment, which consists of one or two smaller veins, runs together with the abducent nerve on the lateral side of the ICA (Fig. 5 b). The network of veins converges towards the inferior petrosal sinus, which represents its continuation. Thus, in the posterior part of the cavernous sinus region, the main compartment of the veins lies superior to the ICA which descends towards the internal carotid canal. The ICA has no intimate contact with the venous plexus, and may be removed without compromising the veins. The same is true for the abducent nerve. The oculomotor nerve, the trochlear nerve, and the ophthalmic nerve run lateral to the venous plexus.

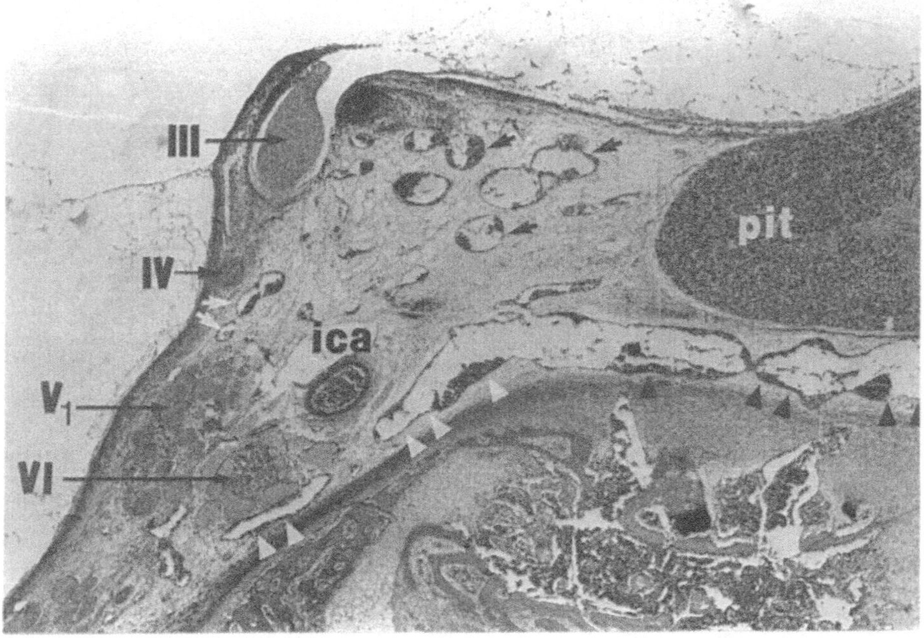

Fig. 4. Histological section through the left parasellar area, posterior to the entrance of the oculomotor nerve (fetus of 20 cm CRL). The cavernous venous plexus clearly consists of individual vessels (black arrows), which are richly surrounded by connective tissue. At this level some vessels of the main compartment of the venous plexus lie superior to the ICA. The inferior intercavernous connection (black triangles) joins the medial compartment of the venous plexus (white triangles). Lateral compartment of the venous plexus (white arrows). Oculomotor nerve (*III*); trochlear nerve (*IV*); ophthalmic nerve (*V/1*); abducent nerve (*VI*); internal carotid artery (*ica*); pituitary gland (*pit*)

In one case the left cavernous venous plexus was completely absent. The left superior ophthalmic vein drained via the anterior intercavernous vein into the contralateral venous plexus (see below). In this specimen the left middle cerebral veins did not join the venous plexus, but left the skull base through the oval foramen.

Intracavernous connections

The cavernous plexuses of both sides are connected across the midline. These interconnecting veins, which are called "intracavernous sinuses" in the adult, pass in front of, inferior to, and dorsal to the pituitary gland. The inferior interconnection was seen in all specimens. In one third of the cases

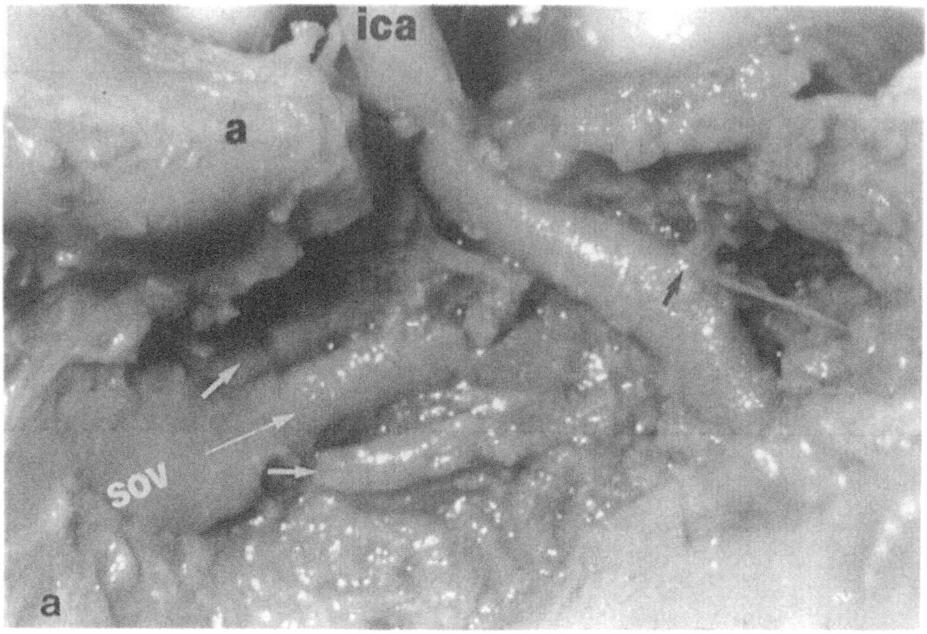
ica
a
sov
a

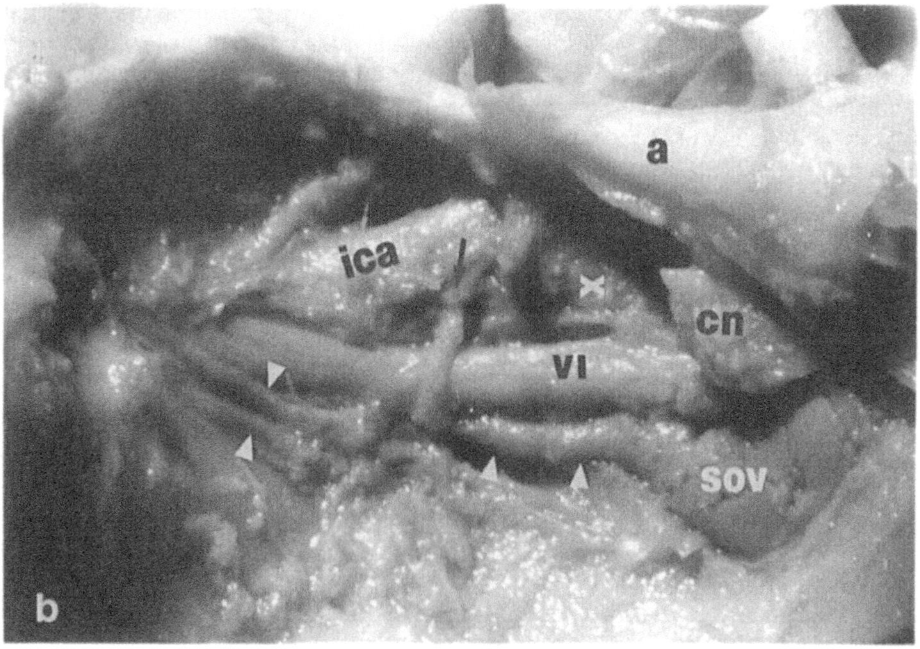
a
ica
x
cn
vi
sov
b

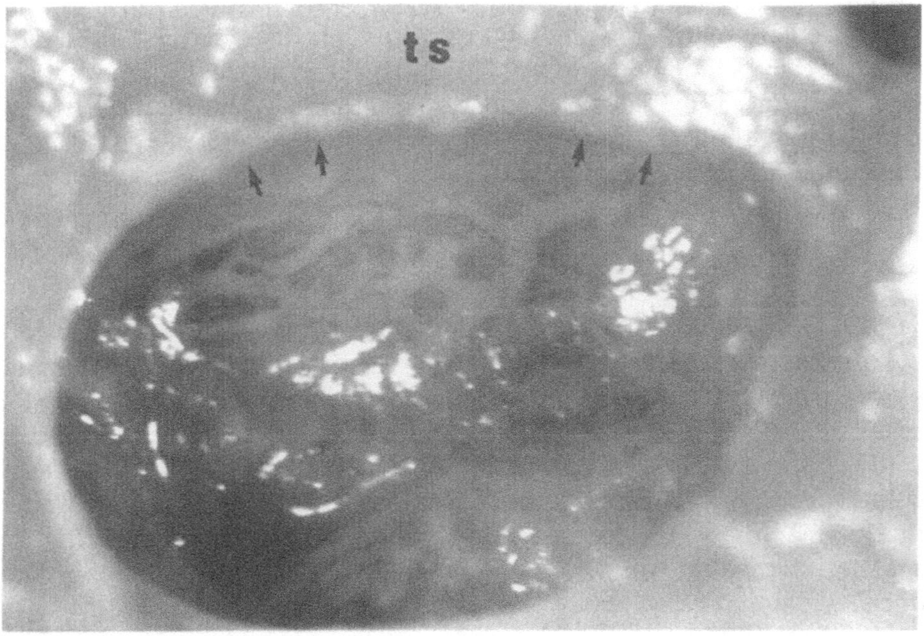

Fig. 6. Hypophyseal fossa after removal of the pituitary gland (fetus of 18 cm CRL). A rich venous network forms the inferior intercavernous connection at the sella floor. The diaphragma sellae is cut open (arrows); tuberculum sellae (*ts*)

Fig. 5. Parasellar area, lateral view (fetus of 22 cm CRL): **a** Left cavernous venous plexus after the removal of the lateral sinus wall and of the cranial nerves. The main compartment of the venous plexus consists of several individual veins (white arrows), which come from the superior ophthalmic vein (*sov*), and take a course medial to the internal carotid artery (*ica*). Note the rather straight course of the fetal ICA and the origin of the meningohypophyseal trunk (black arrow). Anterior clinoid process (*a*). **b** Lateral compartment of a right cavernous venous plexus (white triangles): the veins originate from the superior ophthalmic vein (*sov*), and follow the course of the abducent nerve (*VI*). Medial compartment of the venous plexus (*x*); internal carotid artery (*ica*); inferior lateral trunk (arrow); stumps of cranial nerves III, IV, V/1 (*cn*) within the superior orbital fissure; anterior clinoid process (*a*) the latter represented the main intracavernous connection, sometimes forming an irregular venous network at the sella floor (Fig. 6).

In the case of the missing left cavernous plexus described above, the superior ophthalmic vein crossed the midline as an unusually large anterior intercavernous vein. Thus the superior ophthalmic vein of the left orbit drained into the right cavernous plexus. In this variant no other intercavernous connection was present.

Drainage of the cavernous venous plexus

The inferior petrosal sinus represents the main drainage of the cavernous venous plexus. This sinus is formed by the converging veins of the cavernous plexus, which leave the area of the "cavernous sinus" lateral to the dorsum sellae.

The foramen ovale represents an important pathway for direct transcranial drainage of the cavernous plexus into the pterygoid plexus. Within the foramen the vein is located medial to the mandibular nerve.

The internal carotid venous plexus represents in many cases a very important drainage system of the cavernous plexus. This venous pathway passes through the carotid canal and joins the internal jugular vein. This pathway was generally found to be more prominent in the fetus, when compared to the adult condition.

Occasionally other transcranial drainage pathways were seen to pass through the round foramen as well as through the foramen of Vesal; both join the pterygoid venous plexus.

Discussion

The development of the cranial venous system is described in detail by Padget [14]. According to her work, the cavernous sinus forms, during the 40 mm stage of embryonic development, as a plexiform extension of the prootic sinus and of the ventral myelencephalic vein (Fig. 7 a). Through this process the primitive maxillary vein, which drained into the prootic sinus, now joins the cavernous sinus. Thus this vein, later known as the superior ophthalmic vein, drains the orbit via the cavernous sinus and the inferior petrosal sinus into the jugular system. Padget [14] also emphasizes that the connection of the superficial middle cerebral veins with the cavernous sinus, and the connection of the superior petrosal sinus with the cavernous sinus, usually are not yet established before birth (Fig. 7 b). According to her, only after the establishment of these secondary connections do the cerebral veins, which formerly drained via the tentorial sinus into the transverse sinus, bring cerebral blood to the cavernous sinus system.

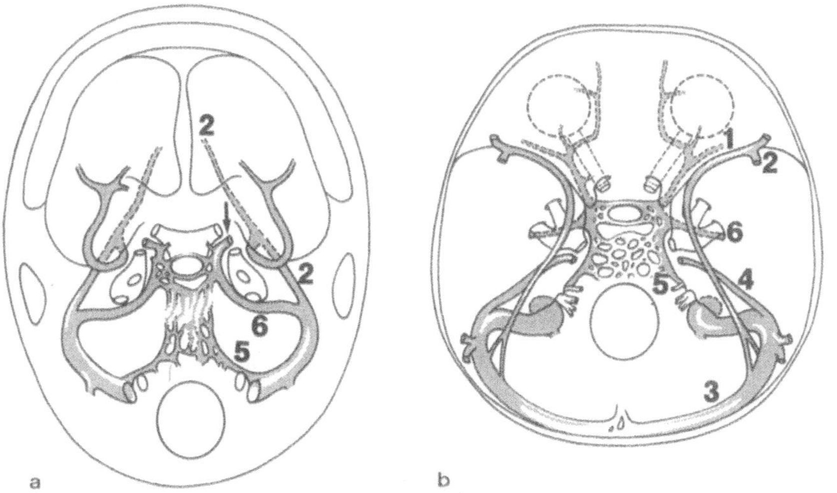

Fig. 7. Developmental stages of the basal cranial veins (after Padget [14]): **a** 40 mm stage of human embryo. The "cavernous sinus" and the inferior petrosal sinus develop as extensions of the prootic sinus (*6*) and the ventral myelencephalic vein (*5*). Tentorial sinus (*2*); superior ophthalmic vein (arrow). **b** Early infant stage. The superior ophthalmic vein (*1*) drains into the internal jugular vein via the cavernous plexus and the inferior petrosal sinus (*5*). The tentorial sinus drains the middle cerebral veins (*2*) into the transverse sinus (*3*). The connection of the superior petrosal sinus (*4*) to the cavernous plexus is not yet formed. Venous drainage through the oval foramen (*6*)

In contrast to Padget's concept, Butler [4] described the cavernous sinus as the expanded remnant to the embryonic vena capitis medialis, and not as the coalescence of a venous plexus.

The findings of our present study of fetal skull base are summarized in Fig. 8. The results are basically in accordance with the developmental concept of Padget [14]. In about 20% of our cases, however, we could demonstrate that either the middle cerebral veins drained directly into the cavernous plexus, or the tentorial sinus had a connection to the cavernous plexus. The superior petrosal sinus was also connected to the cavernous plexus in 60% of the dissected specimens, but only in two cases did this connection seem to be of major functional significance. These findings demonstrate the prenatal existence of cerebral blood drainage through the cavernous plexus, which becomes more pronounced in postnatal life.

Our microanatomical and histological analysis of the cavernous sinus area shows individual venous vessels with endothelial vessel walls. These veins are separated and richly surrounded by loose connective tissue. The main compartment of veins lies medial to the ICA. Thus it is early confirmed that, during the fetal period of the development of the cranial venous system, the so-called cavernous sinus actually is a venous network, consisting of distinct individual veins. We therefore propose to apply the term "cavernous venous plexus" (see Introduction).

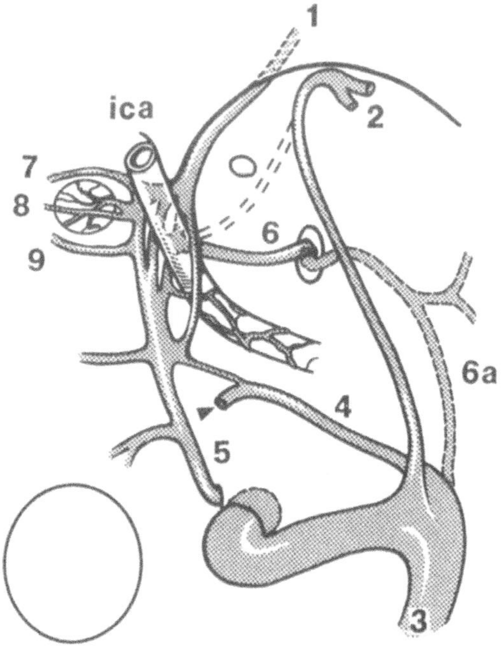

Fig. 8. Diagram of the fetal cavernous venous plexus and associated venous pathways. The superior ophthalmic vein (*1*) represents the main supply to the cavernous plexus. The vein divides into several individual vessels, which form a plexiform network in the space of the cavernous sinus. The main compartment of the veins runs medial to the internal carotid artery (*ica*), and has connections to the contralateral plexus anterior to (*7*), posterior to (*9*), and inferior to (*8*) the pituitary gland. The latter is the largest intercavernous connection in the fetal period. A minor compartment of the veins passes lateral to the ICA. The venous network converges, posterior and superior to the ICA, to form the inferior petrosal sinus (*5*), which brings the blood to the jugular vein. The vessel to the oval foramen (*6*) is a remnant of the former prootic sinus (*6*, together with *6 a*). The middle cerebral veins (*2*) drain cerebral blood into the transverse sinus (*3*), but may also have connections (dotted lines) to the cavernous venous plexus. The pericarotid plexus drains venous blood through the canal of the internal carotid artery (*ica*). The anterior petrosal vein (▶) joins the superior petrosal sinus (*5*)

Our findings are in agreement with Taptas' [21, 22] concept, which proposes a distinction between the "space of the cavernous sinus" and the "parasellar venous pathway". We, however, were not able to confirm Bedford's [1] description of the fetal ICA within a cavernous sinus. In all our cases the ICA was richly surrounded by connective tissue without intimate contact to the venous plexus. The ICA, however, clearly runs within the "space of the cavernous sinus" in the sense of Taptas' [22] concept. Parkinson [17] also emphasizes that it is possible to operate within the cavernous sinus, yet remaining outside of the venous components.

Surgery within the cavernous sinus space has gained importance since the pioneering work of Parkinson, who reported the successful direct repair of a carotid-cavernous fistula [17]. Since the development of more sophisticated endovascular techniques (Serbinenko [20], Debrun et al. [5, 6], Kerber et al. [13]) direct surgical repair of such fistulae should not be necessary any more. Instead, aneurysm and tumor surgery, within and around the cavernous sinus, is becoming a topic of increasing interest (Bonnal et al. [2], Hakuba et al. [10], Dolenc [7, 8], Perneczky et al. [18] and this volume, Sekhar and Moller [19]). Dolenc et al. [9] report the removal of 15 tumors which originated from the cavernous sinus. Low mortality and morbidity seem to justify a more direct approach to lesions in the cavernous sinus area (Sekhar and Moller [19]).

Removal of the anterior clinoid process, with transsection of the fibrous ring around the ICA, enables the surgeon to follow the C 3 segment of the artery along a pericarotid tissue layer, without opening venous compartments (Perneczky et al. [18]). The frequent presence of intercavernous venous connections is of great importance for the transsphenoidal approach to intrasellar and parasellar tumors. While the anterior and posterior intercavernous sinuses are well mentioned in anatomy textbooks, our work supports the study of Kaplan et al. [12], who pointed out that intercavernous connections must be expected at the sella floor.

Traditional anatomy textbooks, as well as many recent anatomical investigations (e.g. Harris and Rhoton [11]), essentially work with a descriptive concept of the adult cavernous sinus. The discussions focus mainly on the presence or absence or trabeculations and compartmentalizations within a single venous space. It is our view that this traditional approach must be replaced by a more dynamic, developmentally based concept of the parasellar area.

References

1. Bedford MA (1966) The "cavernous" sinus. Br J Ophthalmol 50: 41–46
2. Bonnal J, Thibaut A, Brotchi J, Born J (1980) Invading meningiomas of the sphenoid ridge. J Neurosurg 53: 587–599

3. Bonnet P (1955) La loge caverneuse et les syndromes de la loge caverneuse. Arch Ophthalmol 15: 357–372
4. Butler H (1957) The development of certain human dural venous sinuses. J Anat 91: 510–526
5. Debrun G, Lacour P, Caron JP et al (1978) Detachable balloon and calibrated-leak balloon techniques in the treatment of cerebral vascular lesions. J Neurosurg 49: 635–649
6. Debrun G, Lacour P, Viñuela F et al (1981) Treatment of 54 traumatic carotid-cavernous fistulas. J Neurosurg 55: 678–692
7. Dolenc VV (1983) Direct microsurgical repair of intracavernous vascular lesions. J Neurosurg 58: 824–831
8. Dolenc VV (1985) A combined epi- and subdural direct approach to carotid-ophthalmic artery aneurysms. J Neurosurg 62: 667–672
9. Dolenc VV, Kregar T, Ferluga M, Fettich M, Morina A (1986) Treatment of tumors invading the cavernous sinus. In: Berce B, Možina A, Šuc S (eds) Proc int symp on cavernous sinus. Ljubljana, pp 277–289
10. Hakuba A, Nishimura S, Shirakata S, Tuskamoto M (1982) Surgical approaches to the cavernous sinus. Report of 19 cases. Neurol Med Chir (Tokyo) 22: 295–308
11. Harris FS, Rhoton AC (1976) Anatomy of the cavernous sinus. A microsurgical study. J Neurosurg 45: 169–180
12. Kaplan HA, Browder J, Krieger AJ (1976) Intracavernous connections of the cavernous sinuses. J Neurosurg 45: 166–168
13. Kerber CW, Bank WO, Cromwell LD (1979) Cyanocrylate occlusion of carotid-cavernous fistula with preservation of carotid artery flow. Neurosurgery 4: 210–215
14. Padget DH (1956) The cranial venous system in man in reference to development, adult configuration and relation to the arteries. Am J Anat 98: 307–335
15. Parkinson D (1964) Collateral circulation of cavernous carotid artery anatomy. Can J Surg 7/8: 251–268
16. Parkinson D (1965) A surgical approach to the cavernous portion of the carotid artery. Anatomical studies and case report. J Neurosurg 23: 474–483
17. Parkinson D (1973) Carotid cavernous fistula: direct repair with preservation of the carotid artery. Technical note. J Neurosurg 38: 99–106
18. Perneczky A, Knosp E, Vorkapic P, Czech T (1985) Direct surgical approach to infraclinoidal aneurysms. Acta Neurochir (Wien) 76: 36
19. Sekhar LN, Møller AR (1986) Operative management of tumors involving the cavernous sinus. J Neurosurg 64: 879–890
20. Serbinenko FA (1974) Balloon catheterization and occlusion of major cerebral vessels. J Neurosurg 41: 125–145
21. Taptas JM (1949) La loge du sinus caverneux. Rev Otoneuroophthalmol 21: 193–199
22. Taptas JM (1982) The so-called cavernous sinus: a review of the controversy and its implications for neurosurgeons. Neurosurgery 11: 712–717

Histoarchitecture of the cavernous sinus

I. Krivosic

Laboratory of Neuropathology, Hospital B, C.H.R.U., Lille, France

Introduction

It seems to us that the concept of the parasellar region should be evaluated by applied techniques. In classical, exclusively macroscopic dissections reviewed by Bedford (1966) [2] and modern stereomicroscopic dissections [4], there was evidence for the existence of one unbroken trabeculated canal surrounding the horizontal portion of the internal carotid artery and nerve VI. Architectural studies of dura mater foldsrealised by Taptas in [9] showed evidence of the extradural position of the parsellar lodge and favored a conception of the venous plexus as surrounding the ICA. The venous plexus concept was supported also by phlebographic studies and corrosion casts [6, 7, 8].

Nevertheless, the coexistence of large venous cavities and the venous plexus was also proposed reviewed by Duroux (1956) [3].

To avoid an one-sided interpretation we have to combine anatomical and stereomicroscopic dissection with histological, histochemical, transmission electronic microscope and histoarchitectural examinations.

Materials and methods

Three hundred cadaver specimens of the parasellar region (600 cavernous sinuses) were utilized alterantely for different examinations: anatomical and stereomicroscopic dissection, paraffin embedded frontal, sagittal and horizontal sections, frozen macroscopic, histological and histochemical sections and transmission electron microscopy.

Anatomical and microscopic dissection

a) *In situ* dissection of the cavernous sinus.

b) En bloc dissection with the help of a circular saw of a rectangular fragment (8 × 8 cm) of the base of the skull centered on the sella turcica. This was followed by microdissection of the cavernous sinus under a Zeiss stereomicroscope at magnification 8 to 40 ×.

c) En bloc dissection with the help of a circular saw of a rectangular fragment (8 × 8 cm) of the base of the skull centered on the sella turcica. This was followed by serial frontal, horizontal and sagittal sections of the soft part of the cavernous sinus with the help of a razor blade.

Paraffin-embedded sliced sections

a) En bloc dissection with the help of a circular saw of a rectangular fragment (8 × 8 cm) of the base of the skull centered on the sella turcica frozen by isopentane cooled with liquid nitrogen at —70 °C. These fragments were sliced in sections 0.5 cm thick with a saw in a sagittal, horizontal and coronal plane which allowed the taking of photographs and X-rays of sliced sections under conditions which resembled those *in vivo*. After rapid fixation in a alcohol-acetic acid-formalin mixture, the sliced sections were embedded in paraffin. Serial histological sections made on each sliced section were stained with hematoxylin-eosin, trichrome and reticulin, and examined under a Zeiss stereomicroscope (magnification 7 to 70 ×) and a Polyvar Reichert microscope (magnification 40 to 400 ×). For each specimen, standard sliced sections were selected for histoarchitectural studies on montage. (For frontal sections: slices passing in the immediate postorbitary plane, tuberculum sellae, pituitary stalk, dorsum sellae and 0.1 and 0.5 cm posterior to the dorsum sellae. For horizontal sections: slices passing through Merkel's cave and through the bottom of the sella turcica. For sagittal sections: slices passing through the pituitary stalk, at the lateral border of the hypophysis, in the middle of the width of the cavernous sinus as well as the root of nerve V.) The selected histological sections were analysed as follows:

Histotomogram

We call a black and white print made by directly inserting the histological slides H.E. stained into the enlarger a histotomogram. The enlarged print is then a black and white negative of the histological slide similar to an X-ray print but magnified 10 times, which permits histoarchitectural studies.

Histoarchitectural montage

The histological slides were microphotographed in 10 to 40 segments under a Zeiss stereomicroscope or Polyvar Reichert microscope at an initial enlargement of 8 to 40 × and exceptionally for the detail 250 ×. The photographs were assembled to give a montage of 50 to 100 cm in its widest axis, representing the entire histological section in a final enlargement of 20 × permitting comparative topographical anatomical and histoarchitectural studies.

b) En bloc dissection with the help of a circular saw of a rectangular fragment (8 × 8 cm) of the base of the skull centered on the sella turcica. The fragments were then fixed in a alcohol-acetic acid-formalin mixture, embedded in paraffin and then process proceeded as for a).

c) En bloc dissection of the soft part of the cavernous sinus with the help of scissors and scalpel. These fragments were then fixed in a alcohol-acetic acid-formalin mixture, and embedded in paraffin, permitting the realization of histological sections for classical stains.

Frozen tissues

a) En bloc dissection of one basal central cubic segment of brain together with a rectangular fragment of the base of the skull centered on the sella turcica. This fragment (brain + base of skull) was frozen in isopentane cooled with liquid nitrogen at —70 °C cut with a saw in frontal, horizontal and sagittal sections. The projection of color slides of sliced section which permitted us to study these regions without any artefact was carried out at the Institute of Pathology and Surgery Unit at the University Hospital Strasbourg.

b) En bloc dissection using a circular saw of a rectangular fragment (8 × 8 cm) of the base of the skull centered on the sella turcica frozen by isopentane cooled with liquid nitrogen at —70 °C. For one half of the specimens the bony parts were then removed and soft tissue serial histological sections 10 to 20 microns thick of the entire specimens of the cavernous sinus including pituitary gland were performed using a Reichert cryomicrotome. For the other half of the cases, the bony parts were partially removed by means of a drill, leaving intact the cavernous sinus bony limits. In these conditions, the structure, histoarchitectural relationships and histochemical proprietis were preserved as *in vivo* conditions. This permitted the detailed analysis of classical histopathological stained section (hematoxylin-eosin, trichrome, reticulin), classical histochemical stains (oil red, Sudan black B, P. A. S.), histoenzymological reactions (acid and alkaline phosphatase, ATPase, deshydrogenase, phosphorylase) and histoimmunological reactions (vimentine extracted from meningioma, factor VIII). Hemytoxylin-Eosin stained slides were used for histological studies of detail which were retracted and therefore unidentifiable or deformed on paraffin-embedded slides. Histochemical and histoimmunological stained slides were used for identification of the different cells and tissues: adipose tissues, arachnoidal cells, endothelial cells, smooth muscle cells.

c) En bloc dissection of the soft part of the cavernous sinus with the help of scissors and scalpel. These fragments were then frozen in isopentane cooled with liquid nitrogen at —70 °C. The histological sections made with a cryomicrotome permitted classical histological stains as well as histochemical, histoenzymological and histoimmunological stains as for b).

Results

Adipose tissue compartment

Macroscopic and stereomicroscopic examination showed the existence of partial coating of intrasinusal structures with a soft tissue of yellow color, which histochemical examinations permitted us to identify adipose tissue made of typical adipocytes. On histological slides of fresh frozen tissue, this adipose tissue often occupies a large island filling somehow the space between different structures (Fig. 1). Particularly at the level of the anterior aspect, where it is in continuity with extrasinusal adipose tissue. Delicate thin-walled venous ramifications of the anterior and superior part of the cavernous sinus are found surrounded by large islands of adipose tissue. It exists towards the rear surrounding venous ramifications, the internal carotid artery, and the dura mater sheath around the nerves reducing progressively in the trabeculae and the posterior part of the cavernous sinus. In place, particularly under the roof of cavernous sinus, the small islands of arachnoid cells attached to the thin fibrous venous wall are found in adipose tissue.

Arachnoid compartment

Typical arachnoid compartment

In the cavernous sinus the typical arachnoid compartment is developed in relationship with the CSF, typical arachnoidal trabeculae, arachnoidal epithelial covering of a gutter or canals of nerves, particularly nerve V in Merkel's cave. In this latter localization the internal wall of Merkel's cave separates the intracranial CSF from blood in the cavernous sinus (Fig. 2). The typical arachnoidal epithelium covers the surface of nerve root V, and the wall of Merkel's cave including the sheath of the dura mater which separates Merkel's cave from the cavernous sinus. At this topography the arachnoidal epithelial covering develops extensions into dura mater.

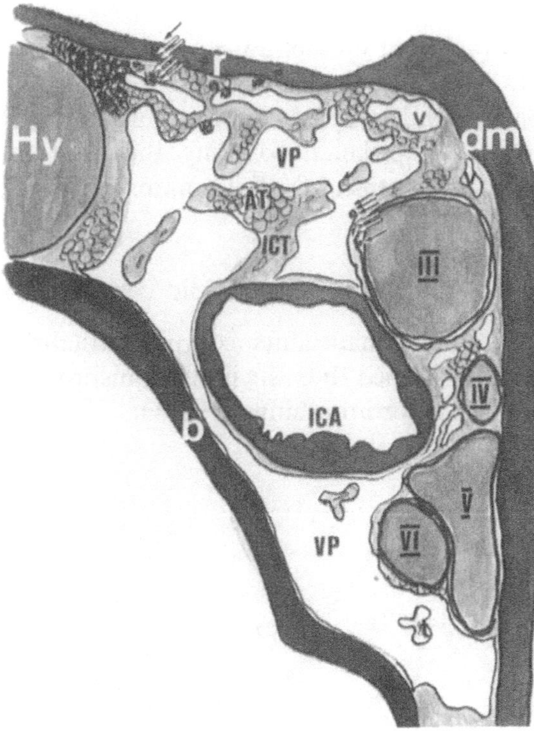

Fig. 1. Scheme of frontal section following enlarged montage of fresh frozen section oil red stained. Islands of adipose tissue (*AT*) are found in interstitial intrasinusal connective tissue. Arachnoidal compartment extends from arachnoidal epithelium of roof (*r*) of cavernous sinus, and sheaths of nerves (↓), penetrates inside of dura mater (↓↓) and riches interstitial connective tissue of cavernous sinus around and appears in venous pathway lumen (↓↓↓). Sometimes anterior external angle in front of hypophysis is filled with large fields of arachnoid cells. Interstitial connective tissue (*ICT*, stained very pale) represents internal skeleton of cavernous sinus in connection with walls. It varies in structure: adipose, loose connective, or fibrocollagenous thick. Venous pathway (*VP*) covered with endothelium (thin line) varies in shape. Ramified but confluent on anterior and superior aspects of cavernous sinus it becomes large open cavity on posterior-internal and inferior aspects. Various number and forms of relics of interstitial connective tissue containing small vascular and nervous ramifications persist even in larger cavities as trabeculae (*t*). Near and in the wall exists individualized venous canals (*v*). Internal carotid artery (*ICA*) is surrounded by connective interstitial tissue of various thickness, in place fibrosclerous. Against this tissue is applied extremely fine wall of venous pathway covered by endothelium (fine line). The nerves are applied against dura mater of lateral wall. The walls are of different structure. Lateral dura mater (*dm*) wall is very thick. The roof (*r*) is much thiner. On the bottom periosteum of bone (*b*) is covered with endothelium of venous pathway. Numerous trabeculae nevertheless are often attached to bone. Cavernous sinus is separated from hypophysis (*Hy*) by hypophyseal capsula doubled by variously developed sheaths of internal connective tissue skeleton

Furthermore this arachnoid epithelium protrudes into the lumen of the cavernous sinus to form a typical arachnoid villi (Fig. 2). Therefore here exists a typical arachnoidal compartment made up to the CSF, arachnoidal trabeculae, arachnoidal epithelial covering the dura mater, islands of arachnoidal cells inside sheaths of the dura mater and arachnoid villi inside the cavernous sinus.

Typical rudimentary arachnoid compartment

It is made up of the same constituants as typical arachnoid tissue but the components are less developed. It exists in relationship with a root of nerve III and the roof of the cavernous sinus (Fig. 1).

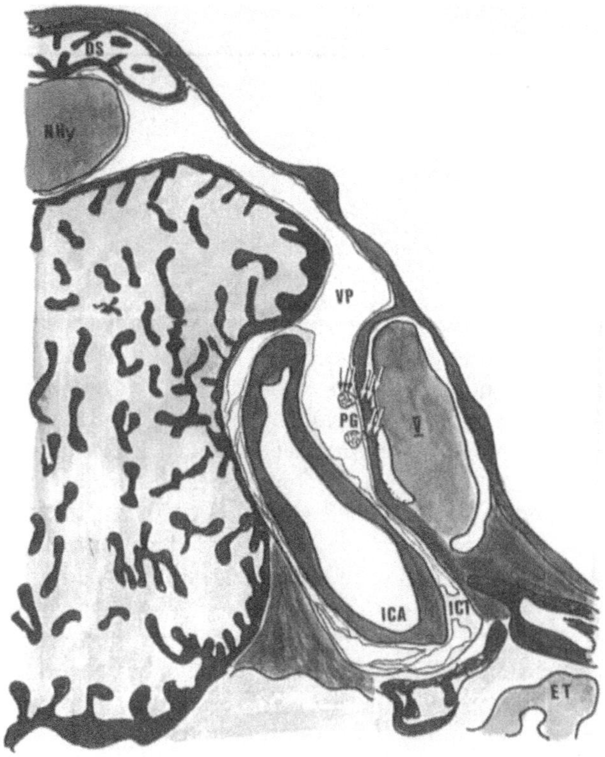

Fig. 2. Scheme of frontal section following enlarged montage of paraffin-embedded section passing through dorsum sellae (*DS*). Venous pathway (*VP*) is a large cavity devoid of trabeculae especially in elderly patients. Nevertheless inferior segment of internal carotid artery (*ICA*) is surrounded by interstitial connective tissue (*ICT*). Typical arachnoid compartment exists here in relation with Merkel's cave. It includes arachnoidal epithelium covering Merkel's cave (↓), islands of arachnoid cells in medial wall of Merkel's cave (↓↓), and typical Pacchianian granulations (*PG*) in lumen of venous pathway of cavernous sinus (↓↓↓); fifth nerve (*V*); Eustachian tube (*ET*); Neurohypophysis (*NHy*)

Atypical arachnoid compartment

This concerns the extension of arachnoid tissue without organization of arachnoid villi. It corresponds to the arachnoid extended under the dura mater covering the sella turcica and was found in front of and at the level of the anterior angles of the pituitary gland. In this later localization there often exist large fields occupied by arachnoid cells. The sheaths and pockets of arachnoid are found also around the ICA at the level of its exit from the cavernous sinus. Arachnoid tissue is therefore largely extended into the cavernous sinus. Although scattered, the island of arachnoid around the sheaths of the dura mater, venous ramifications, hypophyseal capsule, the ICA almost forms a layer inside the cavernous sinus. This intrasinusal arachnoid is in continuity from the left to the right cavernous sinus alongside the sheaths of the dura mater and the pituitary gland capsule. On the other side this intrasinusal arachnoid is in continuity with the arachnoidal epithelial covering of the dura mater and arachnoidal trabeculae on the intracranial surface of the cavernous sinus.

Venous pathways

Ocular and stereomicroscopic examinations of fresh blood free tissue fine sections permits us in particular to check the existence and the extension of the endothelium covering free surfaces inside the cavernous sinus including cavernous, reticular, and trabeculated parts and sheaths around the ICA, nerves and pituitary gland.

All types of examination showed numerous veins in front of the cavernous sinus. At the level posterior to the orbit the wall of ophthalmic veins contained sometimes a layer of typical smooth muscle cells corresponding to vascular media. Going backwards, the layer of smooth muscle cells, if they existed, disappeared rapidly at the level of the tuberculum sellae. The vascular walls are reduced to a layer of fibrous tissue covered by vascular endothelium and surrounded by adipose tissue. Further backwards the veins turn variably. On the lateral aspect the venous walls often become thicker by unification with the sheaths of the dura mater in the lateral wall of the cavernous sinus and the sheaths around the nerves. They run alongside the wall and could be identified. On the medial aspect the venous wall rapidly reduces to a very thin layer of fibrous tissue. The veins are surrounded with adipose tissue which reduces in volume and contain islands of arachnoid cells under the roof of the cavernous sinus. Backwards the number of veins is reduced by unification and retraction of their thin walls. The relics of these walls with interposed collagenous tissue containing adipose cells and collagenous fibers form the membranes, cords trabeculae or "reticular tissue". The venous cavity is delimited by a extremely thin delicate fibrous wall found applied to the internal carotid artery, hypophyseal capsula, the roof and floor of the cavernous sinus and collagenous sheaths around the nerve. It is separated nervertheless very often by relics of intervenous conjunctive tissue (adipose cells and collagen fibers). The large cavity continues at the level of the dorsum sellae into the plexus basilaris and inferior petrous sinus (Fig. 2).

The largest part of the venous structure in the cavernous sinus is extremely delicate, often broken or retracted by the techniques of classical anatomical and histological examinations. Only fresh frozen tissue examination permits the identification and precision of extension of this delicate venous structure (Fig. 1).

Histoimmunological reaction with specific antibodies antifactor VIII is positive on the endothelial cells of ophthalmic veins, individualized veins in lateral sinus wall and the large venous cavity on median and posterior aspects of the cavernous sinus. Electron microscope examination showed flattened endothelial cells covering the luminal surface of these cavities.

Dura mater

The dura mater covers the cavernous sinus endocranialy. This sheath can easily be removed from the lateral wall by dissection on fresh cadaveric preparations without entering the cavernous sinus because it is doubled by dural sheaths of the underlying nerves. At the level of the roof the underlying structures (thin-walled venous canal and adipose tissue) are very delicate and inevitably removed with the dura mater. Dissection of the dura mater of the roof opens the cavernous sinus cavity. Inside the cavernous sinus exists one framework of collagen-sheath, often in connection with the dura mater, girdling all structures, with focal reinforcement and bone attachements making one cavernous sinus internal "skeleton". The origins of these intracavernous sheaths are variable. Some are in connection with the dura mater, this is evident for the dural sheaths around the nerves. Some are relics of collagenous interstitial tissue around different intracavernous structures often containg adipose cells and are unified with the walls of neighboring structures.

Nerves

The nerves are localized on the periphery under the lateral wall of the cavernous sinus (Fig. 1) except for the nerve VI (in 30% of cases this nerve consisted of 2 or more rootlets), which initially, in the posterior aspect of the sinus runs directly through the cavernous sinus and leaves a nerve-free zone of the sinus wall. The nerves have their own sheaths in direct connection with endocranial cavernous sinus sheath of the dura mater. These sheaths surround nerves, alongside a gutter of nerves which then becomes a cannal (when the nerves pierce the sinus roof). The nerves and internal face of the gutters and canals are covered with arachnoid epithelium which extends in a dead end (in a cul de sac) from the cerebral side of nerve roots. On the anterior part of the cavernous sinus, this arachnoidal extension disappears. Here exists a crossing of nerves, the nerve III which is on the posterior aspect on the innermost position will join nerve VI in the lateral position, while the first branch of nerve V will join nerve IV which comes to the medial position passing under nerve III. On the extreme anterior part of the sinus the nerves form the anterior wall of the sinus through which pass the ophthalmic veins and which is somehow closed up with adipose tissue which extends also backwards around the nerve sheats.

Intracranial carotid artery

Comparative histopathological studies of en bloc dissection of the soft part of the cavernous sinus (300 specimens) as well as the study of en bloc paraffin-embedded and frozen sections showed more important athero-sclerotic alterations on intracavernous segments of the internal carotid artery than on the intracranial intradural segment of this artery, as well as on other cerebral arteries. These important atherosclerotic alterations provoke an important widening and lengthening of the carotid artery, which occupies an increasing space in the cavernous sinus. The internal carotid artery was covered in its trajectory by a sheath of conjunctive tissue. Against the ICA wall were thin-walled venous ramifications separated partially by adipose tissue and islands of arachnoid.

Comments

Arachnoid compartment

Normal arachnoid tissue consists of one ill-defined compartment which includes the pia mater applied to the surface of the brain, arachnoidal trabeculae into the CSF, arachnoidal covering of the dura mater, an extension of this covering into dura mater sheaths of sinuses and extensions into venous lumens concerning arachnoidal villis (macroscopic) and Paccionian granulations (macroscopic). Arachnoidal cells therefore normally possess the capacity of extension into conjunctive tissue. The existence of arachnoid tissue inside the cavernous sinus was not mentioned in previous descriptions.

We started the study on structure of arachnoid in this region in 1972 when we observed CSF nasal outflow a day after hypophysialysis carried out by Prof. A. Sibilly (Department of Surgery, CHU, Strasbourg) with radioactive itrium without lesions at the level of the sellar diaphragm examined the following day on postmortem examination. The pathway of the CSF seemed unaccountable. Following this, the histological examination realized on numerous specimens of this region showed us that the arachnoid compartment extended much farther than was noted in classical descriptions. Inside the cavernous sinus, the arachnoid forms an interrupted network made up of islands of arachnoidal cells found around venous structures and in communication from the left to the right cavernous sinus, particularly in front and anterior angles of the pituitary and under the sellar diaphragm. This extension could explain the possibility of CSF outflow through the trocar hole in the bone of sphenoidal sinus.

The existence of the arachnoidal intracavernous sinus network explains the possibility of genuine intracavernous sinus meningioma and its extensions in the opposite cavernous sinus. Natural spontaneous evolution of primary cavernous sinus meningioma seems to be the formation of a bridge meningioma filling both cavernous sinuses. In this case the neoplastic meningioma tissue fills up the spaces of venous ramifications which then progressively collapses. The meningioma extends alongside connective tissue sheaths inside the sinuses and will bridge, alongside dura mater sheaths and pituitary capsule, on the opposite cavernous sinus to form a meningioma on the bridge. On the other hand, the capacity of the extension of arachnoid tissue permits us to understand the possibility of invasion of the cavernous sinus by nearby extracranial and intracranial meningiomas.

Venous pathway

The question was raised whether the cavernous sinus is a canal or a network of small caliber veins. We found venous canals of various caliber traversing laterosellar lodge. Their walls were very thin fibrous without muscle cells, reduced sometimes to endothelium and several collagenous fibers, surrounded by adipose tissue cells. The shape of these veins follows the space between the structure inside the cavernous sinus: ICA, hypophysis and nerves. When the space between elements in cavernous sinus is large, the veins have a tendency to confluence and form a large cavity with some relicts of their walls giving a reticular or septate or trabecular aspect. These relicts are in fact the remains of interstitial space and contain adipose tissue cells, collagen fibers and small vessels which are essentially branches of the ICA and small local veins. We believe that these small veins should be distinguished from veins which traverse the laterosellar region.

Histoarchitectural studies of serial frontal sagittal and horizontal sections are in favor of progressive filling of the interstitial compartment between the carotid artery hypophysis and nerves by venous canals. On the posterior aspect, the transformation of this canal could grow into a structure identical to typical intracranial sinus. This shows the importance of adaptational capacities of venous structure following functional modifications. We observed this kind of phenomenon in studying portal hypertension [1]. In this study the minute 1 mm diaphragmatic inferior veins were transformed into an enlarged enormous venous 30 mm diameter spleno renal communication with a fibrous wall. In an other study concerning modification of venous structures of umbilical vein following closure after birth and reopening following rising of portal hypertension [6], it was shown that there exists a large spectrum of possibilities of the venous wall becoming fibrous or muscular following pressure in the lumen. Nevertheless when smooth muscle cells disappear from the venous wall they will not be reconstitued from fibrous tissue. Concerning cavernous sinus veins it could be reasonably admitted that the fibrous aspect and absence of smooth muscle cells on histological examination of the canal wall is not sufficient to refute the venous origin of the posterior large cavity of the cavernous sinus.

Connective tissue

Analytical studies have shown the existence of two variants of connective tissue: adipose tissue and a network of collagenous sheaths. It seems to represent various aspects of the connective tissue compartment between structures in the cavernous sinus. Classical descriptions did not mention the existence of adipose tissue in the cavernous sinus. We found this tissue somehow closing the anterior aspect of cavernous sinus. It extends posteriorly and fills the space between different structures.

In places, collagenous tissue dominates, forming a reticular, trabeculated, ligamentous or ring-shaped aspect. In these places adipose tissue is reduced or absent. Some of this structure can be very strong and plays a role in the attachment of the ICA to bones by a ligament-like (on horizontal trajectory) or ring-like (near anterior clinoid) processes and could have operating implications. On the other hand, the existence of connective tissue, particularly adipose, will probably have to be taken into account in future in the interpretation of radiological examinations.

Cavernous sinus is delimited by an external sheath of various aspects. The lateral wall is in continuity with the dura mater of the fossa temporalis. It seems different from the floor which is in continuity with the sellar diaphragm. We have seen one case of Arnold Chiari's syndrome treated as a newborn by supraoptic laminectomy. When this patient died at the age of

20, the floor of the cavernous sinus was depressed the underlying cavernous sinus had collapsed while the lateral wall persisted in the normal position. The common oculomotor nerve in this case was free in parasellar trajectory without the dural sheath. Therefore it seems that sella turcica and the cavernous sinus are covered by one particular sheath. This sheath somehow closes the central "hole" in the base of the skull by which some elements enter (adenohypophysis, ICA, plexus of veins), and some elements exit (neurohypophysis, nerves). In definitive organization, these topographical and histological structures could be apparently dissented with their origins. The existence of adipose tissue around the large true sinus-like cavity on the medial and posterior aspect of the cavernous sinus appears contradictory. In fact this large cavity is secondarily formed by coalescence of extradural veins and adipose tissue which represents relics of connective perivenous tissue. In contrast with this on the anterior and superior aspects of the cavernous sinus, the islands of arachnoid are found in adipose tissue around remified veins.

Summary

Combined anatomical stereomicroscopic, histoarchitectural and histochemical analysis of 600 fresh cadaver specimens of the cavernous sinus permitted us to study different compartments. We were able to identify two compartments not mentioed in classical descriptions of the cavernous sinus: adipose tissue compartment and arachnoid compartment.

The adipose tissue compartment filled up the spaces between different structures particularly on the anterior aspect of the cavernous sinus. The existence of adipose tissue will probably have to be taken into acount in future in the interpretation of radiological examinations.

The arachnoid compartment forms an interrupted network. It extends from the arachnoid around the nerves, pituitary stalk and directly through the external dura mater wall of the cavernous sinus. The arachnoid compartment of both sinuses is in communication with islands of arachnoid tissue around the pituitary gland.

The existence of an arachnoid compartment inside the cavernous sinus permits us to conceptualize the formation and extension of cavernous sinus meningiomas, whose natural course is extension on both sinuses to form a "bridge" meningioma.

The existence of the arachnoid compartment in extradural space could permit the development of a CSF fistula by an extradural intracranial lesion of the anterior wall of the sella turcica.

This study supports the conception of extradural topography of cavernous sinus similar to the pituitary gland. The cavernous sinus as well as the sella turcica contains structures of encephalic origin displaced in extradural space (nerves in the parasellar lodge, neurohypophysis in the sellar lodge) and structures entering the intracranial space (the adenohypophysis in the sella turcica, ICA, and veins in the cavernous sinus, the sella turcica and the floor of the cavernous sinus seem to have their own mutual covering of dura mater sheath which closes somehow the central "hole" of passage in the base of the skull).

The veins passing through the cavernous sinus change progressively going backwards and transform finally at the level of the dorsum sellae in the structure identical to the typical intracranial sinus. Anteriorly and laterally, however, they stay individualized.

The veins, as well as the ICA and their intrasinusal branches are surrounded by connective tissue containing adipose cells, nerves, fibrocytes and collagenous fibers. In places, this connective tissue presents reinforcements as cords or ring particularly in relation to the ICA. Connective tissue is found also in trabeculae and reticular structures which represent relics of retracted confluent venous walls. The whole connective tissue constitues one internal framework as a skeleton of the cavernous sinus which could have operative implications particularly concerning liberation of the ICA.

References

1. Batzenschlager A, Krivosic I (1969) Communications veineuses spléno-rénales ou cours des cirrhoses hépatiques. Sem Hop Paris 46: 2891–2989
2. Bedford MA (1966) The "cavernous sinus". Br J Ophthal 50: 41–46
3. Duroux PE, Bouchet A, Bossy J, Calas F (1955) Contribution à l'étude du sinus caverneux. CR Ass Anat 90: 486–490
4. Harris FS, Rhoton AL Jr (1976) Anatomy of the cavernous sinus. A microsurgical study. J Neurosurg 15: 169–180
5. Kaplan HA, Browder J, Krieger AJ (1976) Intracavernous connections of the cavernous sinuses. J Neurosurg 45: 166–168
6. Krivosic A (1976) Das Ligamentum teres hepatis und seine Modifikationen im Verlauf der Leberzirrhose. Histopathologische Studie. Diss Univ, Homburg, (Saar)
7. Papadakis N, Lukl ND (1976) The cavernous sinus. 44th ann meet ame assoc neurosurgical surgeons. San Francisco, California. loc cit [10]
8. Parkinson D, Hunt B, Zeal A (1978) Lateral sellar venous anatomy, "cavernous sinus" (abstract). Anat Rec: 190–503
9. Taptas JN (1949) La loge du sinus caverneux et sinus caverneux, sa constitution et les rapports des éléments vasculaires et nerveux qui la traversent. Sem Hop Paris 25: 1719–1722
10. Taptas JN (1982) The so-called cavernous sinus: a review of the controversy and its implications for neurosurgeons. Neurosurgery 5: 712–717

Diagnostic procedures

Facial reflex examination for assessment of subclinical trigeminal nerve involvement in the cavernous sinus

O. Bynke

Department of Neurosurgery, University Hospital, Linköping, Sweden

Introduction

Encroachments made by a pituitary tumor on the flexible walls of the cavernous sinus are often evident only at the time of transsphenoidal surgery. The effects of lateral tumor extension on the trigeminal nerve in the cavernous sinus have been studied by a neurophysiological test, facial reflex examination.

Mechanical stimulation by tapping the supraorbital region evokes a double response in the orbicularis oculi muscles. The late response (R 2) is the visible blink reflex. It has a multisynaptic reflex arc and its latency is variable and habituation is a normal finding. The early response (R 1) is evoked on the side of tapping by activation of skin receptors [2]. It is a steady response, suitable in studying transmission along its reflex arc, the first trigeminal division, a short connection in the brain stem, and the facial nerve. A test based on the mechanically evoked R 1 has been developed and it is called the facial reflex examination [1].

Methods

Facial reflex examination

The equipment for mechanical stimulation consists of two identical electromagnetic hammers attached to a pair of goggles (Fig. 1). The region just below the eyebrow is tapped one side at a time. The mechanical stimulation is painless and a repetitive mode with in all 100 stimuli in a series of 10 or more taps at a frequency of 1 Hz can be performed on each side with no discomfort or comprehension on the part of the subject. The evoked

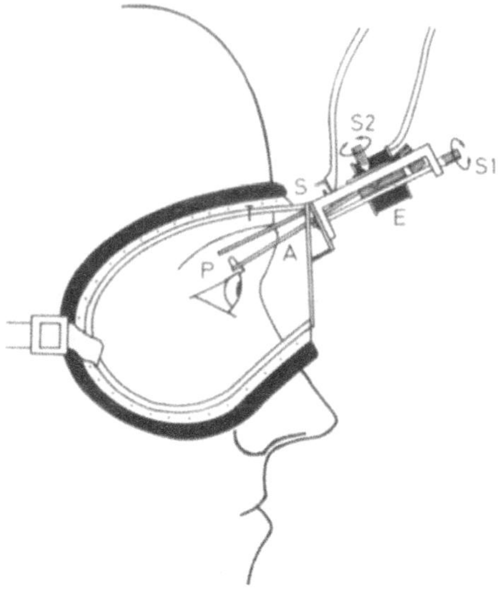

Fig. 1. Diagram illustrating the equipment for mechanical stimulation. The electromagnets (*E*), one on each side, are individually adjusted to a symmetrical position so that the "tentacle" (*T*) is just touching the skin below the eyebrow. This position is maintained by locking the screws (*S 1* and *S 2*). Taps are delivered by driving the pellet (*P*) on the tapping-arm (*A*) through the hole in the "tentacle". A trigger pulse to the recording unit is released by the interrupter-spring (*S*) the instant the pellet contacts the skin

responses are recorded from the orbicularies oculi muscles by the electromyographic technique using subdermal needles. R 1 latency is measured by a latency meter based on the pattern recognition technique (Fig. 2).

The mean latency of R 1 is used to describe the conduction along the trigemino-facial pathway. The difference of the mean latency on the right and left sides is the mean latency difference and a value exceeding 0.25 ms has been established as abnormal. The value of the R 1 latency obtained must also be correlated to the reference value of the corresponding age as R 1 is age dependent [1]. The mean latency distribution (standard deviation) of R 1 describes the quality of the afferent input and/or the central influences. Values above the upper reference limit (0.65 ms), indicate a dysfunction of the first trigeminal division and/or the brain stem.

Patients

Twenty patients with sellar tumors were studied (Table 1). Microadenomas

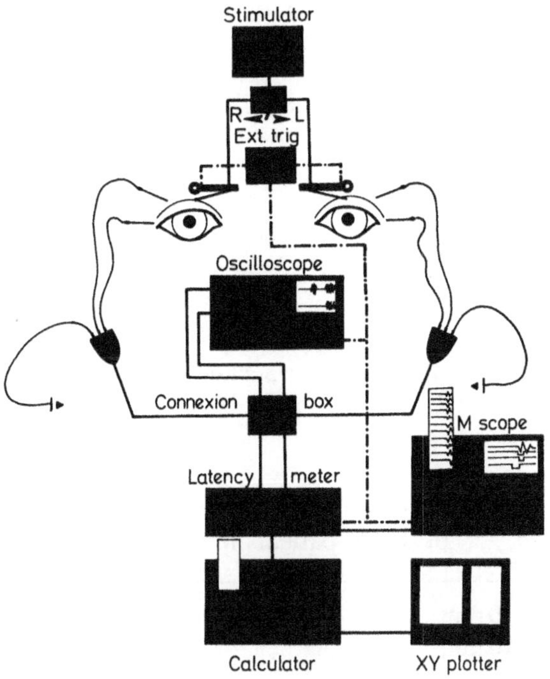

Fig. 2. Diagram illustrating the equipment for facial reflex examination

were present in two patients but the tumor size was larger in the other cases. Partial tumor necrosis occurred in four patients and two of them had oculomotor symptoms. There were no clinical signs of trigeminal nerve involvement in any patient, and no encroachment on the brain stem and the facial nerve (Table 2).

The intrasellar pressure was carefully studied at incision of dura to the sella, and it was graded in three categories (Table 3). The transsphenoidal approach implied also an opportunity to study the encroachment of the tumor on the flexible wall of the cavernous sinus.

Results

The individual results of the preoperative facial reflex examination and the largest lateral intrasellar tumor extension based on CT and intraoperative findings are shown in Table 4. R 1 was delayed or abolished on the side of the largest lateral tumor extension except in two patients (nos. 7 and 17)

Table 1. Data on the patients

Age: 22–68 years; mean 43		
Sex: 7 females and 13 males		
Pituitary adenomas		19
GH-secreting	6	
PRL-secreting	4	
ACTH-secreting	1	
Nonsecreting	8	
Craniopharyngioma		1
Therapy for pituitary insufficiency in $^{2}/_{20}$ cases		

Table 2. The size of sellar tumors and presenting neurological symptoms in the 20 patients in the study

Tumor diameter < 10 mm	2 cases
Tumor diameter > 10 mm	18
Neurological symptoms and signs	
Chiasmal	4
Oculomotor	2 cases
Trigeminal nerve	0 cases
Facial nerve	0 cases

Table 3. The classification of the intrasellar pressure and its occurrence in 20 patients with sellar tumors

Greatly raised	
– intrasellar tissue was squeezed through the dural incision	in 11 cases
Moderately raised	
– intrasellar tissue filled up the dural incision	in 7 cases
Not raised	
– intrasellar content was easily explored with no removal	in 2 cases (microadenomas were present in both)

Table 4. The side of R 1 delay, the mean latency difference (MLD) in ms, and the side of the largest intrasellar tumor extension in patient nos. 1–20

Patient no.	Side(s) of R 1	MLD (ms)	Largest intrasellar tumor extension
1	R	1.2	R
2	R	0.5	R
3	R	0.6	R
4	both	0.1	R = L
5	R	1.7	L
6	L	1.3	L
7	none	0.1	—
8	L	1.1	L
9	R	1.7	R
10	R	1.7	R
11	R	1.6	R
12	L	1.6	L
13	R	> 5.0	R
14	R > L	0.6	R > L
15	L	1.7	L
16	L	> 5.0	L
17	none	0.1	—
18	both	0.1	R = L
19	L	1.6	L
20	R > L	0.7	R > L

R Right side, *L* left side

Table 5. Summary of the results of the preoperative facial reflex examination in patients with raised intrasellar pressure

Greatly raised intrasellar pressure	
– R 1 delay on tumor side—mean (n = 8)	2.25 ms
– R 1 latency distribution raised in	10/11 pat.
Moderately raised intrasellar pressure	
– R 1 delay on tumor side—mean (n = 7)	1.14 ms
– R 1 latency distribution raised in	3/7 pat.

Table 6. The change in R 1 latency after removal of the tumors in the postoperatively examined 12 patients. The intrasellar pressure was greatly raised in the upper 6 cases and moderately raised in the lower 6 cases

Patient no.	Decrease in R 1 latency (ms)		After operation
	Tumor side(s)	Nontumor side(s)	
4	1.0, 0.9	—	1 month
8	1.4	ns	1 week
14	1.9	0.5	6 months
16	> 5.0	ns	3 months
18	2.0, 0.8	—	2 months
20	1.8	0.8	2 months
2	0.5	ns	1 month
3	0.8	0.5	2 months
5	ns	ns	2 months
6	1.0	0.4	5 months
11	2.8	1.9	1 month
12	0.6	ns	2 months

ns Nonsignificant

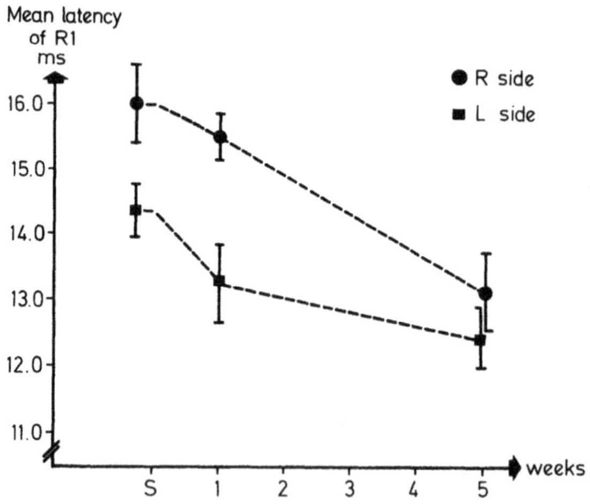

Fig. 3. Change in R 1 latency after removal of a nonsecreting pituitary macroadenoma in patient (no. 11). His intrasellar tumor extension was above all on the right side. Recovery in R 1 latency was shown on both sides but it was not complete five weeks after the tumor removal. The observed decrease in R 1 latency can be ascribed to a recovery in transmission along the first trigeminal division after release of their entrapments in the cavernous sinuses

both with microadenomas. R 1 was significantly delayed on both sides in four patients and their tumors extended bilaterally in a symmetrical way. R 1 was significantly delayed on the least involved side in one patient (no. 5), but sign of prior tumor necrosis was shown during surgery on that side.

R 1 was more delayed and its latency distribution was more elevated in patients with greatly raised intrasellar pressure than in those with moderately raised pressure (Table 5).

Removal of the tumors resulted in recovery in nerve conduction. Twelve patients were reexamined after surgery and their results are shown in Table 6. A significant decrease in R 1 latency was present above all on the tumor side. The decrease was larger in patients with greatly raised intrasellar pressure than in those with moderately raised pressure. Recovery in R 1 latency did not occur in one patient (no. 5). Her age, 68 years, and an earlier tumor apoplexy may explain the failed recovery and the suspicion of permanent nerve damage. The change in R 1 latency after transsphenoidal removal of a nonsecreting pituitary adenoma is shown in Fig. 3.

Discussion

The R 1 delay observed may be ascribed to involvement of the first trigeminal division as careful clinical, radiographic, and electromyographic examination excluded involvement of the remaining part of the reflex arc. Release of the encroachment of the wall of the cavernous sinus resulted, furthermore, in recovery in R 1 latency. Endocrine causes could be eliminated as patients with pituitary insufficiences were substituted before the examination, and as R 1 delay was observed in patients with secreting as well as nonsecreting pituitary tumors.

The cranial nerves of the cavernous sinus are poorly protected from a medially expanding lesion as they are not embedded in the lateral wall [3]. The first trigeminal division passes through the cavernous sinus with the internal carotid on its medial side (Fig. 4). A sellar tumor encroaching on the flexible medial wall of the cavernous sinus may, therefore, compress the first trigeminal division either directly or by the laterally displaced carotid.

Clinical signs of involvement of the trigeminal nerve are rare symptoms in patients with slowly growing pituitary tumors if complaints of headaches are not included. Sudden intrasellar expansion as in tumor apoplexy may produce sensory disturbances within the forehead as a part of a cavernous sinus syndrome. Facial reflex examination can be used to ascertain involvement of the trigeminal nerve in patients with lesions of the cavernous sinus.

In conclusion, the present study has shown that facial reflex examination is a valuable test for detecting subclinical involvement of the trigeminal nerve in patients with laterally extending sellar tumors. The lateral tumor extension seems to be a common but not always noticed feature in patients with lesions enlarging the pituitary fossa. The lateral borders of the sella are often difficult to delineate even with the use of the later generation of CT scanners but in conjunction with the facial reflex examination lateral tumor extension may be clarified.

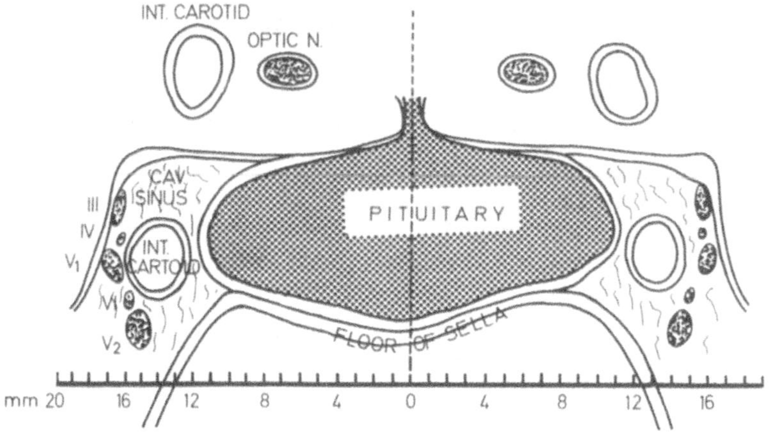

Fig. 4. Diagram illustrating the relation of the cranial nerves to the carotid in the cavernous sinus. An expanding sellar lesion may compress the first trigeminal division either directly by an invasive growth or indirectly by the laterally displaced carotid

References

1. Bynke O (1980) Facial reflex examination. A clinical and neurophysiological study on acoustic tumours and brain displacement at the tentorial notch. Acta Neurol Scand 62 [Suppl] 76: 1–127
2. Lindquist C, Mårtensson A (1970) Mechanisms involved in the cat's blink reflex. Acta Physiol Scand 80: 149–159
3. Umansky F, Nathan H (1982) The lateral wall of the cavernous sinus with special reference to the nerves related to it. J Neurosurg 56: 228–234

Dynamic CT scanning of the cavernous sinus

J. F. Bonneville, F. Cattin, and M. Bouchareb

Department of Neuroradiology, University Hospital of Besançon, Besançon, France

The direct surgical approach to the cavernous sinus either for vascular malformations or invasive tumors treatment is now largely accepted. The need for detailed vascular anatomy including venous anatomy of the parasellar space and for precise diagnosis is obvious: for instance medical management can be completely modified for pituitary adenomas invading the cavernous sinus versus pituitary adenomas displacing the cavernous sinus. Dynamic CT scanning can help to answer these questions.

Material and methods

Our technique for demonstration of the cavernous sinus is slightly modified from that we have used routinely since 1982 for demonstration of the progressive enhancement of the pituitary gland using intravenous contrast.

For dynamic CT of the cavernous sinus, 300 patients were evaluated last year with a General Electric CT/T 9800 scanner using 1.5 mm collimation.

Dynamic CT scan was obtained in direct coronal plane during rapid intravenous bolus of 80 cm^3 of iodinated contrast material. Scan time was 2 seconds and interscan delay time 2.3 seconds authorizing 6 serial cuts at the same midsellar level during the first 30 seconds following the onset of the bolus injection. The use of a special algorithm for reconstruction identical to this for bone detail imaging avoids a partial volume effect and permits precise delineation of all vascular elements.

Results

Apart from demonstration of the pituitary capillary bed, the so-called pituitary tuft [1, 2] and progressive enhancement of the pituitary gland,

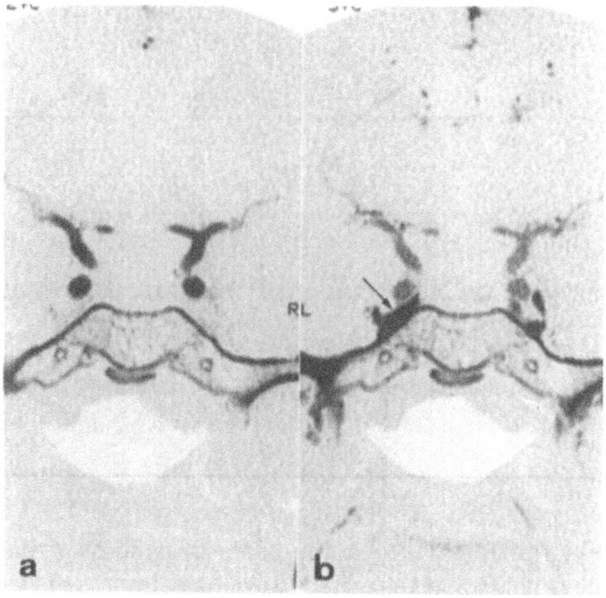

Fig. 1. Dynamic CT scanning of the cavernous sinus. **a** Demonstration of the internal carotid arteries; **b** 5 seconds later, optimal visualization of the parasellar veins. Prominent carotid sulcus vein (arrow)

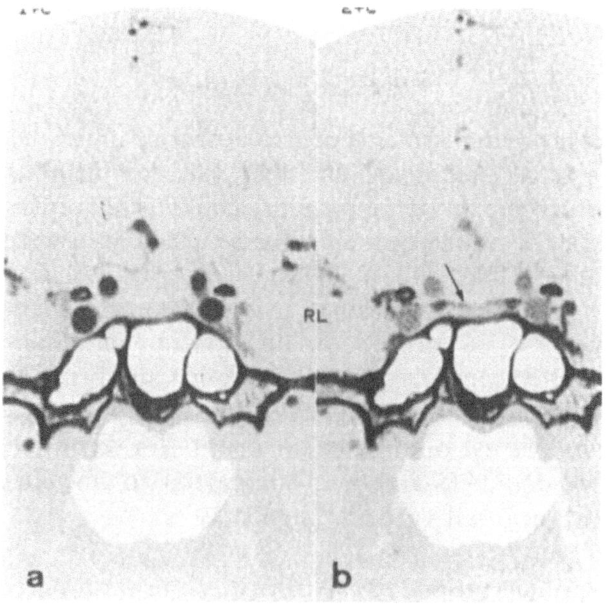

Fig. 2. Dynamic CT scanning of the cavernous sinus. **a** Optimal demonstration of the parasellar veins delineating the intracavernous cranial nerves "in negative". Visualization also of the anterior intercavernous sinus (arrow) (**b**)

dynamic CT scanning nicely demonstrates the exact limit between the pituitary gland and cavernous sinus, the intracavernous internal carotid arteries, the lateral wall of the cavernous sinus, routinely cranial nerve III and most often other intracavernous cranial nerves, between the venous elements of the cavernous sinus.

Dynamic scanning permits the clarification of some controversy and confusion about the exact nature of these veins: the classic description of a blood-filled trabeculated canal completely surrounding the internal carotid artery has to be changed to that of a plexus of various size veins. During dynamic scanning, optimal visualization of these parasellar veins occurs about 15 seconds after the onset to the bolus injection; 5 seconds later venous enhancement becomes too poor and the veins are no longer demonstrated.

The parasellar veins are quite always very asymetrical from one side to the other.

Five groups of veins can be described (Figs. 1 and 2): the lateral group, the inferior group, the vein located between the internal carotid artery and sphenoïd bone, we have called "vein of the carotid sulcus", the vein located between the pituitary gland and the internal carotid artery (unusual), the pericarotid plexus (most often incomplete).

Veins medial to the internal carotid artery (rare) and veins between the sphenoid bone and the internal carotid artery (usual) are more likely to be compressed first in the case of invasive pituitary adenomas.

Conclusion

The need for detailed demonstration of the anatomy of the cavernous sinus is obvious. Magnetic resonance imaging has not totally solved this problem [3, 4]. CT dynamic scanning is very helpful to demonstrate the parasellar veins. In most cases, dynamic CT scanning allows the diagnosis of the initial involvement of the cavernous sinus by pituitary tumors. But anatomical variations can compromise the diagnostic value of the demonstration of cavernous sinus veins.

References

1. Bonneville JF, Cattin F, Moussa-Bacha K, Portha C (1983) Dynamic computed tomography of the pituitary gland: the "tuft sign". Radiology 149: 145–148
2. Bonneville JF, Cattin F, Dietemann JL (1986) Computed tomography of the pituitary gland. Springer, Berlin Heidelberg New York Tokyo, pp 33–46
3. Daniels DL, Pech P, Leighton M, Pojunas K, Williams AL, Haughton VM (1985) Magnetic resonance imaging of the cavernous sinus. Am J Neuroradiol 6: 187–192
4. Ahmadi J, North CM, Segall HD, Zee CS, Weiss MH (1985) Cavernous sinus invasion by pituitary adenomas. Am J Neuroradiol 6: 893–898

Radiological grading of tumor extension of the cavernous sinus

Y. Nakano[1], S. Toya[1], T. Kawase[1], S. Harada[1], and H. Shiga[2]

Departments of [1] Neurosurgery and of [2] Diagnostic Radiology,
Keio University School of Medicine, Tokyo, Japan

One hundred and twenty-three cavernous sinuses (CS) were studied in 72 patients with or without parasellar or intrasellar tumors by conventional cerebral angiography, contrasted with CT findings. Subtraction films were used for the analysis.

The angiographical findings were categorized into four grades according to the visualization of the CS and venous routes from the CS.

In chordomas or meningiomas arising around the CS, all the patients showed abnormality on the angiograms. Inferior petrosal sinus was frequently affected by those tumors, whereas the CS was seldom affected by pituitary adenomas. The angiographical grading was beneficial for the strategy of surgical excision of tumors arising around the CS.

Introduction

Angiographical variations of the CS have been described by several authors in recent years [4, 10].

The possibility of angiographical demonstration of the CS has been considerably improved using subtraction and magnification techniques. But there are few mentions in the literature of angiographical variation of the CS and accessory veins in case of parasellar or intrasellar tumors, and it is sometimes hard to know even by CT scan whether a tumor is invading the CS. In this study angiographical analysis was carried out on patients with parasellar or intracavernous sinus tumor, and the abnormality was graded on angiograms.

Patients and method

We observed 122 CSs in 72 patients between 11 and 68 years of age. Thirty-four patients were males and 38 patients were females. Those patients were classified into 3 groups:

Group 1

Thirty-two patients without lesion around the CS and on the accessory venous route: 3 patients without any findings, 1 patient with epilepsy, 1 patient with oculomotor nerve palsy, 1 patient with aqueduct stenosis, 1 patient with trigeminal neuralgia, 9 patients with cerebral aneurysm, 2 patients with arterio-venous malformation, 4 patients with meningioma, 2 patients with metastatic tumor, 4 patients with astrocytoma, 1 patient with trigeminal neurinoma, 2 patients with lymphoma, and 1 patient with lacrimal gland carcinoma.

Group 2

Seventeen patients with intrasellar or suprasellar tumors: 13 patients with pituitary adenoma, 2 patients with tuberculum sellae meningioma, 2 patients with craniopharyngioma.

Group 3

Twenty-three patients with parasellar tumor affecting the venous route of the CS: 18 patients with meningioma, 2 patients with chordoma, 2 patients with von Recklinghausen disease, and 1 patient with fibrous dysplasia.

Angiographical findings were classified into the following 4 grades (Fig. 1):

Grade 0: normal CS.

Grade 1: almost normal CS or partially defective CS, with disappearance of one or two main venous routes (except for ophthalmic veins).

Grade 2: the CS is not clearly depicted while venous outflow canals are still preserved through dural collaterals.

Grade 3: the CS is not depicted and the collaterals are established through cortical veins to the intracranial sinuses.

All cases of group 3 were classified into 2 classes in terms of tumor invasion of the CS on CT scans.

1. There is no invasion into the CS on the CT finding.
2. There is some invasion into the CS on the CT finding.

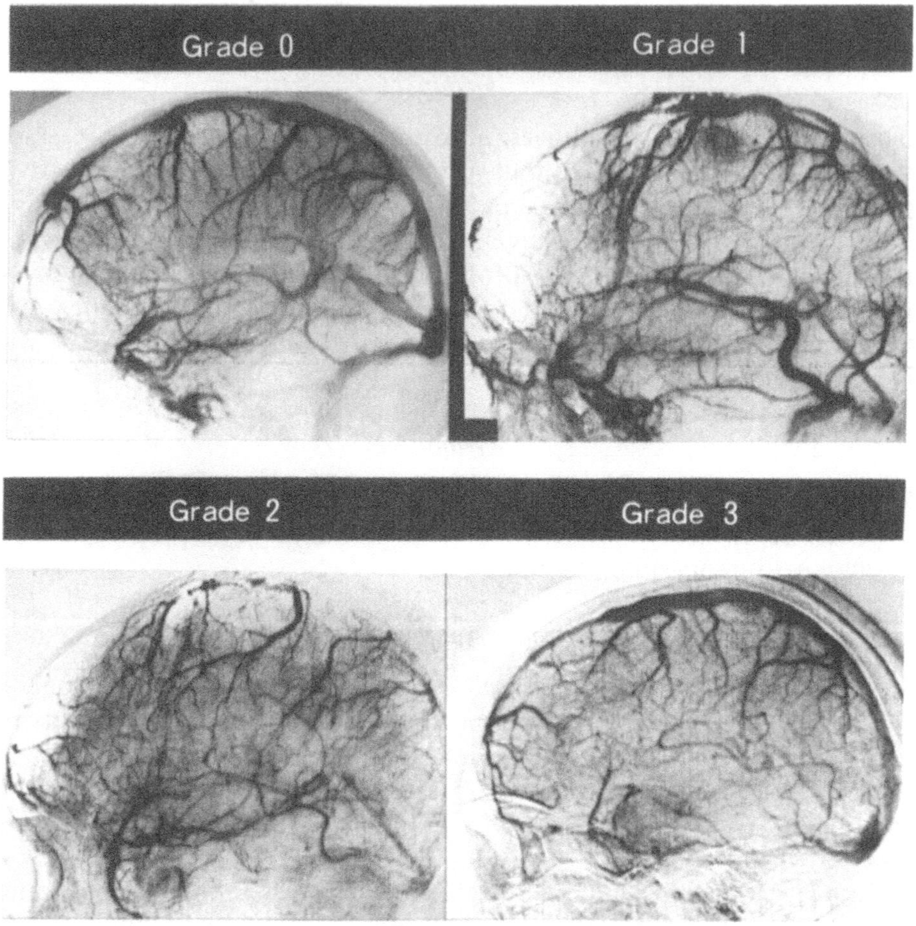

Fig. 1. Angiographical grading. Grade 0: Normal cavernous sinus; Grade 1: almost normal cavernous sinus or partially defective cavernous sinus, with disappearance of one or two main venous routes (except for ophthalmic veins); Grade 2: cavernous sinus is not clearly depicted but venous outflow channels are still preserved through dural collaterals; Grade 3: cavernous sinus is not depicted and the collaterals are established through cortical veins to the intracranial sinuses

Table 1. The existence of the venous route in group 1 and group 2

	Group 1		Group 2	
	Cases	Rate (%)	Cases	Rate (%)
Orbital veins	2	3.2	4	11.8
Pterygoid plexus	46	74.2	24	70.6
Superior petrosal sinus	53	85.5	27	79.4
Inferior petrosal sinus	39	62.9	15	44.1
Cortical anastomoses				
Labbé	45	72.6	24	70.6
Trolard	29	46.8	10	29.4
Others	7	11.3	4	11.8
Total number of CS	62		34	
Total number of patients	32		17	

Table 2. The existence of the venous route in group 3

	Group	
	Cases	Rate (%)
Orbital veins	3	11.5
Pterygoid plexus	14	53.8
Superior petrosal sinus	18	69.2
Inferior petrosal sinus	4	15.4
Cortical anastomoses		
Labbé	21	80.8
Trolard	12	46.2
Others	2	7.7
Total number of CS	26	
Total number of patients	22	

Results

Tables 1 and 2 and Fig. 2 indicate the existence of the venous routes in the 3 groups.

In group 1 orbital veins were less evident (3.2%) than other venous routes. The following three veins were highly evident: pterygoid plexus (74.2%), superior petrosal sinus (85.5%), and inferior petrosal sinus (62.9%), being common outflow canals. Cortical venous communications were present even in those patients without lesion in the CS. The most common route was between the Sylvian vein and the vein of Labbé (72.6%).

Group 2 had almost the same tendency as group 1. The following veins were highly evident: pterygoid plexus (70.6%), superior petrosal sinus (79.4%), Labbé (79.4%), whereas the rate for the inferior petrosal sinus (44.1%) is lower than that of group 1.

In group 3, the rate for the main venous routes were lower than that of group 1 or 2, that of the inferior petrosal sinus (15.4%) especially being much lower than the others. On the other hand the rates of cortical anastomoses were slightly higher than the other veins (i.e. Labbé 80.8%).

Table 3 and Fig. 3 indicate the distribution of abnormality according to the angiographical grading.

Group 1 has 20 CSs of grade 0, 40 CSs of grade 1, and 2 CSs of grade 2. Even in the group with no tumor around the CS, two thirds of the CSs in group 1 were invisible.

Group 2 had almost the same tendency as group 1 except for a slightly higher rate of grade 2.

In group 3, the rate of grade 1 was about half, and there was none in grade 0.

Table 4 indicates angiographical grading compared to CT findings. All patients without a tumor around the CS on CT were classified in grade 1 on the angiograms. But most patients with a tumor invading the CS are classified as grades 2 or 3.

Table 3. The distribution abnormality according to the angiographical grading

Angiographical grading	0	1	2	3	Total
Group 1	20	40	2	0	62
Group 2	11	19	4	0	34
Group 3	0	15	3	8	26
Total number of CS	31	74	9	8	122

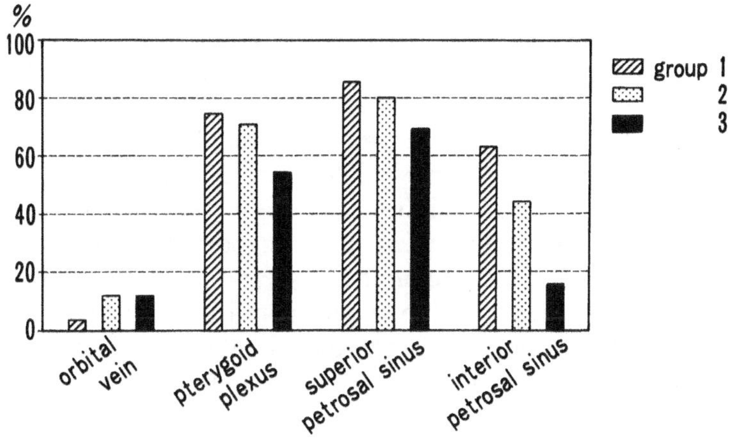

Fig. 2. Existence of venous routes

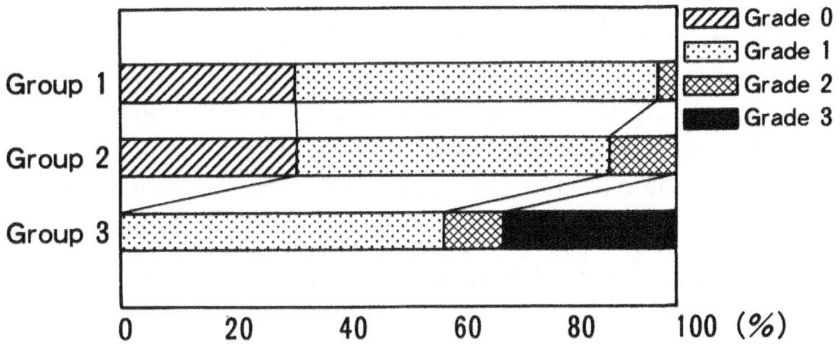

Fig. 3. Distribution abnormality according to the angiographical grading

Table 4. Angiographical grading compared to CT findings

Invasion into CS on CT	Angiographical grading	0	1	2	3	Total
No		0	13	0	1	14
Yes		0	2	3	8	13
Total		0	15	3	9	27

Discussion

The CS are paired structures, roughly rectangular in shape, one lying adjacent to each side of the body of sphenoid bone. Each CS is a trabeculated venous network forming a plexus interconnected in several distinct planes. The CSs are united with each other by anterior and posterior intercommunicating sinuses beneath the dura of diaphragma sellae. The anterior intercommunicating sinuses is usually larger, and the posterior intercommunication is often absent. Further posteriorly the two CSs are connected by the basilar or occipital transverse sinuses or plexus.

Anteriorly the CS receives the superior and inferior ophthalmic veins and the sphenoparietal sinus. The sphenoparietal sinus, which varies greatly in caliber, drains blood from the region of the planum sphenoidale and the Sylvian fissure.

Posteriorly the CS drains into the petrosal sinuses and then into the internal jugular vein [3].

In our study, the venous route varies even in patients without a lesion around the CS. Half of the patients had one or two venous routes missing (grade 1). In the analysis of each venous route, the ophthalmic vein was seldom demonstrated in all cases. The reason is that the ophthalmic vein is the outflow vein from the facial veins to the CS, and most of the patients received a selective internal carotid angiography [7]. That resulted in a difficulty in angiographical diagnosis if the tumor had slightly invaded the CS. However, when the inferior petrosal sinus was pointed out, there was a considerable difference in the visualization between normal and abnormal. The reason for the lower rate for the inferior petrosal sinus is the following:

1. In anatomical tests, the sphenoparietal sinus easily establishes a collateral flow to the pterygoid plexus without a CS route. When venous flow from the cortical middle cerebral vein is blocked in the CS, it easily bypasses to the pterygoid plexus through the emissary veins.

2. The superior petrosal sinus runs along the tentorial edge, so it is hard to compress. When the inferior petrosal sinus is invisible in the tumor around the CS, it suggests an early sign of tumor invasion in the CS. Simultaneously it must be considered, however, that it is not uncommonly demonstrated as one of normal variation.

This studies indicates that angiographical granding can offer a strategy for surgery around the CS. The grade 2 patients may have some risk of venous circulation disturbance when the remaining dural outflow is sacrificed at surgery. Dural emissary veins should not be cut during craniotomy in those patients. In grade 3 patients, any craniotomy may be carried out, because draining veins are all on the cerebral hemisphere. However, one of the main collaterals, subtemporal bridging veins, must be preserved, especially on the subtemporal approach.

References

1. Baker HL Jr (1972) The angiographic delineation of sellar and parasellar masses. Neuroradiology 104: 67–78
2. Carpenter MB, Sutin J (1983) Blood supply of the central nervous system. In: Tracy TM (ed) Human neuroanatomy, 8th edn. Williams and Wilkins, Baltimore, pp 733–734
3. Doyon DL, Aron-Rosa DS, Ranee A (1974) Orbital veins and cavernous sinus. In: Newton TH et al (eds) Radiology of the skull and brain angiography. Mosby, Saint Louis, pp 2220–2254
4. Miyazaki H (1981) The "cavernous" sinus. No Shinkei Geka 9: 1131–1138
5. Nagata K et al (1983) Tolosa-hunt syndrome: report of two interesting cases similar to the syndrome, one histologically, the other clinically. No Shinkei Geka 35: 719–726
6. Post MJD et al (1979) The radiographic diagnosis of cavernous meningiomas and aneurysm with a review of the neurovascular anatomy of the cavernous sinus. CRC Cr Rev Diagn Imaging 12: 1–34
7. Servo A (1982) Visualization of the superior ophthalmic vein on carotid angiography. Neuroradiology 23: 141–146
8. Taptas JN (1982) The so-called cavernous sinus. A review of the controversy and its implications on neurosurgeons. Neurosurgery 11: 712–717
9. Umansky F, Nathan H (1982) The lateral wall of the cavernous sinus with special reference to the nerves related to it. J Neurosurg 56: 228–234

MR imaging: normal and invaded cavernous sinus studied with and without Gd-DTPA

M. Komiyama[1], T. Yasui[1], M. Baba[1], A. Hakuba[2], S. Nishimura[2], Y. Nemoto[3], and Y. Inoue[3]

[1] Department of Neurosurgery, Baba Memorial Hospital, Sakai, Osaka, and Departments of [2] Neurosurgery and of [3] Radiology, Osaka City University Medical School, Osaka, Japan

Clinical efficacy of MR imaging for demonstrating the normal and abnormal cavernous sinus (CS) was evaluated. Six normal CS and six CS invaded by pituitary adenomas were studied with a 0.5 T MR scanner using T 1-weighted SE sequences. Furthermore, all normal CS and one invaded CS were studied with gadolinium (Gd)-DTPA. The internal carotid artery (ICA) was shown as low intensity and not enhanced with Gd-DTPA. Venous flow in the CS could be divided into two compartments, *i.e.*, rapid and slow flows. Both flows were demonstrated as lower intensity than the white matter and higher than ICA. Slow flow was markedly enhanced with Gd-DTPA, but rapid flow was enhanced to a lesser degree than the slow. Invasion of the CS was demonstrated as follows: the engulfment of the ICA by the tumor; lack of relatively low intensity of venous flow; the extension of the tumor to the lateral wall of the CS; and the marked displacement of the ICA. MR imaging was useful for the recognition of the blood flows and the tumor invasion in the CS.

Introduction

Recent advances in magnetic resonance (MR) imaging have brought a new era in diagnostic neuroradiology. Most advantages are due to lack of ionizing radiation, high contrast resolution, lack of artifacts from the adjacent bony structures, and multiplanar imaging capabilities. Pituitary adenomas are readily diagnosed with MR imaging since it enables the recognition of the suprasellar extension of the tumors and visual pathways which are difficult to visualize with X-ray computed tomography (CT) [2, 7, 9, 11]. The recognition of a tumor invasion of the cavernous sinus (CS) still remains as a diagnostic problem even with high resolution X-ray CT with contrast media. Here, normal CS and CS invaded by pituitary adenomas were studied and visualization of the CS was described and the clinical efficacy of MR for CS pathology was discussed.

Patients and methods

Six brain tumor patients (group A), who had a normal CS clinically and radiologically, and six pituitary adenoma patients (group B), 4 of whom were operated on and diagnosed histopathologically and 2 of whom were diagnosed clinically and radiologically, underwent MR examinations. In

Table 1. Case Summary

Group A: Normal cavernous sinus

Case no.	Age	Sex	Diagnosis
1	35	M	Occipital glioma
2	50	M	Frontal glioma
3	34	M	Frontal glioma
4	35	F	Falx meningioma
5	20	F	Parietal cavernoma
6	48	F	Frontal metastasis

Group B: Cavernous sinus invaded by pituitary adenomas

Case no.	Age	Sex	Producing hormone	CS invasion on MRI		Operation	CS invasion confirmed	
7	54	M	non	R−	L+	+	R?	L?
8	55	M	non	R?	L+	+	R?	L?
9	63	M	non	R+	L−	−	−	−
10	79	F	non	R+	L−	−	−	−
11	24	F	GH	R?	L+	+	R−	L+
12	37	F	PRL	R+	L−	+	R+	L−

CS cavernous sinus. In cases 7 and 8, CS were not explored group B, in two pituitary adenoma cases (cases 11 and 12), CS invasion by pituitary adenomas was confirmed by surgery and in the remaining 4 cases CS invasion was diagnosed clinically and/or radiologically. The case summary is presented in Table 1. The MR scanner was a 0.5 T superconductive MR system (Picker International, Cleveland, OH). T 1-weighted spin echo (SE) sequences, i.e., SE 600–1,000/40 (repetition time/echo time, msec) were used. Slice thickness was 1.0 cm and coronal images were obtained. The data collection matrix was 256 by 256 and averaging was carried out once. In all patients in group A and in case 11 in group B, the CS was examined by intravenous administration of gadolinium-diethylenetriamine pentaacetic acid (Gd-DTPA) in a dose of 0.1 mmol/kg. MR signal intensity is expressed as intensity relative to the normal white matter.

Results

Normal CS images

Arterial flow in the internal carotid artery (ICA) (Fig. 1) was always demonstrated as low signal intensity on both plain and enhanced images with Gd-DTPA. Venous canals were recognized as two compartments. Both compartments showed lower signal intensity than the normal white matter and higher than the ICA. However, one was enhanced markedly with Gd-DTPA and the other was enhanced to a lesser degree. Although neural structures in the CS were not always visualized, enhanced images with Gd-DTPA were superior than nonenhanced images for the demonstration of neural structures in the CS.

Images of CS invaded by pituitary adenomas

Pituitary adenomas showed isointensity or slightly high intensity compared with the normal white matter (Figs. 2, 3, 4, 5). CS invasion by pituitary adenomas was demonstrated as follows: the engulfment of the ICA by the tumor; lack of relatively low signal intensity of venous flow; the extension of the tumor to the lateral wall of the CS; and the marked displacement of the ICA. In case 11, the pituitary adenoma was enhanced heterogeneously with Gd-DTPA and the tumor invading the CS was also enhanced.

Discussion

In MR imaging of the normal CS, arterial flow in the ICA usually shows low or negligible signal intensity due to the high velocity of the blood flow [10] unless the flow velocity is low due to stenosis or obliteration of the ICA.

Angiographically, there are two ways to demonstrate the venous canals in the CS. One is carotid angiography and the other venography. As regards venography, there are two methods, i.e., orbital venography and jugular venography. It is of great interest that opacification of venous canals in the CS is different between the venous phase of carotid angiography and venography. Visualized venous canals in the CS are always larger in venography than in carotid angiography. We think that there are principally two kinds of venous flows in the CS, *i.e.*, rapid flow and slow flow. In the venous phase of carotid angiography, only rapid venous flow is visualized and slow flow in scarcely visualized. However, in venography both rapid and slow flows are visualized. This is the reason why there are differences regarding sizes of opacified venous canals between carotid angiography and venography.

In MR images, these two venous flows showed relatively low signal intensities, which were dependent on their flow velocities and imaging parameters (pulse sequences, repetition times, and echo times). They were easily recognized as relatively low intensity on T 1-weighted SE images. However, they were not absolutely low or of negligible intensity like an arterial flow in the ICA since they were enhanced by the flow-related enhancement (paradoxical enhancement) [3, 10] even without Gd-DTPA. Gd-DTPA has the property of reducing the relaxation times (T 1 and T 2) of surrounding protons due to proton relaxation enhancement [4, 14]. Its enhancement effect on images is very similar to that of iodinated contrast enhancement in X-ray CT. Venous flows imaged with Gd-DTPA show various signal intensities due to the combination of flow-related enhancement and proton relaxation enhancement. Slow venous flow was always enhanced with Gd-DTPA due to these two enhancement mechanisms, while rapid venous flow was enhanced to a lesser degree than slow flow.

Pituitary adenomas showed isointensity or sightly high intensity in comparison to the normal white matter and were enhanced with Gd-DTPA. Slow venous flow showed lower intensity than those of pituitary adenomas. Intracavernous nerve structures were not identified probably due to the thickness of the image slices, so visualization of neural structures in the CS was poor and is not discussed extensively in this paper. Gd-DTPA enhanced the pituitary glands, stalks, and venous flows in the CS, but did not enhance the optic chiasm and nerves in the CS. Gd-DTPA could facilitate demonstrating venous flows and nerve structures in the CS.

It is difficult to diagnose invasion of the CS by pituitary adenomas definitely at present. In order to evaluate CS pathology with X-ray CT, the CS is studied with high resolution, thin-section, and direct coronal

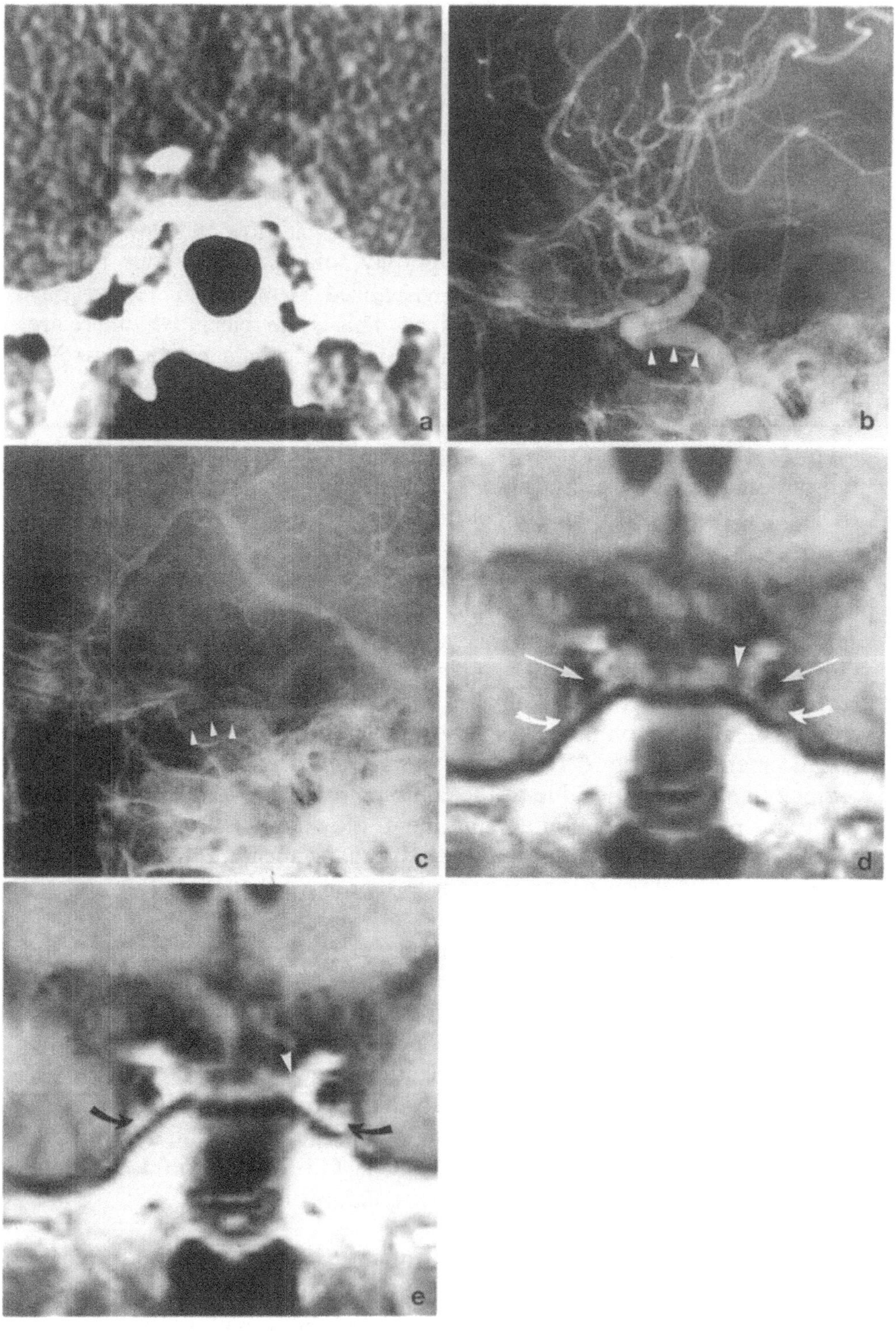
a
b
c
d
e

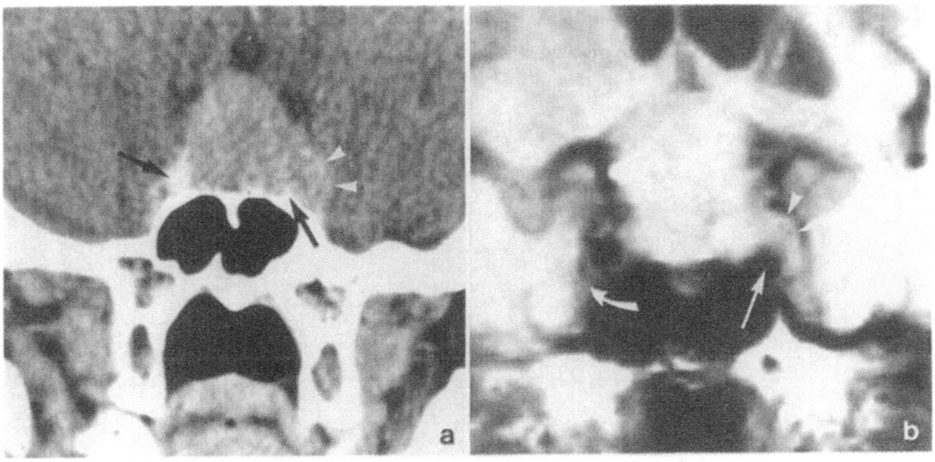

Fig. 2. A 54-year-old male with nonfunctioning pituitary adenoma (case 7). **a** Enhanced CT demonstrates the high density of internal carotid arteries (arrows). Bulging of the left cavernous sinus may be noted (arrowheads). **b** T 1-weighted SE image. Left carotid artery (straight arrow) is displaced infero-laterally and engulfed by the tumor. The tumor extends to the lateral wall of the cavernous sinus (arrowheads). Relatively low intensity of venous flow (curved arrow) is noted on the right side and it is not observed on the left side due to the invasion of the tumor

techniques, in which intravenous bolus and/or continuous administration of iodinated contrast media is mandatory [6, 8, 12, 13]. With these techniques, the CS is markedly enhanced and pituitary adenomas usually show slightly less enhancement than the CS. Invasion of pituitary adenomas into the CS was demonstrated in X-ray CT as follows: CS expansion; visible encasement of the ICA; intracavernous cranial nerve compression, obliteration, or displacement; invasion of the lateral wall of the CS, and diffuse

---

Fig. 1. Normal cavernous sinus in an occipital glioma patient (case 1). **a** Enhanced CT can not demonstrate internal carotid arteries. **b** Arterial phase of the left carotid angiography. Arrowheads indicate internal carotid artery. **c** Venous phase of the left carotid angiography. Arrowheads indicate rapid venous flow in the cavernous sinus. **d** T 1-weighted SE image without Gd-DTPA. Carotid arteries are clearly demonstrated as a low intensity area (straight arrows) and rapid venous flow is demonstrated just medial to the left internal carotid artery (arrowhead) in the cavernous sinus as a slightly low intensity area. The relatively low signal intensity of slow venous flows by may noted (curved arrows). **e** T 1-weighted SE image with Gd-DTPA. Slow venous flows are markedly enhanced (curved arrows), whereas fast venous flow (arrowhead) shows lower signal intensity than slow venous flow

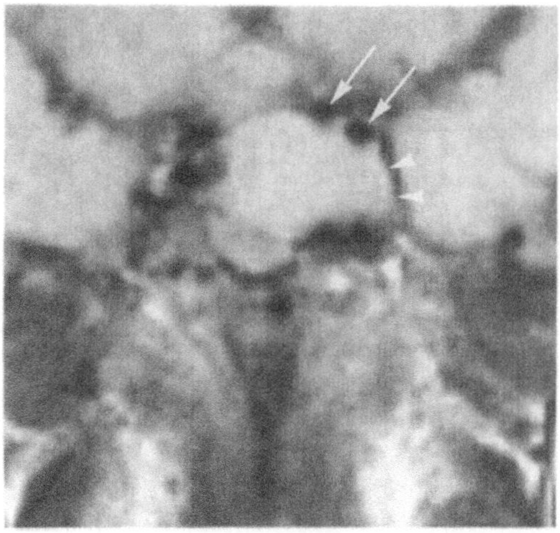

Fig. 3. A 55-year-old male with nonfunctioning pituitary adenoma (case 8). T 1-weighted SE image. The internal carotid artery (arrows) is markedly displaced superiorly and the tumor extends to the lateral wall of the cavernous sinus (arrowheads)

bone destruction [1]. However, it is sometimes difficult to diagnose the invasion of pituitary adenomas into the CS and it is impossible to differentiate rapid and slow flows in the CS with X-ray CT even with the above-mentioned techniques.

To obtain coronal images, MR imaging can be performed with the neck of the patient in the neutral position. This is a great advantage over X-ray CT. Although Daniels et al. [5] demonstrated good MR images of the normal CS, there has not been an extensive description of CS invasion by pituitary adenomas so far. CS invasion by pituitary adenomas is strongly suggested by the following findings: the engulfment of the ICA by the tumor; lack of relatively low signal intensity of venous flow on T 1-weighted SE images; the extension of the tumor to the lateral wall of the CS; and marked displacement of the ICA. These findings help us to recognize CS invasion by pituitary adenomas.

In conclusion, MR imaging is useful for the recognition of tumor invasion of the CS as well as for the demonstration of the relationships between the visual pathways and the tumor, and suprasellar extension of the tumor. MR imaging can give us a lot of information for the determination of the appropriate therapy for pituitary adenomas.

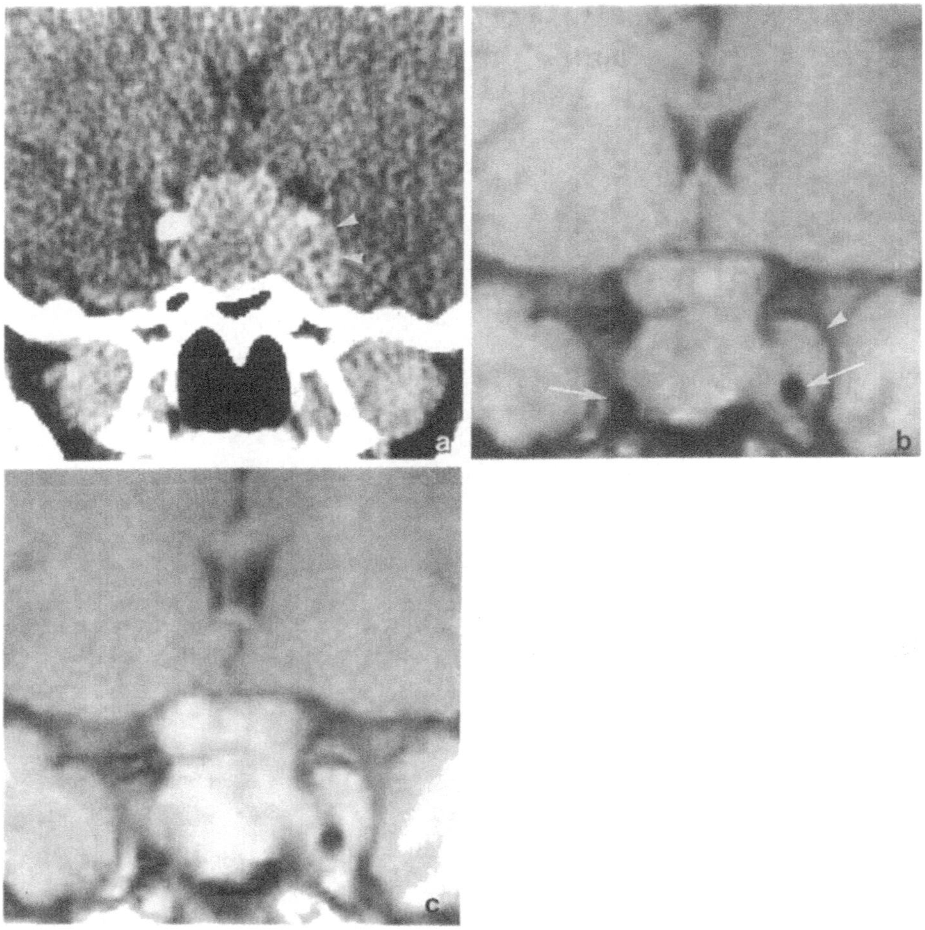

Fig. 4. A 24-year-old female with human growth hormone producing pituitary adenoma (case 11). **a** Enhanced CT demonstrates the bulging of the left cavernous sinus (arrowheads). However, it is difficult to differentiate internal carotid arteries from the tumor. **b** T 1-weighted SE image without Gd-DTPA. Internal carotid arteries are clearly demonstrated as low intensity area (arrows). The left internal carotid artery is markedly displaced laterally and engulfed by the tumor. The tumor extends to the left lateral wall of the cavernous sinus (arrowhead). **c** T 1-weighted SE image with Gd-DTPA. The tumor is enhanced with Gd-DTPA

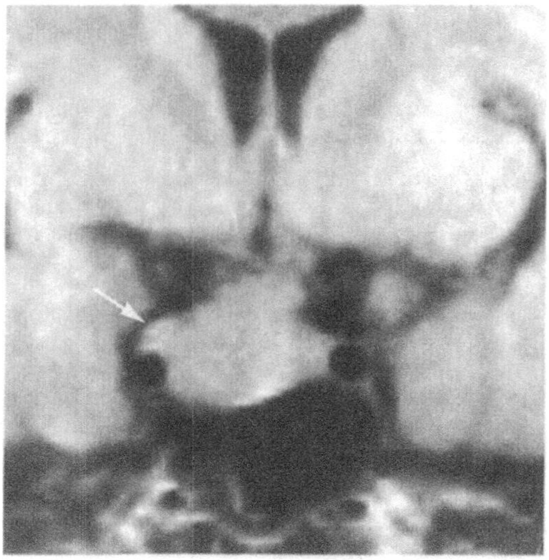

Fig. 5. A 37-year-old female with prolactinoma (case 12). T 1-weighted SE image. The tumor extends to the right lateral wall of the cavernous sinus (arrow) and engulfs the right internal carotid artery, which is displaced laterally. Lack of relatively low intensity of venous flow is noted on the right side

References

1. Ahmadi J, North CM, Segall HD, Zee CS, Weiss MH (1985) Cavernous sinus invasion by pituitary adenomas. ANJR 6: 893–898
2. Bilaniuk LT, Zimmerman RA, Wehrli FW, Snyder PJ, Goldberg HI, Grossman RI, Bottomley PA, Edelstein WA, Glover GH, MacFall JR, Redington RW (1984) Magnetic resonance imaging of pituitary lesions using 1.0 to 1.5 T field strength. Radiology 153: 415–418
3. Bradley WG, Waluch V, Lai KS, Fernandez EJ, Spalter C (1984) The appearance of rapidly flowing blood on magnetic resonance images. AJR 143: 1167–1174
4. Carr DH, Brown J, Bydder GM, Steiner RE, Weinmann HJ, Speck U, Hall AS, Young IR (1984) Gadolinium-DTPA as a contrast agent in MRI: initial clinical experience in 20 patients. AJNR 143: 215–224
5. Daniels DL, Pech P, Mark L, Pojunas K, Williams AL, Haughton VM (1985) Magnetic resonance imaging of the cavernous sinus. AJR 6: 187–192
6. Hasso AN, Aubin ML, Pop PM, Bar D, Thompson JR, Becker TS, Hinshaw DB Jr, Vignaud J (1982) High resolution thin section computed tomography of the cavernous sinus. RadioGraphics 2: 83–100
7. Hawkes RC, Holland GN, Moore WS, Corston R, Kean DM, Worthington BS (1983) The application of NMR imaging to the evaluation of pituitary and juxtasellar tumors. AJNR 4: 221–222

8. Kline LB, Acker JD, Post MJD, Vitek JJ (1981) The cavernous sinus: A computed tomographic study. AJNR 2: 299–305
9. Lee BCP, Deck MDF (1985) Sellar and juxtasellar lesion detection with MR. Radiology 157: 143–147
10. Mills CM, Brant-Zawadzki M, Crooks LE, Kaufman L, Sheldon P, Norman D, Bank W, Newton TH (1984) Nuclear magnetic resonance: principles of blood flow imaging. AJR 142: 165–170
11. Oot R, New PFJ, Buonanno FS, Pykett IL, Kistler P, Delapaz R, Davis KR, Taveras JM, Brady TJ (1984) MR imaging of pituitary adenomas using a prototype resistive magnet: preliminary assessment. AJNR 5: 131–137
12. Swartz JD, Russell KB, Basile BA, O'Donnell PC, Popky GL (1983) High resolution computed tomography of the intrasellar contents: normal, near normal and abnormal. RadioGraphics 3: 228–247
13. Taylor S (1982) High resolution computed tomography of the sella. Radiol Clin North Am 20: 207–236
14. Weinmann HJ, Brasch RC, Press WR, Wesbey GE (1984) Characteristics of gadolinium-DTPA complex: a potential NMR contrast agent. AJR 142: 619–624

The utility of intravenous DSA for cavernous sinus venography

S. Harada[1], S. Toya[1], T. Kawase[1], Y. Nakano[1], and H. Shiga[2]

Departments of [1] Neurosurgery and of [2] Diagnostic Radiology,
Keio University School of Medicine, Tokyo, Japan

Intravenous DSA (IVDSA) applied to an intracranial lesion, especially tumors around cavernous sinuses, can reveal the laterality of the sinus with minimal invasiveness. In this study, a total of 30 patients who had parasellar tumors were examined and preoperative information concerning the extent of tumor invasion was obtained. Pituitary adenomas and craniopharyngiomas seldom invade the cavernous sinus, whereas meningiomas and chordomas often invade it. IVDSA can offer information as a routine venogram of the cavernous sinus with a minimally invasive technique.

Introduction

Tumors growing around the cavernous sinus, such as pituitary adenoma, chordoma, meningioma etc. occasionally invade the sinuses. Although cavernous sinus syndrome is a clinically typical manifestation of the destruction or occlusion of the sinuses, neuroradiological examination of conventional angiography often fails to show bilateral cavernous sinuses if comparison with the opposite site is necessary. One of the reasons why bilateral cavernous sinuses can not be seen simultaneously by conventional angiography is laminar flow in the sinuses.

Intravenous digital subtraction angiography (IVDSA) applied to intracranial vessels is new technique sufficient to give the information of dural sinuses simultaneously [2]. We can see bilateral cavernous sinuses with ease by means of IVDSA applied to intracranial vessels and know the extent of invasion of the tumors to cavernous sinuses when we compare both sites.

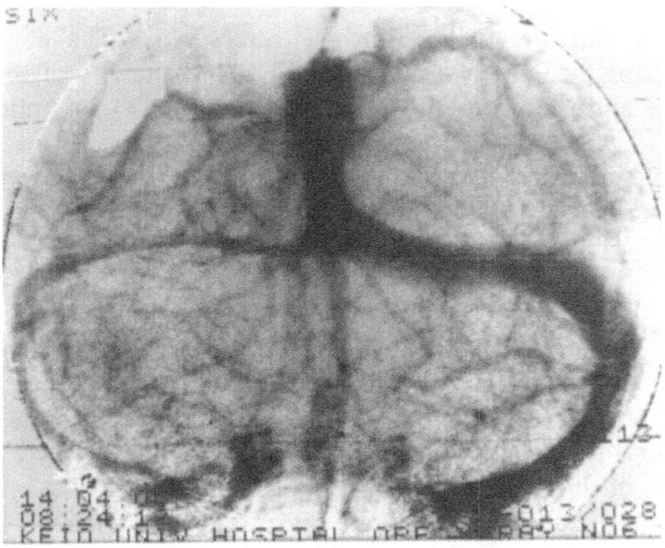

Fig. 1. Normal IVDSA on Towne's view

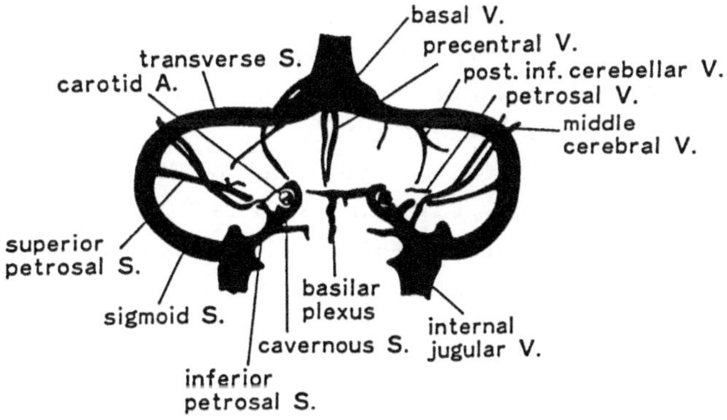

Fig. 2. Diagram of IVDSA

Method and cases

A Siemens Angiotron II was used for this study. The procedure is described below.

1. The cubital or femoral vein was punctured and a guide wire was inserted. Using the guide wire, an eight French catheter was inserted to the central vein and the tip of the catheter was lodged there under an image intensifier.

2. 20 cm^3/min (total 40 cc) of angiographin was injected by an automatic injector and lateral, axial and 25° Towne's views were taken for the projection.

Materials

During the last three years, thirty patients who were suspected to have a tumor around the cavernous sinus have all been studied by IVDSA.

Nineteen of those had a pituitary adenoma, six cases had meningioma, three cases had craniopharyngioma, two cases chordoma.

Figures 1 and 2 show an example of the normal picture and illustration of dural sinuses on Towne's view.

Results

In order to identify each side of cavernous sinuses, lateral projection was inadequate because both sides of the cavernous sinus were overlapped on one film. On the axial projection, a laryngeal motion artifact which frequently appeared in the center of the picture was a considerable problem which decreased the spatial resolution.

Towne's view was used to compare the width of each side of the cavernous sinus. On this view, cavernous sinuses are clearly shown without overlapping. When the maximum width of the cavernous sinus was smaller than 50% of that of the contralateral cavernous sinus, laterality was regarded as being present. When laterality was present, we considered that the tumor attached to cavernous sinus had invaded or compressed the whole or partial lumen of the sinus. The angiographical laterality was present only in one case out of 19 pituitary adenomas and 3 craniopharyngiomas, whereas in the case of meningioma and chordoma, seven out of eight cases showed laterality of cavernous sinus (Table 1):

Table 1.

Diagnosis	Number of patients	Laterality > 50%	Laterality < 50%
Pituitary adenoma	19	1	18
Craniopharyngioma	3	0	3
Meningioma	6	5	1
Chordoma	2	2	0

Case Report

Case 1

This 49-year-old woman had been well until March 21, 1984, on which date, when she got up in the morning, she felt double vision. She consulted a nearby ophthalmologist and neurosurgeon, but no abnormality was pointed out.

Then she consulted our hospital and left abducens nerve palsy was pointed out. No other neurological abnormality was found. CT scan showed a right parasellar high density mass (Fig. 3). IVDSA was then performed, the finding of which was obstruction of the right cavernous sinus. It was suspected that the tumor had invaded the cavernous sinus and obliterated its lumen (Fig. 4). The opposite site of the cavernous sinus was intact. Surgery was performed by the middle fossa approach on August 24, 1984. The histology of the tumor was meningioma.

Case 2

This 57-year-old woman felt sudden diplopia which disappeared 1 month later. In September 1982, she had a severe headache on the left side. She was hospitalized for precise examination.

CT scan revealed a left parasellar mass extending to the posterior fossa (Fig. 5) and she was admitted to our hospital for surgery. Abnormal neurological findings on admission were left abducens palsy and trigeminal (V/1, V/3) palsy. IVDSA showed obstruction of the left cavernous sinus (Fig. 6). Pituitary function based on hormonal examinations were within normal limits. Surgery was carried out on February 15, 1983, by subtemporal approach and the tumor was removed subtotally; then irradiation of 50 Gry was carried out. Her complaints of left palsy in nerves V and VI still remained but slightly improved on discharge.

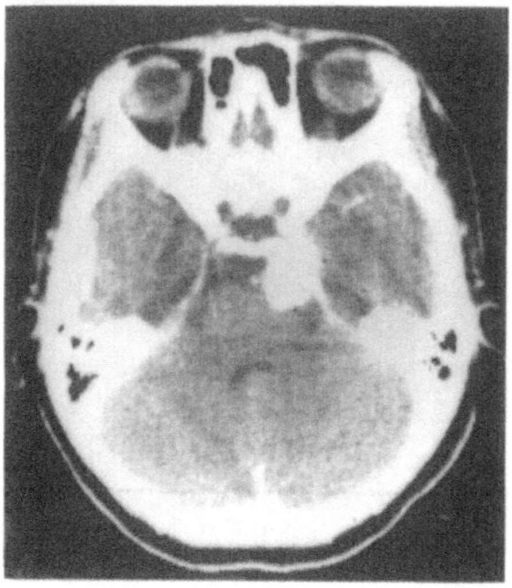

Fig. 3. CT scan showing high density mass attached to right tentorial notch or clivus

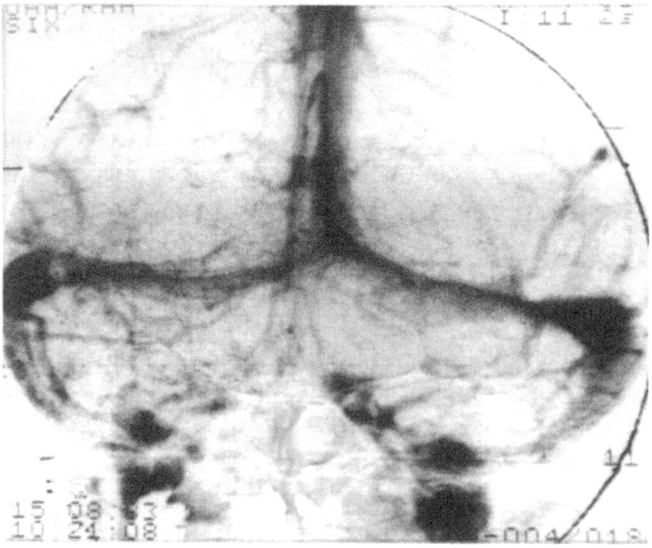

Fig. 4. IVDSA film showing obliteration of right cavernous sinus compared with left side. It is demonstrable that the tumor invaded or compressed the right cavernous sinus

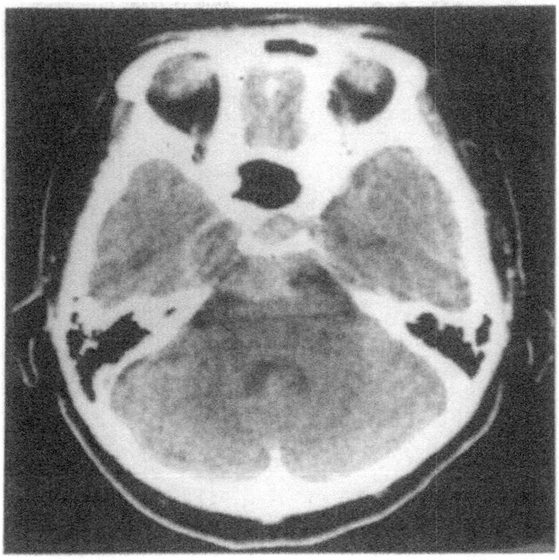

Fig. 5. CT scan showing parasellar mass extending to posterior fossa

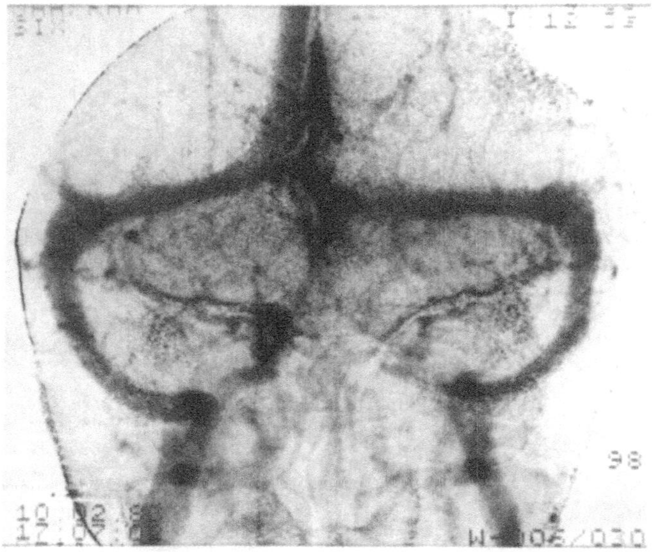

Fig. 6. IVDSA showing obliteration of left cavernous sinus

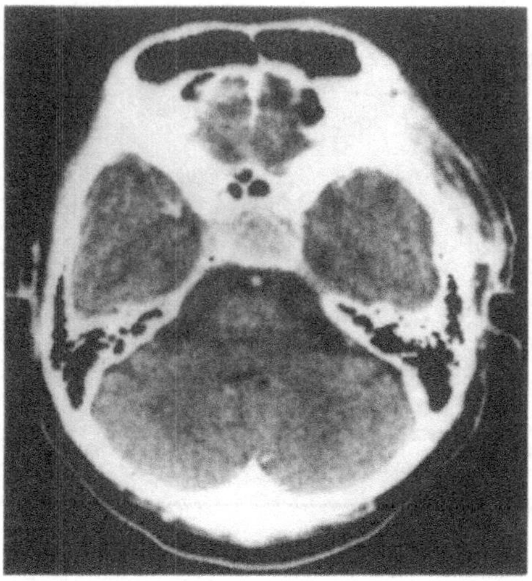

Fig. 7. CT scan showing intrasellar high or isodensity mass of pituitary adenoma

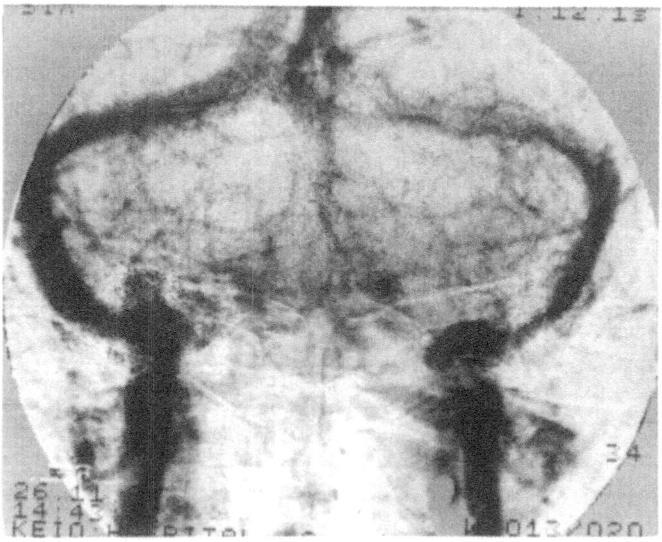

Fig. 8. IVDSA showing almost the same size of bilateral cavernous sinus. It was suspected that the tumor did not invade or expand the extrasellar space

Case 3

This 16-year-old woman noticed an increase in body weight and facial flushing over a one-year period. Laboratory data revealed findings of diabetes mellitus and diet therapy was carried out. Then she consulted the Pediatric Department of our hospital and a hormonal examinations were performed. Laboratory data showed a Cushing syndrome of high level of ACTH (105–270) and cortisol (50–170), urine sugar more than 100 g/day. CT scan revealed she had a pituitary adenoma (Fig. 7).

On admission, she had a moon face, weakness of the extremities, central obesity, and moreover was herself bothered by her psychological instability. IVDSA was performed and the bilateral cavernous sinuses looked intact (Fig. 8). The tumor was surgically removed by the transcranial approach. By the surgical view, no mass lesion seemed to have invaded the cavernous sinuses.

Discussion

IVDSA has the advantage of utility and capability on demonstrating the arterial structure via venous injection of contrast media [1, 3, 4]. They are, in short, noninvasive to patients and allow investigation of out-patients. It has been emphasized by certain investigators that IVDSA has the advantage of showing cerebral veins and dural sinuses [3]. Both sides of cavernous sinus are demonstrable simultaneously on one Towne's view, which offers a comparable venogram with one shot of contrast media.

On the other hand, IVDSA has a disadvantage concerning spatial resolution compared with the conventional angiography [2]. Although in this study, IVDSA has given us satisfactory results regarding the venous structure, a lateral view of IVDSA has resulted in overlapping of the bilateral structure. This overlapping is one of the disadvantages on IVDSA venography. In the case of pituitary adenomas and craniopharyngiomas, they showed a small incidence of abnormality, suggesting that they seldom invade cavernous sinuses. In contrast, meningiomas and chordomas often invade cavernous sinuses. In those parasellar lesions, IVDSA has the possibility of offering information as a routine venogram of the cavernous sinus, with a minimally invasive technique.

References

1. Mistretta CA et al (1981) Digital angiography a perspective. Radiology 139: 273–276
2. Modic MT, Weinstein MA, Chilcote WA, Pavlicek W, Furlan AJ, Duchesneau PM, Little JR (1982) Digital subtraction angiography of the intracranial vascular system; comparative study in 55 patients. AJR 138: 299–306
3. Modic MT, Weinstein MA, Starnes DL, Kinney SE, Duchesneau PM (1983) Intravenous digital subraction angiography of the intracranial veins and dural sinuses. Neuroradiology 146: 383–389
4. Seeger JF, Weinstein PR, Carmody RF, Ovitt TW, Fisher D, Capp MP (1982) Digital video subtraction angiography of the cervical and cerebral vasculature. J Neurosurg 56: 173–179

Occlusion techniques

Embolization techniques in the treatment of vascular lesions involving the cavernous sinus

G. M. DEBRUN

Interventional Neuroradiology, The Johns Hopkins Medical Institutions, Baltimore, Maryland, U.S.A.

It is interesting to see that the treatment alternatives that we offer to patients suffering from carotid cavernous fistula or cavernous aneurysm greatly depend on our background. The neurosurgeon who has great experience in the surgical approach of the cavernous sinus will offer surgical techniques. The neuroradiologist who has experience with superselective catheterization of cerebral vessels will offer endovascular techniques with balloon catheter. From which technique does the patient benefit the most? Rather than considering that these two different therapeutic approaches are in conflict with each other, it is probably more positive to consider which is most appropriate to use in each particular case, to compare the overall results of each. In fact, it should be a team effort between neurosurgeon and neuroradiologist, and it is already proven that a certain number of these cases can be treated by association of surgical exposure and embolization techniques.

Reported here are the overall results of the treatment of 131 carotid cavernous fistulae and 24 cavernous aneurysms. The indication for treatment has always been discussed with my neurosurgeon colleagues, and they have always agreed to share with me the responsibility in the management of these patients, even when they were personally referred to me. I am also indebted to my neuroradiologist colleagues who have assisted me in the treatment of these patients. The different institutions where these patients were treated are:

1974–1978 Hospital Henri Mondor, 94000 Creteil, France (a);

1978–1981 University Hospital, London, Ontario, Canada (b);

1981–1985 Massachusetts General Hospital, Boston, Massachusetts (c);

1985–1986 The Johns Hopkins Medical Institutions, Baltimore, Maryland (d).

Experience from 131 carotid cavernous fistulae, 94 traumatic cases and 37 spontaneous.

a) Neurosurgeons: Drs. J. P. Caron, M. Hurth, Y. Keravel, J. P. Comoy, M. Djindjian. Neuroradiologists: Drs. G. M. Debrun, P. Lacour.

b) Neurosurgeons: Drs. C. Drake, S. Peerless, J. Girvin, G. Ferguson. Neuroradiologists: Drs. G. M. Debrun, A. Fox, F. Viñuela.

c) Neurosurgeons: Drs. N. Zervas, R. Heros, R. Ojeman, R. Martuza, P. Black, P. Chapman. Neuroradiologists: Drs. G. M. Debrun, K. Davis.

d) Neurosurgeons: Drs. D. M. Long, H. Nauta, N. Miller. Neuroradiologists: Drs. G. M. Debrun, H. S. Ahn.

Traumatic carotid cavernous fistulae (CCF)

There were 61 males and 31 females. Two patients had bilateral CCF. Therefore, 94 CCFs are considered. All these patients had severe head injury and the symptomatology was obvious. We were asked to treat them usually at the peak of the ocular symptoms. Proptosis and chemosis were most of the time prominent. A huge systolo-diastolic bruit was present over the eye. However, in three patients who had symptoms of an active CCF the day before treatment the fistula closed spontaneously during the night and the bruit was no longer audible over the eye. It is worth noting that these patients had a long flight the day before.

The angiographic work-up included in each case a selective homolateral internal carotid angiography. Before using intraarterial digital subraction angiography, a selective homolateral external carotid angiogram was taken, which is almost always normal in these traumatic CCFs (91 out of 94 cases). Since we routinely use digital arterial subtraction angiography, we simply check on our real time subtracted pictures that there is no participation of the external carotid branches. The contralateral internal carotid angiography is done with cross compression in antero-posterior projection only. It shows if the anterior communicating artery is patent or not. The vertebral angiography (left side usually) was always done with compression of the carotid ipsilateral to the fistula. It demonstrated the patency of the posterior communicating artery and the size and location of the fistula in most cases.

Treatment alternatives

Three treatment alternatives were used, alone or associated. The endoarterial route with the detachable balloon technique was used in 82 cases. The endovenous route was attempted in 17 cases. Fourteen patients had a surgical procedure associated with embolization.

The endoarterial route with detachable balloon

The detachable balloon technique pioneered by Serbinenko is elegant and effective in a high number of cases. The goal is to manipulate the balloon catheter inside the internal carotid artery, until we see the balloon under fluoroscopy aspirated into the cavernous sinus through the tear of the carotid siphon. When the inflated balloon in the cavernous sinus closes the fistula, it is detached. The internal carotid blood flow is preserved.

This goal is not achieved in every case. The principle is very simple, but many technical details and also the anatomy of the fistula, which varies tremendously from case to case, explain why the carotid blood flow cannot always be preserved. In this group of 94 CCFs, the internal carotid artery was preserved in 64 cases (68%) and was permanently occluded in 30 patients (32%). However, the results improved with more experience and in the last 36 cases treated, the carotid blood flow was preserved in 80% of the cases.

Occasional users of the technique should be discouraged if one wants to avoid catastrophies. The patients do not represent a frequent disease and they should be concentrated in a few experienced centers. It will never be possible to have 100% of carotid arteries patent at the end of the treatment because the tear of the internal carotid as well as of the cavernous sinus is sometimes very large. Sometimes many balloons have to be detached into the cavernous sinus and the last one occludes the fistula but bulges through the wide tear and stenoses the carotid artery. Several cases with this situation ended with complete thrombosis of the carotid artery. Direct surgical repair of these large tears would probably have been difficult as well. There are also three patients in this group who had surgical ligation of the internal carotid artery in the neck many years previously. In ten cases, the patient had more than one therapeutic stage. This occurred in two situations. In the first, there was early modification in the inflation or the position of the detached balloon and there was recurrence of the fistula. Usually, a second balloon closed the fistula. The second situation happens when several balloons have been already detached in a large cavernous sinus, but the last one cannot enter the cavernous sinus in spite of a still active fistula. In this case, it is wise to wait one or two weeks. It is usually possible to enter the cavernous sinus again when the previously detached balloons have slightly deflated. However, some of these patients deteriorate after partial filling of their cavernous sinus and incomplete closure of the fistula. In this situation, they should be treated immediately.

The endovenous route with detachable balloon

The endovenous route has been used in 17 cases, with excellent result in two cases. One or two balloons could be detached in six cases but did not occlude the fistula. One of these patients was an 83-year-old lady. We could not enter the fistula through the arterial route. The balloon was blocking the posterior venous drainage of the cavernous sinus, and was detached when we tried to advance it close to the tear. She developed extensive proptosis and swelling of the eye with decreased vision. The cavernous sinus was surgically exposed the next day. One balloon was detached into the cavernous sinus with cure of the fistula. She had a normal carotid angiography five days later, but ultimately died from a subdural empyema. One patient had surgical exposure of the angular vein but we could not reach the cavernous sinus with our balloon catheter.

In nine cases, we could not advance into the inferior petrosal sinus with our balloon. The venous route through the internal jugular vein is indicated when the venous drainage of the cavernous sinus is mainly postero-inferior through the inferior petrosal sinus. Usually the fistula is posterior and low on the carotid siphon.

Surgical techniques

Fourteen surgical procedures were carried out in this group, either allowing a successful embolization in nine, through surgical exposure of the cavernous sinus or completing an unsuccessful embolization in five. The first group includes one case where cyanoacrylic glue was injected into the cavernous sinus and five cases where balloons were detached in the cavernous sinus at surgery. In three cases, the patient had had the internal carotid artery ligated in the neck many years before. The second group includes five failures of embolization with detachable balloons. The fistula as well as the internal carotid artery were occluded during the procedure, but after partial deflation or dislodgement of the balloon, the fistula recurred, stealing blood from the intracranial circulation above the fistula. This complication can induce ischemic neurological deficit and should be treated promptly by intracranial ligation of the internal carotid and the ophthalmic artery.

Overall results of these 94 traumatic CCFs

Eighty-nine out of 92 patients were clinically cured from their fistula.

There were three deaths in this group. One patient was the 83-year-old lady who died several weeks after cure of her fistula from septic complications. The two other patients died from multiple injuries and brain damage after the accident. Both of them were comatose in grade IV.

Transient oculomotor nerve palsies were noted in 31 cases (30%) with final complete recovery after several weeks or months.

Transient neurological deficit occurred in two patients. One had injection of cyanoacrylic glue in the cavernous sinus at surgery under compression of the carotid artery in the neck (it was probably a mistake). A small amount escaped through the carotid tear and embolized the internal capsule. Hemiparesis and motoraphasia occurred but totally subsided in two weeks.

One patient with severe contusion of the brain had residual stenosis of the carotid artery after closure of the fistula. He had an infarct in the middle cerebral artery territory.

Angiograms were done in most of these patients several days or months after treatment. This survey revealed that the healing of the internal carotid artery was often imperfect leaving a residual bulging into the cavernous sinus or venous pouch. These patients remained asymptomatic whenever the pouch was small. Only a few patients with a giant venous pouch needed to be treated a second time because of persistance of symptoms, either retroorbital pain or oculomotor palsy.

Spontaneous carotid cavernous fistulas

Among 37 cases of spontaneous CCFs, four were associated with cavernous aneurysms. one was purely internal in a child and was probably congenital while 32 were dural arteriovenous malformations (AVMs) of the cavernous sinus. Three in this last category healed spontaneously.

32 dural AVMs—22 females, 10 males

Three patients who had red eye, proptosis and bruit over the eye the day before the procedure had a normal angiogram and recovered a normal looking eye a few weeks later. The ipsilateral external carotid was involved in 29 cases and the contralateral external in 19 cases. The ipsilateral internal carotid artery was involved in 25 cases. The contralateral internal carotid was involved in 17 cases. Only four cases were purely ipsilateral external carotid and were invariably a single fistula between the middle meningeal artery and the cavernous sinus.

Treatment consisted in the association of different modalities

Fourteen cases had embolization with particles of polyvinyl alcohol foam (PVA). Eleven cases had embolization with isobutyl cyanoacrylate (IBCA). Ten cases had both PVA and IBCA. Four cases had embolization with balloons. Two cases had embolization and surgery, one had plugging of both cavernous sinuses after embolization of both external carotid feeders, the other had surgical exposure of the superior ophthalmic vein at the superomedial angle of the orbit and detachment of one balloon at the junction of the vein and cavernous sinus.

Two patients in this group had permanent occlusion of the internal carotid artery, one secondary to premature detachment of the balloon and the second because the patient was referred to us as a purely internal carotid. In fact, these cases where an attempt was made to enter the cavernous sinus were rare. Most of the time the feeders from the internal carotid siphon are so obviously multiple and small that it is useless to try to catheterize them with any size of balloon. Today these two patients could probably be cured by embolization of the cavernous sinus after surgical exposure and they would not end with permanent occlusion of their internal carotid artery. The overall result in this group is not as good as the traumatic cases group. The reason is that these patients are often old, only embolization of the external feeders can be done and they are left with untreated feeders from one or two internal carotid arteries. This disease is also often bilateral and the recurrence rate is high. Twenty-three patients were cured including the three spontaneous cures. These patients were asymptomatic with normal angiograms six months after treatment. Nine patients had persistence of symptoms or insufficient follow up. The morbidity in this group was limited to a transient hemiparesis after IBCA embolization and one patient with persistent dysesthesia in the trigeminal distribution, also after IBCA embolization.

Four cavernous aneurysms presented as a CCF in patients 30, 70, 85, and 89 years of age. The 30-year-old female developed her symptoms after delivery and had in fact a giant varix of the cavernous sinus communicating with the internal carotid artery through a small hole. This case is not included in the group of cavernous aneurysms. The three other patients were 70, 85, and 89 years old. A balloon was detached into the aneurysm with preservation of the carotid artery in all of them. The 30-year-old patient was cured and has a normal internal carotid artery. The 70-year-old male is asymptomatic with incomplete occlusion of this aneurysm. The 85-year-old lady developed a middle cerebral artery infarct three days after treatment and died. The 89-year-old lady is clinically cured but we did not repeat the angiogram. Those three patients are included in the group of cavernous aneurysms.

One case in a five-year-old boy was probably congenital. There was a single tear of the internal carotid artery anteriorly with absence of posterior venous drainage. One balloon was detached in the cavernous sinus with excellent clinical results.

Experience from 24 cavernous aneurysms—16 females and 8 males

Three cases were traumatic aneurysms, two of them associated with a CCF, spontaneously closed in one case, treated with detachable ballon in the other. The third case had the metallic top of an umbrella lodged into the cavernous sinus. For safer surgical removal of this foreign body, the internal carotid was permanently occluded before surgery.

Three cases in elderly people were associated with a spontaneous CCF. They have already been included in this group of patients. One of them, 83 years old, developed a MCA infart three days after treatment and died. This is the only death in the whole group of cavernous aneurysms.

The internal carotid artery was permanently occluded with detachable balloons in fifteen out of 21 cases (3 traumatic cases exluded). The reasons for not preserving the carotid blood flow are the usually broad neck of these giant aneurysms. Even a big balloon inflated in the pouch buldes through the neck and often stenoses the lumen of the carotid siphon. These giant aneurysms are detected because they induce a mass effect on the oculomotor nerves and on the fifth nerve with frequent trigeminal neuralgia. It is not logical to increase the mass effect with an inflated balloon. When these aneurysms contain clots, it is dangerous to navigate inside the pouch with a balloon which risks dislodging a piece of clot and inducing an embolus. Finally, because of the frequent tortuosity, elongation and partial stenosis of the internal carotid artery below the aneurysm, it is sometimes impossible to move the balloon forward, beyond the level of the neck of the aneurysm. When permanent occlusion of the internal carotid is contemplated, it would be nice to be able to detach one balloon above and one below the neck of the aneurysm. When it is impossible the balloon occludes the carotid artery at the level of or immediately below the neck of the aneurysm.

This treatment alternative seems to many neurosurgeons no different from the ligation of the internal carotid artery with a Selverstone clamp in the neck, or even worse because they think that the progressive occlusion of the internal carotid is more physiological and can be reversed if the patient does not tolerate the total occlusion of the internal carotid artery. In fact, it is probably safer to detect the category of patients who will not tolerate the permanent occlusion of the internal carotid artery before tying off the clamp. Test occlusion with the balloon inflated for ten minutes before detachment in a patient systematically heparinized seems to be a very safe way to appreciate tolerance of permanent occlusion of the internal carotid artery. The only imperative precaution is to monitor carefully the blood pressure and to maintain the systolic blood pressure at least at its base line level, specially in elderly patients. It is also postulated that occlusion of the internal carotid as close as possible to the neck of the aneurysm reduces the length of the thrombosis, and decreases the risk of recanalization of the internal carotid through anastomosis with the risk of distal migration of clot emboli.

When the internal carotid is permanently occluded with a detachable balloon, it is a good precaution to detach one and preferably two balloons below the first in order to avoid distal migration of the first in case of premature deflation. Also the third balloon can be detached very close to the origin of the internal carotid artery in the neck which decreases the length of stump of the origin of the internal carotid artery. In this group of 24 patients, only one patient had an EC–IC bypass prior to permanent occlusion of the internal carotid artery. The need for the bypass in this case was detected when the diagnostic angiographic work up was accomplished. An occlusion test of the internal carotid artery with a balloon catheter induced an hemiplegia after ten seconds of inflation, with total immediate recovery after deflation of the balloon. All the other patients perfectly tolerated the 10-minute test occlusion of the internal carotid artery. The patient who developed a MCA infarction three days after treatment had had the carotid artery preserved and had an embolic complication. She finally died and she is the only death in this group of 24 cavernous aneurysms.

The morbidity is limited to two transient neurological complications, one in a patient who had preservation of the internal carotid artery but a severe narrowing of the internal carotid artery. She had an embolus with transient hemiparesis and complete recovery. The second patient had an enormous aneurysm of six centimeters in diameter. A mistake of asepsis was made during the preparation of the balloons. This patient developed a temporal lobe and cavernous sinus abscess which was evacuated with final good recovery. The follow up of this whole group of patients shows excellent clinical results in 23 of them. Even the patients who have their carotid artery patent but with incomplete occlusion of their aneurysm have remained asymptomatic so far.

Conclusion

The tremendous improvement of superselective catheterization of the branches of the external carotid artery and of the intracranial vesssels have opened up new and safe treatment alternatives which were unthinkable fifteen years ago. Simultaneously, microvascular neurosurgery of the cavernous sinus area has added another approach in the treatment of vascular lesions involving the cavernous sinus. Cardiac arrest and deep hypothermia are no longer mandatory and the potential results of intracavernous surgery versus embolization should be kept in mind. The surgical approach of the cavernous sinus will be used more often in the future whenever embolization techniques cannot be done safely and easily. We should also consider that stereotaxic radiotherapy can be a useful tool in the treatment of dural AVMs of the cavernous sinus, especially in elderly patients difficult to treat by any other technique.

These new modalities of treatment are difficult even if the procedure seems very simple. In order to maintain the mortality and morbidity rate at as low a level as possible, these patients should be referred to centers which have the appropriate equipment and the experts in microvascular neurosurgery, interventional neuroradiology and stereotaxic radiotherapy. The improvements of our results will come from a team effort. The different approaches between these three specialties are not antagonistic but complementary.

Endovascular therapy of vascular lesions of the cavernous sinus. Experience with 129 cases

F. Viñuela and P. Lylyk

Interventional Neuroradiology, U.C.L.A. Medical Center, Los Angeles, California, U.S.A.

The relationship of the cavernous sinus with the brain, orbit, sella turcica, mastoid, and middle ear makes this structure of special interest to the neurologist, neurosurgeon, ophthalmologist, otholaryngologist and endocrinologist.

The cavernous sinus is a confined venous structure covered by the dura and containing the internal carotid artery, cranial nerves III, IV and VI and the first and second divisons of cranial nerve V. The presence of fibrous trabeculae was first noted by Winslow in 1732. Bedford showed that the laminae present in the sinuses were indeed trabeculae and not walls of adjacent veins [1]. These trabeculae may become important for the final location of a detachable balloon when positioned through an arteriovenous fistula.

The walls and contents of the cavernous sinus receive their blood supply from external carotid and intracavernous internal carotid branches. These branches anastomose to each other and function as a balanced circuit. Most vascular lesions in this region show this dual blood supply. The angiographer should analyze this particular blood supply by performing external and internal carotid angiograms. Not infrequently, both cavernous sinuses may show a similar pathology, especially in dural AVMs of the cavernous sinus. A bilateral blood supply to a single cavernous sinus lesion may also be depticted.

Several therapeutic procedures have been described to treat intracavernous vascular lesions, including surgical and intravascular occlusive techniques. Not infrequently, the combination of endovascular and surgical therapy is the best alternative to a specific intracavernous vascular pathology.

The aim of these procedures is to occlude and/or resect the vascular pathology while preserving the lumen of the intracavernous internal carotid artery and the blood supply of the cranial nerves.

One hundred and twenty-nine intracavernous vascular lesions were diagnosed and treated using the endovascular route at University Hospital, London, Ontario, Canada, between 1978 and 1986. 89 patients had a carotid-cavernous fistula (69 traumatic and 20 spontaneous) and 40 had a giant intracavernous aneurysm. The diagnostic protocol included a thorough clinical and ophthalmological evaluation, examination of the bilateral external and internal carotid, and vertebral angiography using the transfemoral technique and standard #4 or #5 French catheters. In some cases of dural AVMs, superselective catheterization of specific external carotid artery feeders was performed using calibrated leak balloons [2].

Traumatic carotid cavernous fistulas (69 cases)

Carotid cavernous fistulas have an approximate incidence of one per 10 000 to one per 20 000 hospital admissions [3]. Trauma is the etiology in 75% of cases. Their clinical presentation is determined by involvement of the different venous pathways which drain the arterialized blood flow away from the cavernous sinus. The largest and most frequently utilized pathway is through the superior and inferior ophthalmic veins. Ipsilateral neuro-ophthalmological symptoms are thus produced by orbital and ocular venous enlargement and congestion. The most frequent complaints are bruit 85%, exophthalmos (79%), swelling and redness of the eye and face (70%), double vision (34%), headaches (31%), and visual deterioration (29%) [4].

Ophthalmoplegias are most frequently seen with involvement of the abducens nerve (59%), oculomotor (41%), or trochlear nerve (53%) [4]. The trigeminal nerve (29%), optic nerve (39%), and facial nerve (35%) involvement can also be detected. The age range in our series was between 12 and 46 years, with an average age of 23 years. 34 patients were female and 35 were males. 66 fistulas were unilateral and three were bilateral.

All traumatic fistulas were occluded using a Debrun detachable balloon [5]. In 54 cases a transfemoral arterial approach was used. In 12 cases a venous approach was utilized. A combined endovascular and surgical approach was performed in three cases.

In 47 cases (69%) the carotid cavernous fistula was occluded with preservation of the intracavernous internal carotid artery (Fig. 1). In 19 cases (29%) the fistula was occluded with concomitant obliteration of the internal carotid artery. In three cases an unusual spontaneous thrombosis of the traumatic fistula was seen. In eight patients (11%), postembolization angiography showed an intracavernous pseudoaneurysm due to early

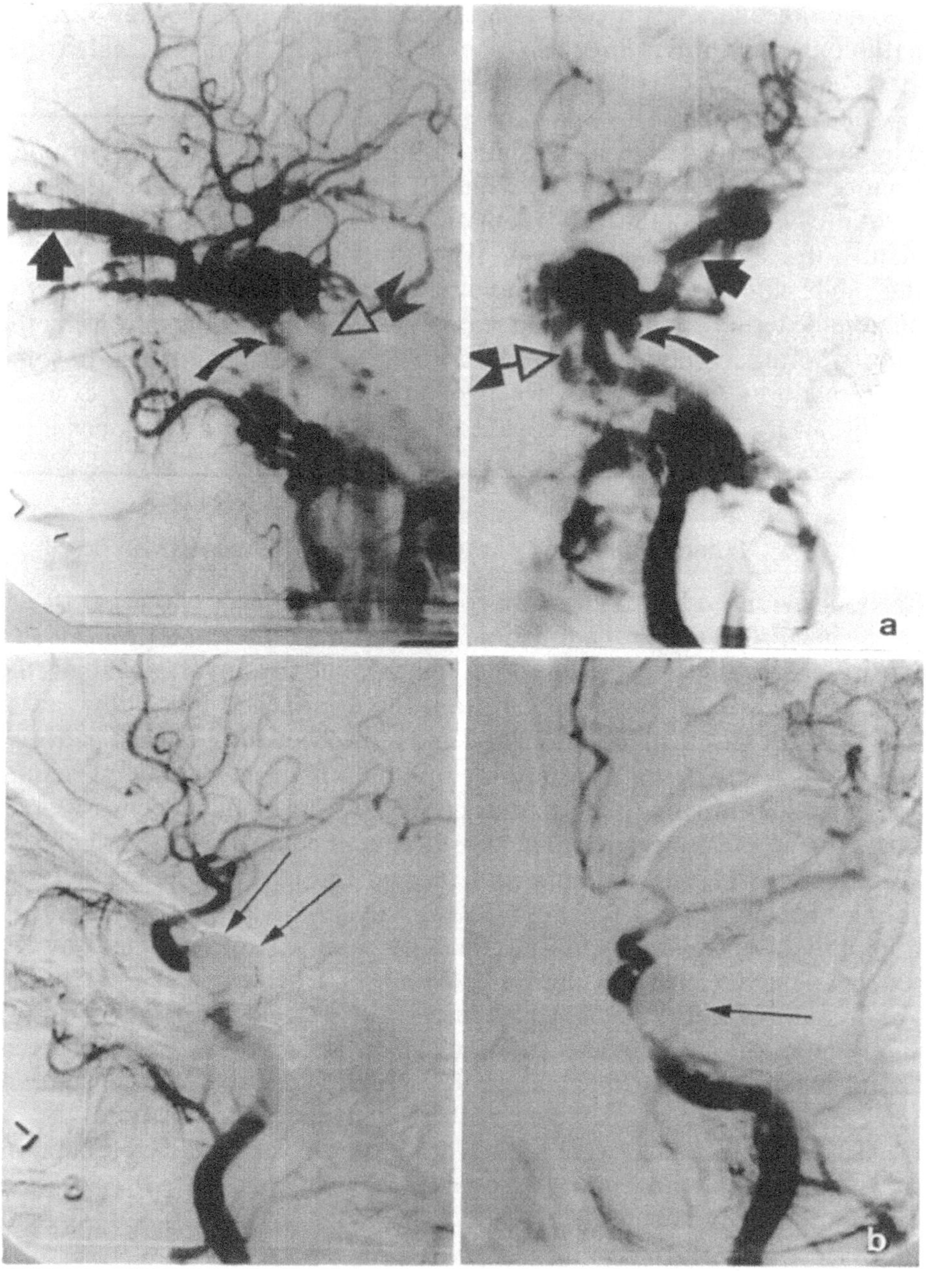

Fig. 1. a Lateral and AP views of left internal carotid angiogram demonstrates a large traumatic c-c fistula. The arterialized cavernous sinus drains through the superior ophthalmic vein (straight arrow), inferior petrosal sinus (open arrow), and sphenopalatine sinus (curved arrow). **b** Postembolization demonstrates two Debrun balloons in the cavernous sinus (straight arrows) occluding the c-c fistula. The lumen of the intracavernous internal carotid artery is preserved

deflation of the balloon (Fig. 2). Only three of these eight patients developed clinical evidence of a cavernous sinus syndrome due to a mass effect produced by the pseudoaneurysm. Balloon occlusion of the internal carotid artery was performed in these three cases with complete clinical recovery. Seven of 69 patients developed an immediate neurological deficit after balloon occlusion of the traumatic carotid cavernous fistulae. All had a full clinical recovery with the exception of one patient, who developed a hemiparesis 12 hours postembolization due to delayed internal carotid artery occlusion (Fig. 3). In one case, surgical exposure of the cavernous sinus and intraoperative balloon occlusion of the fistula and intracavernous carotid artery was performed.

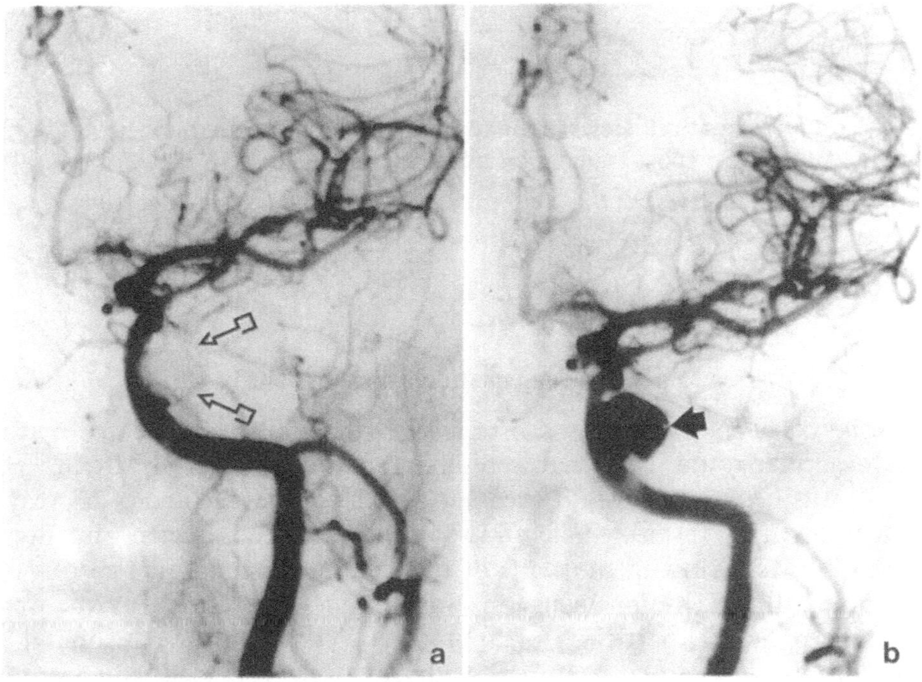

Fig. 2. a Case of traumatic c-c fistula. Immediate postembolization angiogram shows successful obliteration of the fistula by a single detachable balloon (square arrows). **b** Postembolization angiogram performed two months later demonstrates intracavernous pseudoaneurysm induced by early deflation of the balloon. The straight arrow shows the metallic clip located in the tip of the deflated balloon

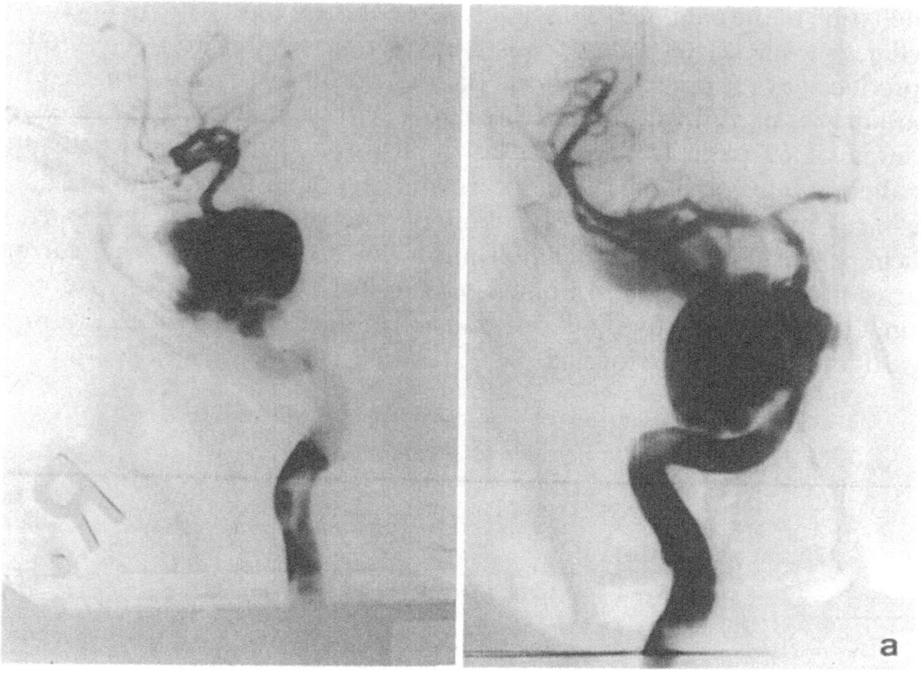

a

Fig. 3 a. Lateral and AP views of right internal carotid angiogram shows a large post-traumatic carotid cavernous fistula

Spontaneous carotid cavernous fistula

A total of 20 spontaneous c-c fistulas were diagnosed and treated by the endovascular route. Fourteen were unilateral and six were bilateral. Age range was between 22 and 83 years old with an average age of 63 years. Thirteen patients were female and seven were male. Eighteen cases were dural AVMs involving the walls of the cavernous sinus. In two cases a rupture intracavernous aneurysm was found. The dural AVMs were embolized with particles of polyvinyl-alcohol and/or isobutyl-2-cyanoacrylate. The two ruptured aneurysms were occluded with Debrun detachable balloons. In one case, the internal carotid artery lumen was preserved. In 14 out of 19 cases a satisfactory angiographic and/or clinical result was obtained (Fig. 4). Three patients developed immediate postembolization neurological deficit, two of them fully recovered. One patient had a long-term hemiparesis and aphasia produced by intracranial IBCA embolization through an external carotid-internal carotid anastomosis.

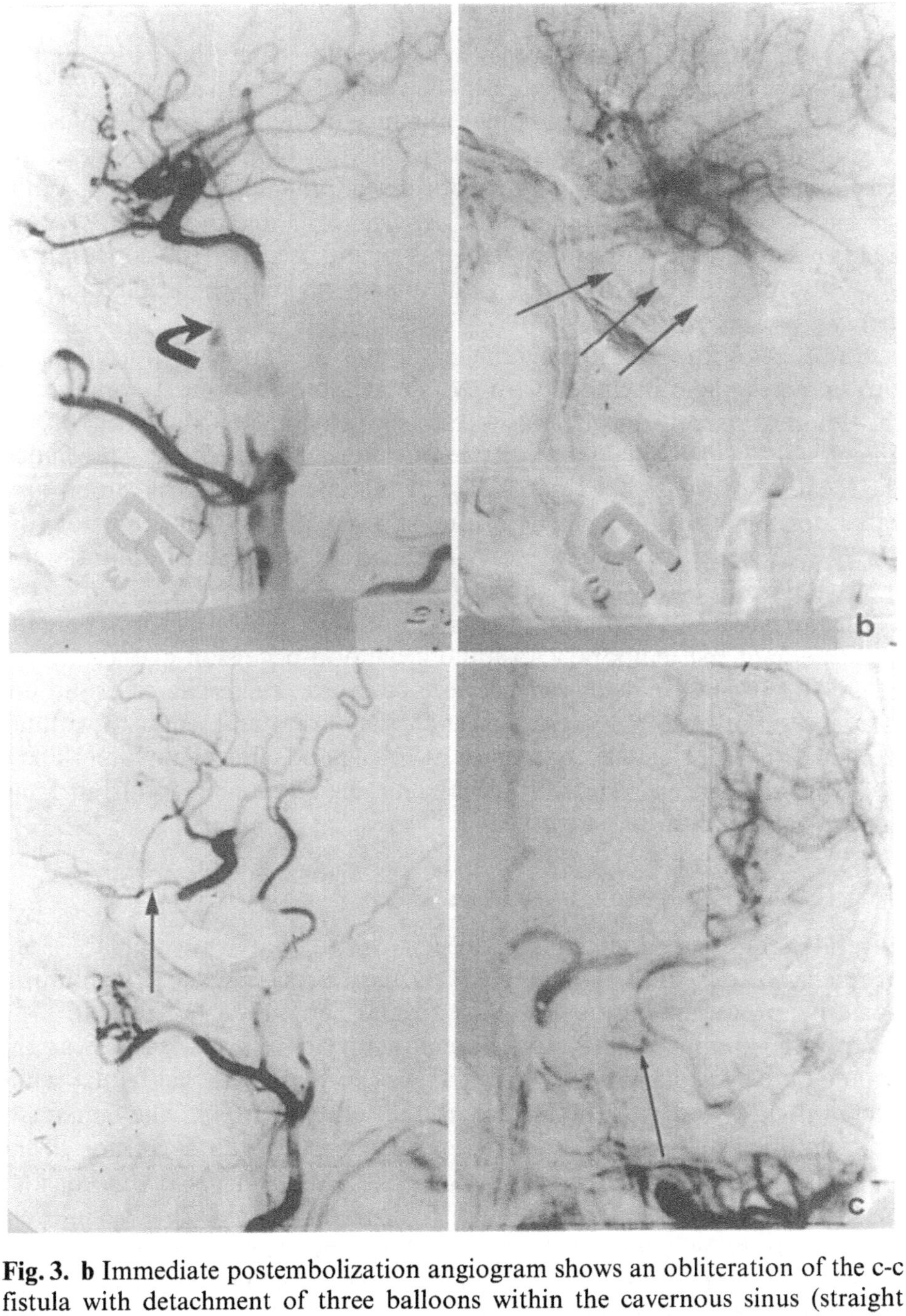

Fig. 3. b Immediate postembolization angiogram shows an obliteration of the c-c fistula with detachment of three balloons within the cavernous sinus (straight arrows). Note the stenosis of the proximal intracavernous carotid artery produced by the largest intracavernous balloon (curved arrow). **c** Left, carotid angiogram postdevelopment of hemiparesis and aphasia. The left internal carotid artery is now occluded and there is reconstitution of the supraclinoid carotid artery through external carotid-ophthalmic collaterals (straight arrows)

Intracavernous giant aneurysm

Forty intracavernous aneurysms were treated using the endovascular approach. The age range was from 15–83 years of age with an average age of 52. There was a strong female predominance (33 females and 7 males). A preembolization ECIC bypass was performed in 11 cases. This procedure was done in those cases showing a poor development of the circle of Willis on angiography and/or abnormal CBF Xenon Inhalation Study [6]. A Debrun detachable balloon system was again used for the concomitant occlusion of the intracavernous giant aneurysm and the internal carotid artery.

In 31 cases, the neck of the aneurysm and the intracavernous internal carotid artery were occluded with two detachable balloons. In nine cases, the internal carotid artery was occluded proximal to the neck of the aneurysm. The proximal tortuosity of the internal carotid artery precluded the location of the balloon at the site of the aneurysmal neck. In all nine cases, postembolization angiograms showed nonvisualization of the aneurysm from the ipsilateral external carotid circulation or contralateral internal carotid artery circulation (Fig. 5).

In two patients, a temporary ischemic event was observed. Both patients had tolerated the temporary 15 minute balloon occlusion of the internal carotid artery before detachment of the balloons. These two cases did not have preembolization bypass surgery. They were treated with volume expansion and antiplatelet aggregation with a good clinical outcome. These two episodes were presumably related to distal branch occlusion from emboli arising from the aneurysm.

Discussion

Several therapeutic procedures have been used to treat intravascular lesions of the cavernous sinus. They include surgical procedures and/or multiple occlusive procedures using the endovascular route [7, 8, 9, 10, 11].

In our experience, the most common intracavernous lesion was the traumatic c-c fistula (53%). Our goal was to obliterate the fistula while preserving the lumen of the intracavernous carotid artery. The fistula site was identified by vertebral arteriogram with concomitant occlusion of the ispilateral internal carotid artery in the neck [5] (Fig. 6). The fistula can also be identified using a double lumen balloon catheter [12]. The internal carotid artery is temporarily occluded in the neck with concomitant injection of contrast material distal to the occlusion. The contrast material so injected advances slowly until it meets the fistula site.

In 47 out of 69 cases one detachable balloon was sufficient to occlude the fistula. This is an ideal situation because a single balloon does not increase significantly the pressure within the cavernous sinus. When more than one balloon needs to be used, the sudden increase of the intracavernous pressure intensifies the cavernous sinus syndrome (Fig. 7). Cranial nerves III and VI were the most commonly involved. The detached balloons in the cavernous sinus were all filled with contrast material. They all had a slow but steady deflation in the following weeks with a decrease pressure within the cavernous sinus and substantial clinical recovery. We did not use either silicon or Hema because we did not want to produce a permanent mass effect within the cavernous sinus.

In selective cases with a dominant venous drainage through the inferior petrosal sinus, a venous approach was used [13]. A #16 balloon was then advanced retrogradely through the inferior petrosal vein into the posterior aspect of the cavernous sinus. The balloon was positioned as close as possible to the fistula site. The overall experience using this methodology indicates that it may be difficult to reach the fistula using this approach. The numerous partitions of the cavernous sinus often prevent the balloon getting closer to the fistula site. The selective catheterization of the inferior petrosal sinus may also be difficult because of the anatomical variations at the junction of the inferior petrosal sinus and internal jugular vein. We have not used the transvenous approach using the superior ophthalmic vein reported by Uflacken et al. [14].

Most traumatic carotid cavernous fistulas may be treated as elective cases. There are two situations in which an urgent therapy may be needed. One is the visualization of prominent arterialized draining veins in the subarachnoid space (Fig. 8). In this situation, those arterialized veins may produce an intracranial brain hematoma. The second indication of an emergency therapy is a progressive loss of vision due to venous hypertension within the orbit.

In our experience, the most frequent technical complications were: internal carotid artery occlusions (19 over 69 patients), and pseudo-aneurysm formation due to early deflation of the balloon (8 over 69). It is very important to try to preserve the internal carotid artery, if this artery is not severely damaged. The presence of marked irregularity of its walls or the visualization of an intimal flap on angiography may be an indication for internal carotid artery occlusion. The impact of a partially inflated balloon in an intimal flat produces a sudden retroorbital pain that disappears as soon as the balloon is withdrawn from the area. The balloon also hesitates to enter the fistula in the cavernous sinus. If the internal carotid artery is not severely damaged, the endovascular therapist should be reluctant to occlude it.

Direct surgical approach of the cavernous sinus with direct clipping of the fistula [7], thrombosis induced by electrical currents [15], introduction of thrombogenic wires [16], and direct injection of fibrant sealants [17] are methods that have been successfully used to preserve the lumen of the

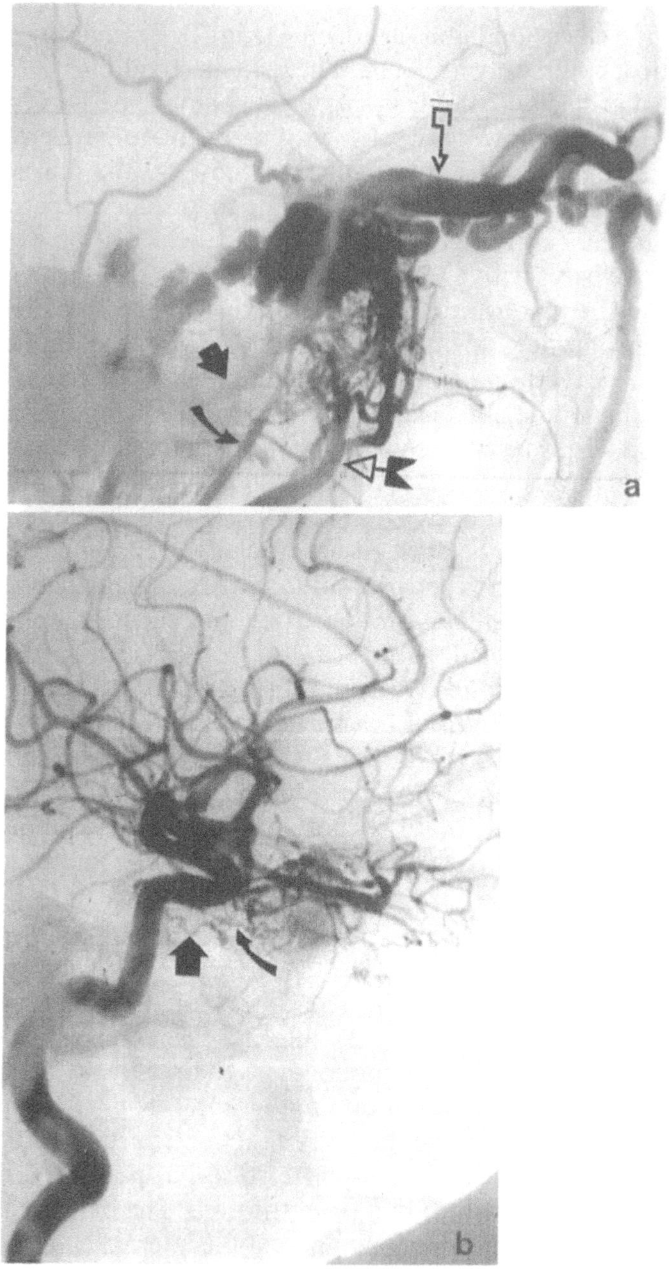

Fig. 4. a Lateral view of internal maxillary arteriogram demonstrates a retroorbital-anterior cavernous sinus dural AVM. The lesion is supplied by middle meningeal (straight arrow), accessory meningeal (curved arrow), and internal maxillary artery branches (open arrow). The venous drainage is mainly through the superior ophthalmic vein (square arrow). **b** Lateral view of internal carotid angiogram demonstrates blood supply to the dural AVM from meningo-hypophyseal trunk

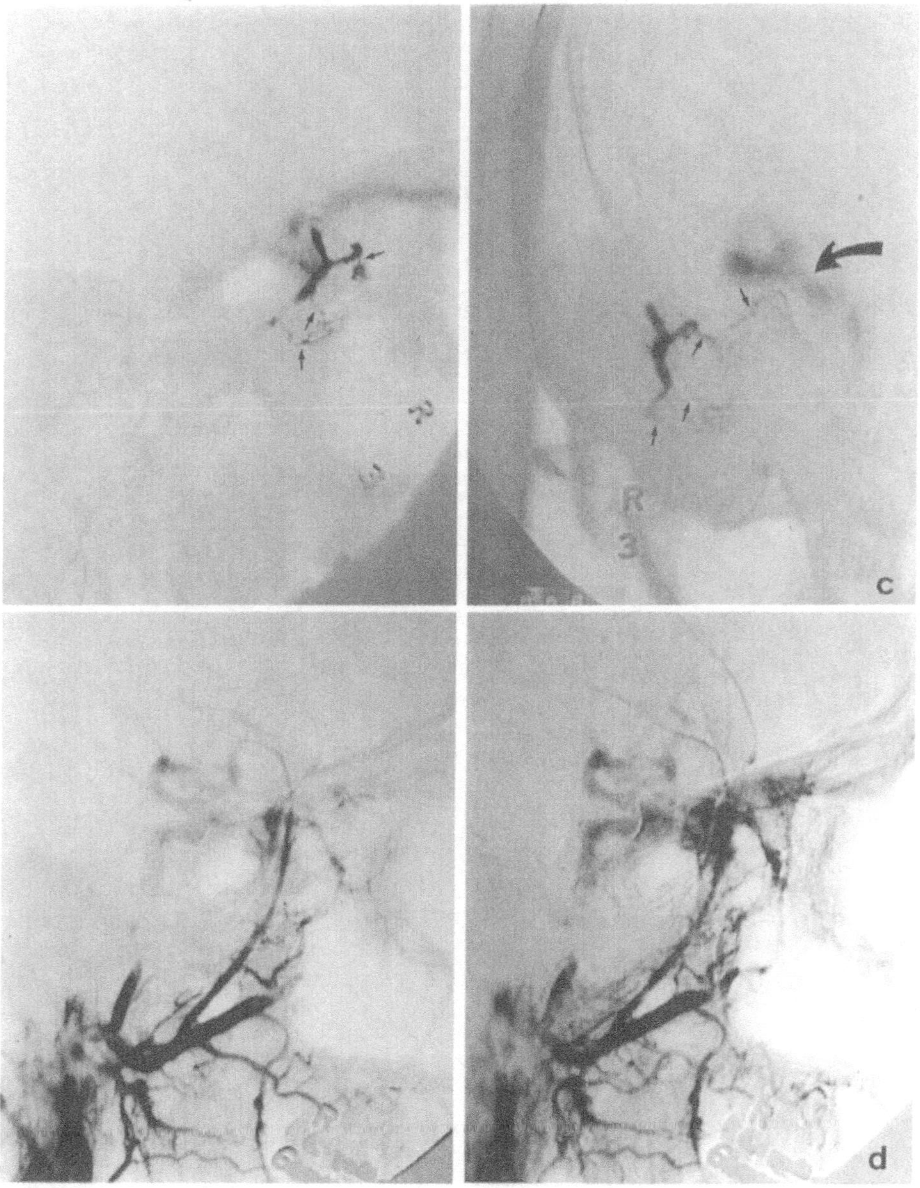

(straight arrow) and inferolateral trunk (curved arrow), branches of the intra-cavernous internal carotid artery. **c** Lateral and AP view of superselective middle meningeal angiogram demonstrating the arterial feeders (straight arrows) and draining veins (curved arrows). The AVM nidus is not well identified. **d** Postembolization internal maxillary arteriogram demonstrates marked reduction in the size of the AVM nidus and the arteriovenous shunting. The normal branches of the external carotid artery have been preserved

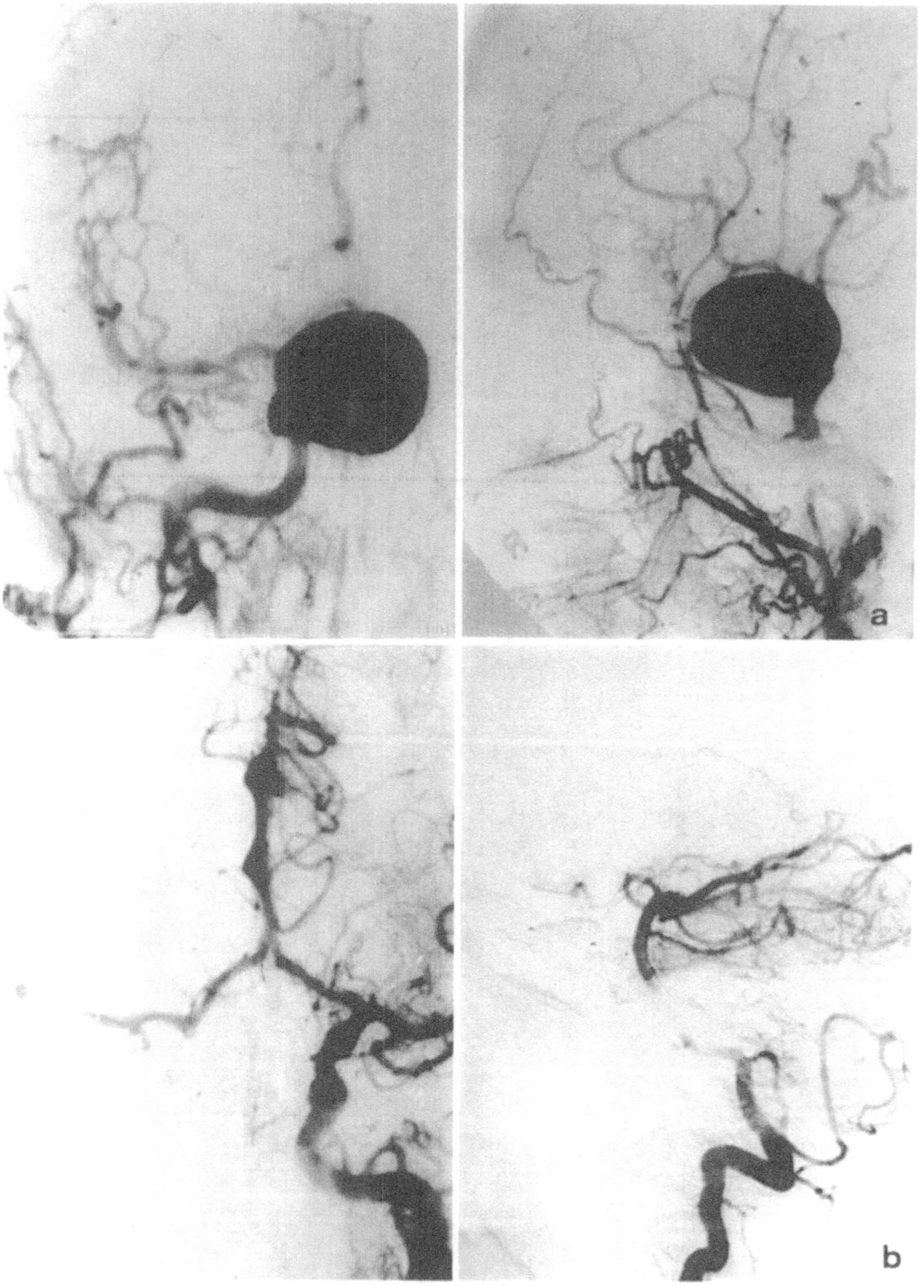

Fig. 5. a AP and lateral view of right, carotid angiogram demonstrates a giant intracavernous aneurysm. **b** Postembolization left carotid, and left vertebral angiograms demonstrate no retrograde filling of the giant intracavernous aneurysm after balloon occlusion of the right internal carotid artery in the region of the cavernous sinus

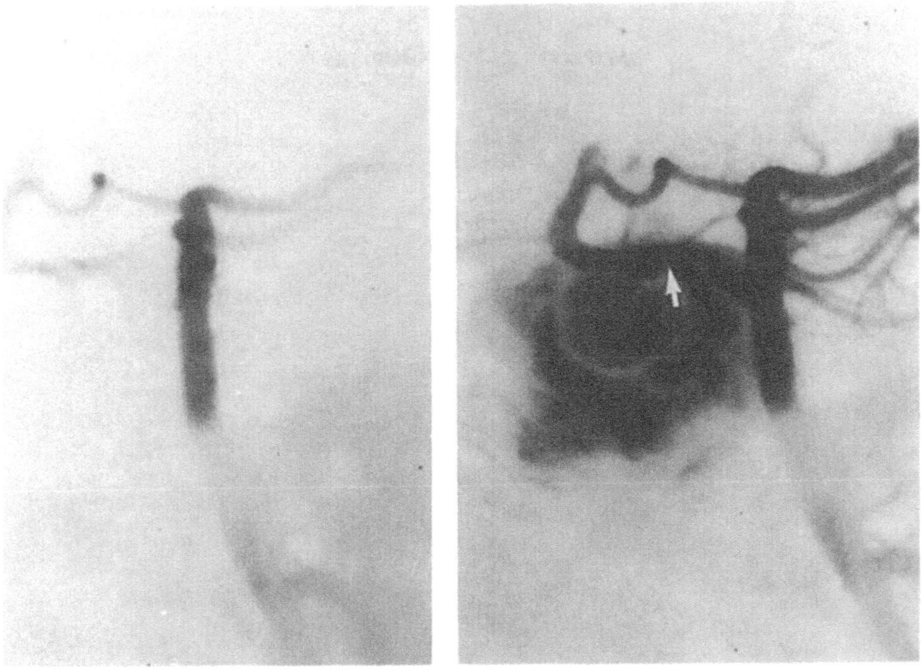

Fig. 6. Lateral view of vertebral angiogram with compression of the internal carotid artery in the neck demonstrates a retrograde filling of the intracavernous carotid artery and the site of the c-c fistula (straight arrow). The walls of the intracavernous internal carotid artery cannot be identified beyond this point

internal carotid artery. They are valuable alternatives to the endovascular balloon techniques, when this procedure fails to preserve the lumen of the internal carotid artery.

Three of the 69 cases with traumatic c-c fistula had spontaneous thrombosis of the fistula. This is an unusual outcome because most of these lesions show a high arteriovenous shunting. This phenomenon is probably related to progressive thrombosis of the cavernous sinus, a phenomenon which is not unusually observed in spontaneous c-c fistulas [18].

A dural AVM in the walls of the cavernous sinus was the most common etiology of spontaneous carotid cavernous fistula in our experience. Their treatment of choice, in contrast to traumatic fistulas, is the endovascular occlusion of the numerous dural feeders arising from the external carotid artery (ascending pharyngeal, middle meningeal, accessory meningeal and internal maxillary arteries) [19]. Endovascular embolization of the meningohypophyseal trunk, inferolateral trunk and branches of the internal carotid artery was not attempted.

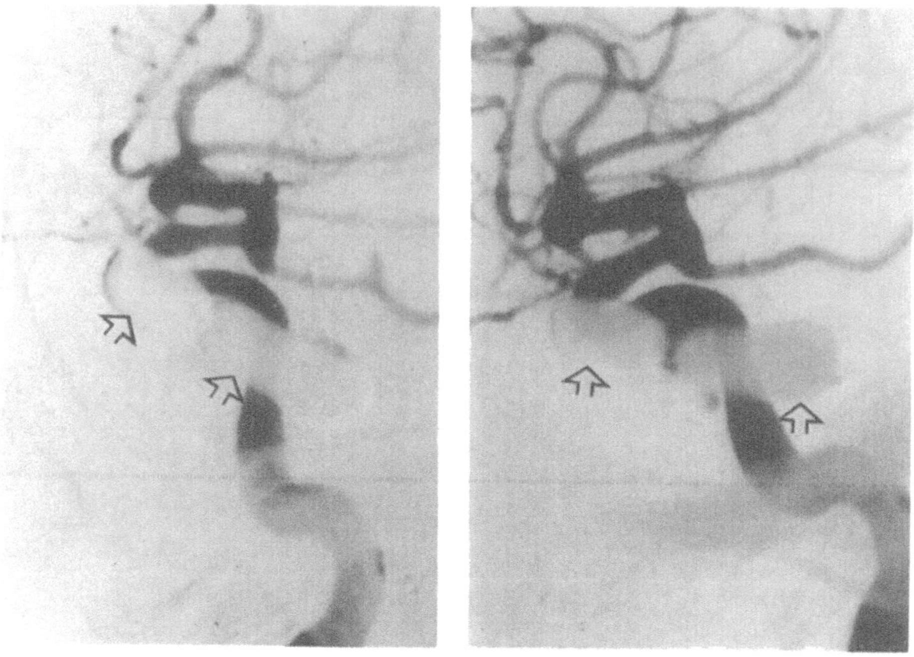

Fig. 7. Postembolization carotid angiogram shows satisfactory occlusion of the traumatic c-c fistula with detachment of two Debrun balloons in the cavernous sinus (straight arrows). This patient had worsening of the cavernous sinus syndrome for two months due to increased pressure produced by the inflated balloons

Barrow et al. [20] reported an anatomical-angiographic classification of carotid-cavernous fistulas. Type A is the most frequently observed in traumatic c-c fistulas. Types B, C and D are dural AVMs in the walls of the cavernous sinus and are related to the dominant blood supply from the external and internal carotid arteries. In our experience, type D (dual blood supply) is the most common. This type of blood supply makes the complete occlusion of the AVM by endovascular embolization very difficult. Partial embolization of these dural AVMs can be sufficient to promote substantial hemodynamic changes and marked clinical improvement [2]. In only one case of a dural AVM of the cavernous sinus, the internal carotid artery was occluded with a detachable balloon. The patient complained of progressive visual loss due to increased intraorbital pressure. The patient had a remarkable clinical recovery after the internal carotid artery occlusion. One patient developed a right hemiparesis and aphasia after superselective embolization of the artery of the foramen rotundum. Only 0.1 cm^3 of IBCA was injected into the feeder. The occlusion of the AVM diverted the IBCA into the intracranial circulation through the A-inferolateral trunk.

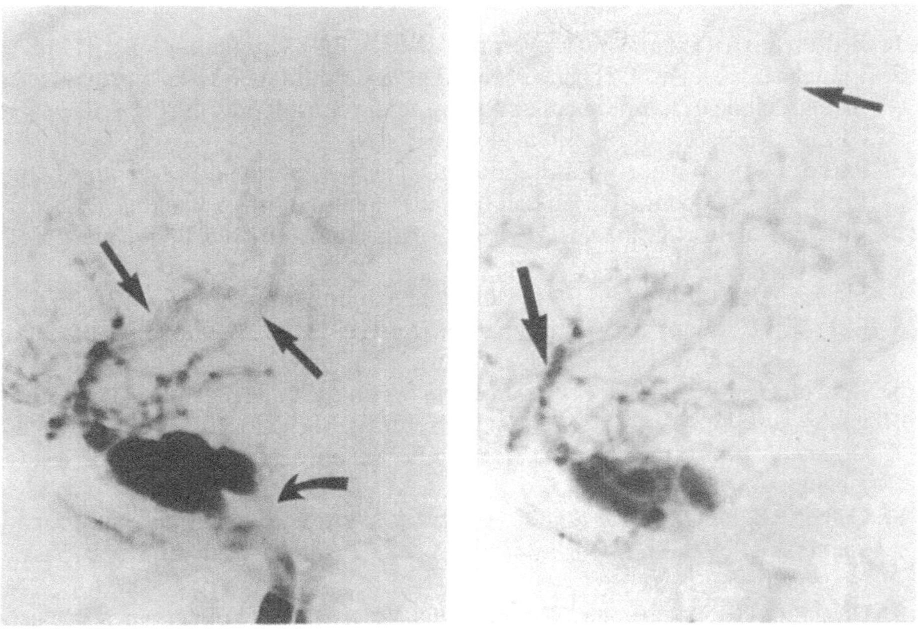

Fig. 8. Posttraumatic c-c fistula. Note retrograde filling prominent Sylvian and frontal cortical veins (straight arrows). Venous drainage through the inferior petrosal sinus is also noted (curved arrow). Emergency treatment of this fistula should be considered because of the possibility of intracranial hemorrhage from arterialized cortical veins

In selected cases of dural AVMs of the cavernous sinus, conservative therapy should be followed. It is well known that they may thrombose spontaneously [21]. In some cases, the symptoms are related to the progressive thrombosis of the cavernous sinus rather than to the arterio-venous shunting [18].

All giant aneurysms in these series were occluded with concomitant obliteration of the intracavernous internal carotid artery. This is a simple method and it has a low rate of morbimortality [22]. A satisfactory clinical result is then achieved, although this method involves the occlusion of a very important artery. Recent experience with detachable balloons have achieved occlusion of intracranial unclippable aneurysms with preservation of the parent vessels [23]. The internal carotid artery should be occluded if the aneurysm has a very wide neck and if the aneurysm cannot hold a balloon within its lumen. Dolenc et al. [7] have reported satisfactory results in preserving the internal carotid artery in small and middle size intra-cavernous aneurysms. Johnston has also reported successful direct surgical treatment of bilateral intracavernous internal carotid artery aneurysms [24].

References

1. Bedford MA (1966) The "cavernous sinus". Br J Ophthalmol 50: 41–45
2. Viñuela F, Fox AJ, Debrun GM et al (1984) Spontaneous carotid-cavernous fistulas: clinical, radiological and therapeutic considerations. Experience with 20 cases. J Neurosurg 60: 976–984
3. Parker L (1982) Neuro-ophthalmological aspects of carotid cavernous fistula. In: Smith R, Armin F, Russell W (eds) Seminars in neurological surgery. Vascular malformations and fistulas of the brain. Raven Press, New York, pp 181–198
4. Martin JD, Mabon RF (1943) Pulsating exophthalmos. JAMA 121: 330–334
5. Debrun G, Jacour P, Viñuela F, Fox AJ (1981) Treatment of 54 traumatic carotid-cavernous fistulas. J Neurosurg 55: 678–692
6. Debrun G, Fox AJ, Drake CG, Peerless SJ, Girvin J, Ferguson G (1981) Giant unclippable aneurysms: treatment with detachable balloons. AJNR 2: 167–173
7. Dolenc V (1983) Direct microsurgical repair of intracavernous vascular lesions. J Neurosurg 58: 824–831
8. Gelber RB, Sundt TM Jr (1980) Treatment of intracavernous and giant carotid aneurysms by combined internal carotid ligation and ECIC bypass. J Neurosurg 52: 1–10
9. Hieshima GB, Mehringer CM, Grinnell VS et al (1978) Emergency occlusive technics. Surg Neurol 9: 293–302
10. Isamat F, Ferrer E, Twose J (1986) Direct intracavernous obliteration of high-flow carotid cavernous fistulas. J Neurosurg 65: 770–775
11. Serbinenko FA (1974) Balloon catheterization and occlusion of major cerebral vessels. J Neurosurg 41: 125–145
12. Cares HL, Roberson GH, Grand W et al (1978) A safe technic for the precise location of carotid-cavernous fistula during balloon obliteration. Technical note. J Neurosurg 49: 146–149
13. Manelfe C, Berenstein A (1980) Treatment of carotid cavernous fistulas by venous approach. J Neuroradiol 7: 13–20
14. Uflaker R, Limas S, Ribas GC, Piske RL (1986) Carotid-cavernous fistulas: embolization through the superior ophthalmic vein approach. Radiology 159: 175–179
15. Hosobuchi Y (1975) Electrothrombosis of carotid-cavernous fistula. J Neurosurg 42: 76–85
16. Mullan S (1979) Treatment of carotid-cavernous fistulas by cavernous sinus occlusion. J Neurosurg 50: 131–144
17. Hasegawa H, Bitoh S, Obashi J (1985) Closure of carotid-cavernous fistulae by use of a fibrin adhesive system. Surg Neurol 24: 23–26
18. Seeger JF, Gabrielson TO, Giannotta SL et al (1980) Carotid cavernous sinus fistulas and venous thrombosis. AJNR 1: 171–178
19. Newton TH, Hoyt WF (1970) Dural arteriovenous shunts in the region of the cavernous sinus. Neuroradiology 1: 71–81
20. Barrow DL, Spector RH, Braun IF et al (1985) Classification and treatment of spontaneous carotid-cavernous sinus fistulas. J Neurosurg 62: 248–256
21. Voigt K, Saver M, Dichgans J (1971) Spontaneous occlusion of a bilateral

carotid-cavernous fistula studied by serial angiography. Neuroradiology 2: 207–211
22. Fox AJ, Viñuela F, Pelz DM, Peerless SJ, Ferguson G, Drake CG (1987) Use of detachable balloons for proximal artery occlusion in the treatment of unclippable aneurysms. J Neurosurg 66: 40–46
23. Hieshima GB, Higashida RT, Wapenski JW et al (1987) Intravascular balloon embolization of a large mid-basilar artery aneurysm. J Neurosurg 66: 124–127
24. Johnston I (1979) Direct surgical treatment of bilateral intracavernous internal carotid artery aneurysms. Case report. J Neurosurg 51: 98–102

The detachable balloon technique in the treatment of direct carotid-cavernous fistulas

A. J. M. van der Werf and F. L. M. Peeters

Departments of Neurosurgery and Diagnostic Radiology,
A.M.C., University of Amsterdam, Amsterdam, The Netherlands

This paper describes our [1, 9] further results in 26 patients treated for a direct carotid cavernous fistula.

It is follow-up to our previous communications where we described the results in our first 7 patients and 12 patients respectively.

The fistulas were occluded by intraarterial detachable balloon as described by Serbinenko and later modified by Debrun.

The aim of this treatment is to close the fistula, leaving carotid patency intact. We succeeded in this respect in 20 of our patients.

Introduction

Fistulas between the carotid artery and the cavernous sinus can be either direct communications between the intracavernous segment of the internal carotid artery and the cavernous sinus (direct fistulas) or communications between the internal or external carotid arteries or both and the cavernous sinus via meningeal vessels. The latter can be interpreted as arteriovenous malformations draining directly into the cavernous sinus, so-called dural fistulas. Direct fistulas usually develop as a result of a severe head injury, but can also be the result of the bursting of an intracavernous carotid aneurysm.

The classical clinical features are pulsating exophthalmus, chemosis, continuous murmur, arterialization of the orbital veins, headache, impaired eye movements.

Differentiation of the various type of cavernous sinus fistulas did not use to be essential for treatment by carotid ligation, which in fact, was the only treatment in the past.

However, in view of recently developed methods of treatment, determination of the kind of fistula and in direct fistulas the exact localization of the fistula is imperative. Fistulas between meningeal branches of the external carotid and the cavernous sinus can be closed by gel-foam embolization [2, 3]. Direct fistulas between the internal carotid and the cavernous sinus can be closed with the aid of one or several balloons [1, 4, 5]. As yet, there are no reports on closure of fistulas between meningeal branches of the internal carotid and the cavernous sinus by catheterization techniques. Closure of these fistulas is possible by deposition of a balloon at the site of origin of these meningeal branches or electrothrombosis [6]. This article describes our experiences in the treatment of direct carotid-cavernous fistulas using a detachable balloon catheter in 26 patients.

Material and methods

We treated direct carotid-cavernous fistulas in 26 patients, ranging in age from 16 to 76 years. In 21 patients the fistula was posttraumatic in origin, while in 5 patients the fistula developed spontaneously as a result of rupture of an intracavernous-carotid aneurysm (pat. 10, 14, 20, 23, 26). The balloon catheter (Ingenor, Paris, France) and the method used were largely those described by Debrun et al. [4) and were the same as described in our previous communications [1, 9].

As far as possible all patients underwent control carotid angiography one month and one year after closure of the fistula. In 8 patients the follow-up was not performed for the following reasons. The fifth patient died as a late sequela of his accident. The tenth, fourteenth, twentieth and twenty-third patient had no check-up after one year because of their age being 76, 73, 67 und 63 years respectively. The seventh, ninth and twenty-fourth patient refused the check-up angiography.

Results

In our first communication about our first seven patients we were able to mention a success rate of 100%, which means closure of the fistula with one or more balloons leaving the carotid artery involved patent. But this time we have to report some disappointments too. In 6 patients we did not achieve our goal. Tables 1 and 2 summarize the clinical data and results in this series of patients.

Let us discuss the 6 patients in whom we did not succeed in closing the fistula and preserving the patency of the carotid artery involved. In patient 2 it was impossible to close the fistula using a balloon with a maximum volume of 1 ml. Consequently two balloons were inserted. The contrast medium in the first balloon (0.4 ml) was not replaced by silicone so that, in accordance with the suggestion made by Debrun et al. [7], its deflation could be compensated for by shrinking of the cavernous sinus. This mechanism failed to develop in our patient.

The balloon's deflation led to development of a large pseudo-aneurysm that increased during the following year. To prevent the induction of retroorbital pain or oculomotor nerve palsy by this growing pouch, the carotid artery was occluded by ligation. The patient has now been free of symptoms for more than 3 years. In patient 8, in whom closure of the fistula required introduction of four balloons, the contrast medium in all balloons was replaced with silicone. Despite the enlargement of the cavernous sinus no dysfunction of the oculomotor nerve has developed. In this patient, however, the inflation of the last balloon with an excess of 0.1 ml silicone resulted not in carotid stenosis but in total occlusion. In patient 11 the balloon ruptured after filling with silicone well beneath capacity. The top of the balloon came off at the moment the catheter was pulled, entered the cerebral circulation and blocked one of the smaller branches of the gyri angularis artery, fortunately without any clinical symptoms. We decided to discontinue the procedure. Within the next 24 hours the clinical status deteriorated quickly resulting in progression of exophthalmus, papilledema and loss of vision. Most probably the rupture of the balloon had caused enormous widening of the fistula. An emergency Hamby procedure was carried out which resulted in complete recovery but meant ipso facto interruption of the flow in the internal carotid artery.

In patient 15 the cavernous sinus showed such a large cavity that it seemed impossible to fill this sinus with a limited number of balloons, therefore we decided at the beginning to occlude the internal carotid artery and the fistula by inflation of a balloon, positioned in the internal carotid artery at the origin of the fistula.

Patients 19 and 22 are the only patients in our series with a direct carotid cavernous fistula in whom we did not succeed in floating the balloon within the cavernous sinus. For a number of reasons, among which the most important was the mildness of subjective complaints we decided to wait for the moment in these cases and eventually to make a new attempt in the future in case of progression of the complaints.

Patient 18 developed a false aneurysm, despite the fact that we injected an excess volume of 0.1 ml silicone in the second balloon.

At the check-up angiography after one year the size of the false aneurysm was markedly reduced, but a carotid stenosis had developed.

The patient is free of symptoms. Perhaps the stenosis will progress until total closure in the future.

Table 1. Summary of cases

Patient no.	Age	Sex	Preexisting impaired nerve function	Nerve function 1 month post-closure	Nerve function 1 year post-closure
1	58	F	N III and VI	unchanged	unchanged
2	22	M	N III and VI	N VI unchanged N III healed	N VI unchanged
3	54	F	not impaired	not impaired	not impaired
4	30	M	N VII and VIII	N VII and VIII unchanged	N VII and VIII unchanged
5	29	M	comatous	comatous	died
6	47	F	not impaired	not impaired	not impaired
7	16	M	not impaired	not impaired	not impaired
8	28	M	N VII R + L	N VII R + L	improved
9	30	M	N III, IV and VI vision 1/10	N III, IV and VI improved vision 10/10	not improved
10	76	F	N VI vision 1/60	N VI unchanged vision 10/10	
11	25	M	not impaired	not impaired	not impaired
12	42	F	not impaired	not impaired	not impaired
13	19	M	vision 2/60	vision 1/3	not impaired
14	73	F	not impaired	not impaired	not impaired
15	28	M	N III and VI vision 0	unchanged	
16	40	F	N III and VI vision 1/300	N III and VI vision 1/10	improved vision 1/10
17	34	M	N VI vision 1/10	unchanged	not impaired vision 1/10
18	21	M	not impaired	N VI palsy	improved
19	73	F	vision 0		
20	67	M	N III R + L	N III L	not impaired
21	20	M	N III and VI vision 1/60	improved vision 5/10	not impaired
22	45	M	vision 1/60 hemiparesis		
23	63	F	N III and VI	much improved	normalized
24	31	M	N III, IV and VI R vision 1/60 VI L	improved	too early to say
25	20	F	N III, IV and VI R vision 1/300	eye movements improved vision 2/60	too early to say
26	60	F	N III, IV and VI R vision 2/60	too early to say	too early to say

Table 2. Results

Patient no.	Number of balloons	Results		Remarks
		at 1 month	at 1 year	
1	1	fistula closed small false aneurysm	unchanged	
2	2	fistula closed large false aneurysm	growing flase aneurysm	carotid ligation
3	1	fistula closed	unchanged	
4	1	fistula closed	unchanged	
5	1	fistula closed carotid stenosis	died	patient comatous since trauma
6	2	fistula closed	unchanged	
7	1	fistula closed	refuses check-up	patient asymptomatic
8	4	fistula closed carotid closed	unchanged	
9	1	fistula closed small false aneurysm	refuses check-up	patient asymptomatic
10	1	fistula closed	because of age no check-up	patient asymptomatic
11	—	—	—	emergency Hamby operation
12	1	fistula closed	unchanged	
13	1	minimal leak	fistula closed	
14	1	fistula closed	because of age no check-up	patient asymptomatic
15	2	fistula closed carotid closed		
16	1	fistula closed small false aneurysm	unchanged	
17	1	fistula closed	unchanged	
18	2	fistula closed large false aneurysm	false aneurysm reduced, carotid stenosis	
19	—	—	—	impossible to float ballon into fistula
20	1	fistula closed	because of age no check-up	patient asymptomatic
21	1	fistula closed	fistula closed	
22	—	—	—	impossible to float ballon into fistula
23	1	fistula closed	because of age no check-up	patient asymptomatic
24	2	refuses check-up		patient asymptomatic
25	1	fistula partially occluded	too early to say	
26	1	too early to say	too early to say	fistula closed at first attempt

Table 3. Comparison of results of endoarterial treatment

Author	Cases	Exclusion of fistula	Arterial axis		False aneurysm
			Patent	Nonpatent	
Debrun et al.	51	48	27	21	19
Scialfa et al.	19	18	16	3	14
Our series	26	23	20	3	4

Discussion

Since our previous publications [1, 9] a number of articles dealing with the detachable balloon technique in the treatment of direct carotid-cavernous fistulas have been published. The largest series described were those from Debrun et al. [7] and from Scialfa et al. [8]. They treated 51 and 19 patients respectively via an arterial approach with one or more detachable balloons. A summary of the results of these two series and of our own series is listed in Table 3. Comparing these results it is obvious that the number of false aneurysms in our series is rather small. A possible explanation for this could be the fact that we tried to prevent the development of a false aneurysm by the injection of 0.1 ml more silicone in the balloon than the amount of contrast medium required to close the fistula. This larger volume entails a risk of carotid stenosis, which proved to be transient in most of the patients. In the Debrun series the development of a large false aneurysm was the main reason for a secondary surgical closure of the internal carotid artery, which explains the relatively high frequency of the nonpatent arterial axis in his series. In our series the development of such a large false aneurysm also led us to ligate the internal carotid artery in the second patient.

As evidenced by comparison of these three larger series the endoarterial treatment with detachable balloons results in occlusion of the fistula and preservation of the patency of the carotid artery in 54–84%.

In none of the series was there an irreversible complication when the detachable balloon technique was successful.

In the Debrun series one patient developed a middle cerebral artery infarction after surgical intracranial ligation of the carotid artery. In the Scialfa series one patient died on an acute occlusion of the internal carotid artery caused by the impossibility of deflating the balloon during the procedure. This has to be considered as a technical failure.

As can be seen in our Table 1 in one patient (no. 18) a reversible abducens palsy developed after closure of the fistula. There were no other neurological complications in our series.

To estimate the risk for the patient before treatment it seems worthwhile to test the collateral capacity from the healthy carotid artery by EEG registration during compression of the carotid artery on the side of the fistula.

In conclusion we maintain the statement of our previous publications [1, 9] that in the treatment of direct carotid-cavernous sinus fistulas the detachable balloon technic has to be preferred to other more conventional methods.

References

1. Peeters FLM, Werf AJM van der (1980) Detachable balloon technique in the treatment of direct carotid-cavernous fistulas. Surg Neurol 14: 11
2. Gilsbach J, Seeger W (1977) Embolisation in der Neurochirurgie. Radiologe 17: 514
3. Peeters FLM (1982) Vascular malformations as the cause of unilateral exophthalmus. Diagnostic and therapeutic considerations. Diagn Imag Clin Med 51: 1–7
4. Debrun G, Lacour P, Caron JP (1977) Balloon arterial catheter techniques in the treatment of arterial intracranial diseases. In: Krayenbühl H et al (eds) Advances and technical standards in neurosurgery. Springer, Wien New York, pp 131–145
5. Benati A, Maschio A, Perini S, Beltramello A (1980) Treatment of posttraumatic carotid-cavernous fistula using a detachable balloon catheter. J Neurosurg 53: 784
6. Ishikawa M, Handa H, Taki W, Yoneda S (1982) Management of spontaneous carotid-cavernous fistulas. Surg Neurol 18: 131
7. Debrun G, Lacour P, Viñuela F, Fox A, Drake CG, Caron JP (1981) Treatment of 54 traumatic carotid-cavernous fistulas. J Neurosurg 55: 678
8. Scialfa G, Vaghi A, Valsecchi F, Bernardi L, Tonon C (1982) Neuroradiological treatment of carotid and vertebral fistulas and intracavernous aneurysms. Technique problems and results. Neuroradiology 24: 13
9. Werf AJM van der, Peeters FLM (1982) Preliminary observations of balloon occlusion technique in carotid cavernous fistulas. In: Smith RR, Haerer A, Russel WF (eds) Seminars in neurological surgery. Vascular malformations and fistulas of the brain. Raven Press, New York, pp 231–239

Criteria for the differentiation of high-, moderate-, and low-flow carotid-cavernous sinus fistulas and their treatment with balloon catheters

F. Brassel, J. Wappenschmidt, and L. Solymosi

Department of Neuroradiology, University Hospital of Neurosurgery, Bonn, Federal Republic of Germany

It is well-known that carotid-cavernous sinus fistulas (CCSF) may influence the entire cerebrovascular circulation [1, 2, 4, 6, 7, 8, 9, 12]. We therefore wanted to know what information can be derived from angiographic data. The most important factor which influences the hemodynamics and the course of the disease is the size of the fistula. It determines not only the shunt volume, but also the increase in intracavernous sinus pressure, implicating a considerable interference in cerebrovenous drainage. In addition, the size of the fistula's opening influences the internal carotid artery (ICA) pressure distal to the lesion. Significant changes in the arterial blood supply may result.

Angiographically we are able to demonstrate three types of CCSFs: small, moderate and large fistulas.

A small fistula (Fig. 1) shows no decrease in arterial pressure distal to the lesion. All branches of the ICA are filled orthogradely. There is, however, a minimal increase in the intracavernous sinus pressure. The shunted blood is mainly drained by the superior opththalmic vein (SOV).

In moderate-sized fistulas (Fig. 2), there is a small decrease in arterial pressure distal to the fistula's opening. Nevertheless, the pressure is adequate for the maintenance of an orthograde circulation. However, compared to that of the contralateral supraclinoid carotid, the pressure is relatively low. Anterior and posterior portions of the circle of Willis may contribute blood to the affected supraclinoid carotid. The fistula thus causes a steal syndrome.

In the case of large fistulas (Fig. 3), the entire blood flow is directed through the fistula's opening into the cavernous sinus. The ispilateral supraclinoid ICA is filled retrogradely, additionally feeding the fistula. Because of the enormous increase in intracavernous sinus pressure, all veins passing into the cavernous sinus are involved in draining the shunted blood. There is no orthograde filling of the ipsilateral ICA. The dilated sinus is as a tumor on surrounding structures.

Drainage pathways are by:

1. the superior petrosal sinus into the sigmoid sinus;
2. the enlarged superior and inferior ophthalmic vein through anastomotic veins into the angular vein;
3. the basal vein of Rosenthal into the great vein of Galen and the straight sinus.

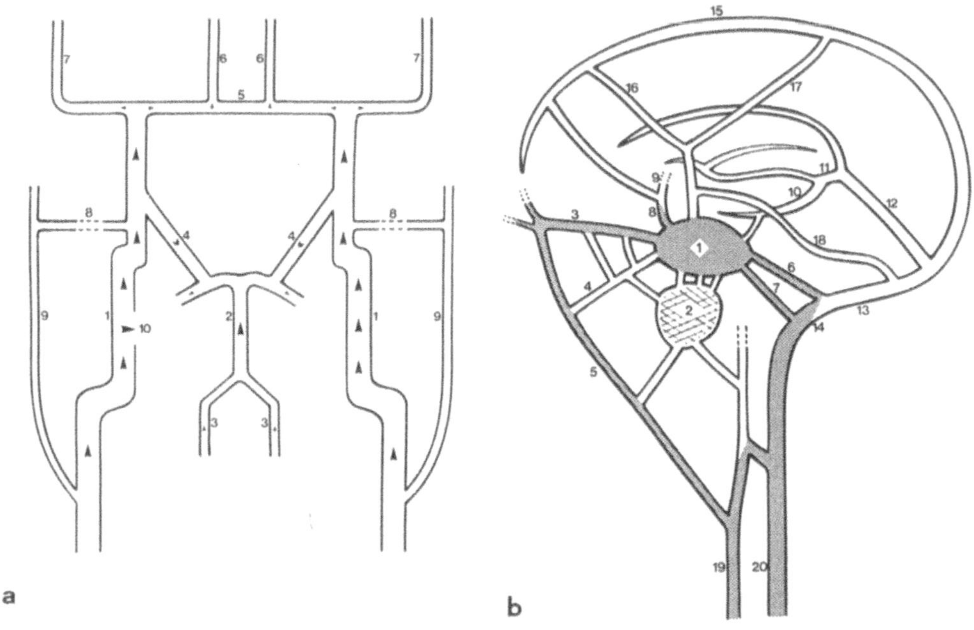

Fig. 1. Circulation of low-flow CCSF. **a** Arterial system in CCSF: *1* Internal carotid artery; *2* basilar artery; *3* vertebral artery; *4* posterior communicating artery; *5* anterior communicating artery; *6* anterior cerebral artery; *7* middle cerebral artery; *8* anastomosis of the internal carotid and the external carotid artery via the ophthalmic artery; *9* facial artery; *10* CCSFs opening. **b** Venous system: *1* Cavernous sinus; *2* pterygoid plexus; *3* superior opththalmic vein; *4* inferior ophthalmic vein; *5* facial vein; *6* superior petrosal sinus; *7* inferior petrosal sinus; *8* sphenoparietal sinus; *9* superficial middle cerebral vein; *10* basal vein of Rosenthal; *11* great vein of Galen; *12* straight sinus; *13* transverse sinus; *14* sigmoid sinus; *15* superior sagittal sinus; *16, 17* superior cerebral veins; *18* inferior anastomotic vein; *19* external jugular vein; *20* internal jugular vein

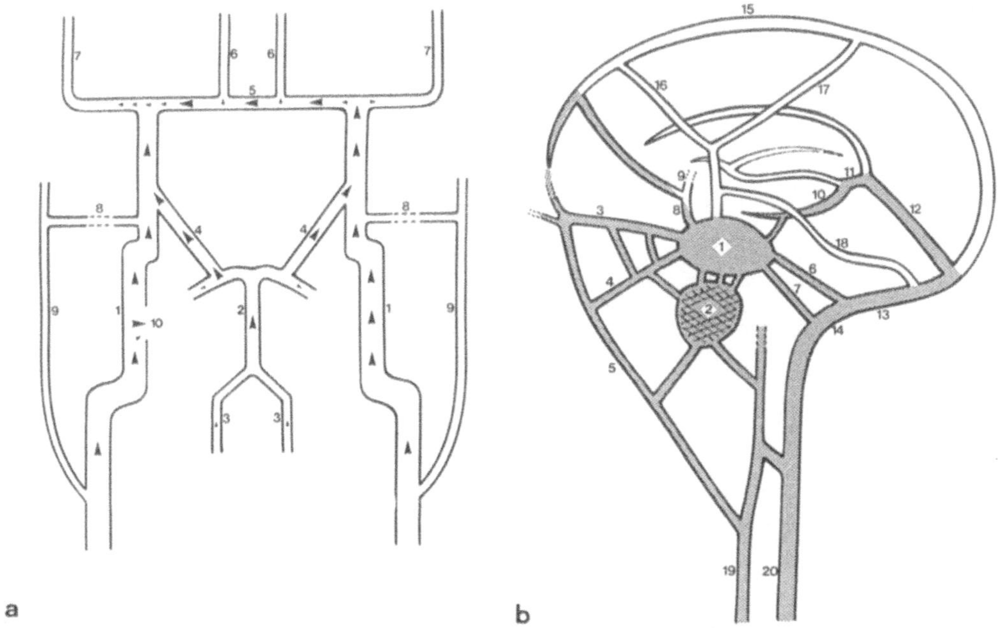

Fig. 2. Circulation of moderate-flow CCSF. Key to the schemes in legend of Fig. 1

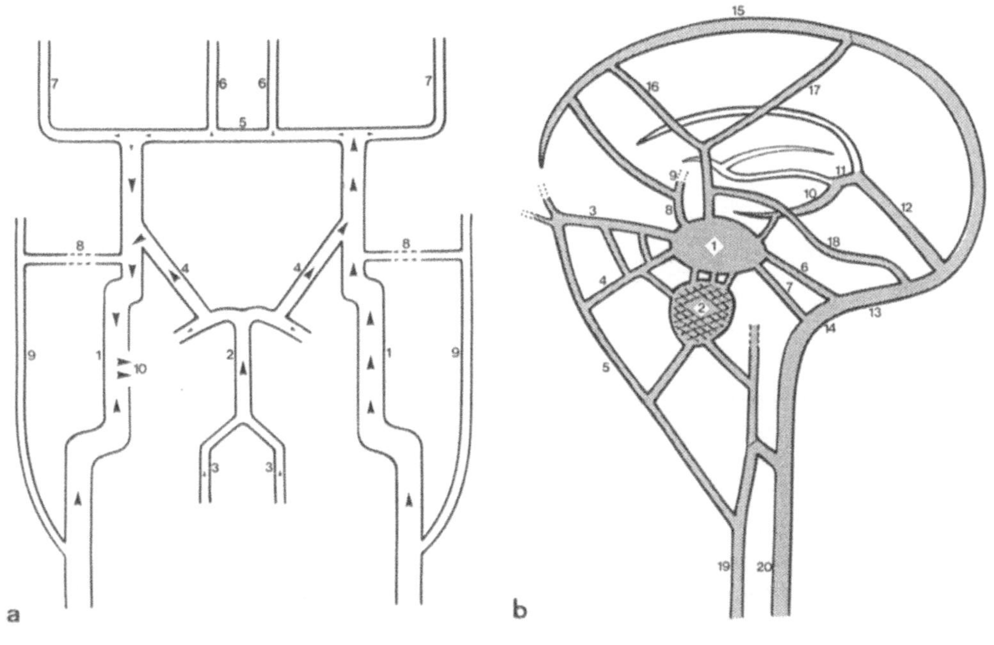

Fig. 3. Circulation of high-flow CCSF. Key to the schemes in legend of Fig. 1

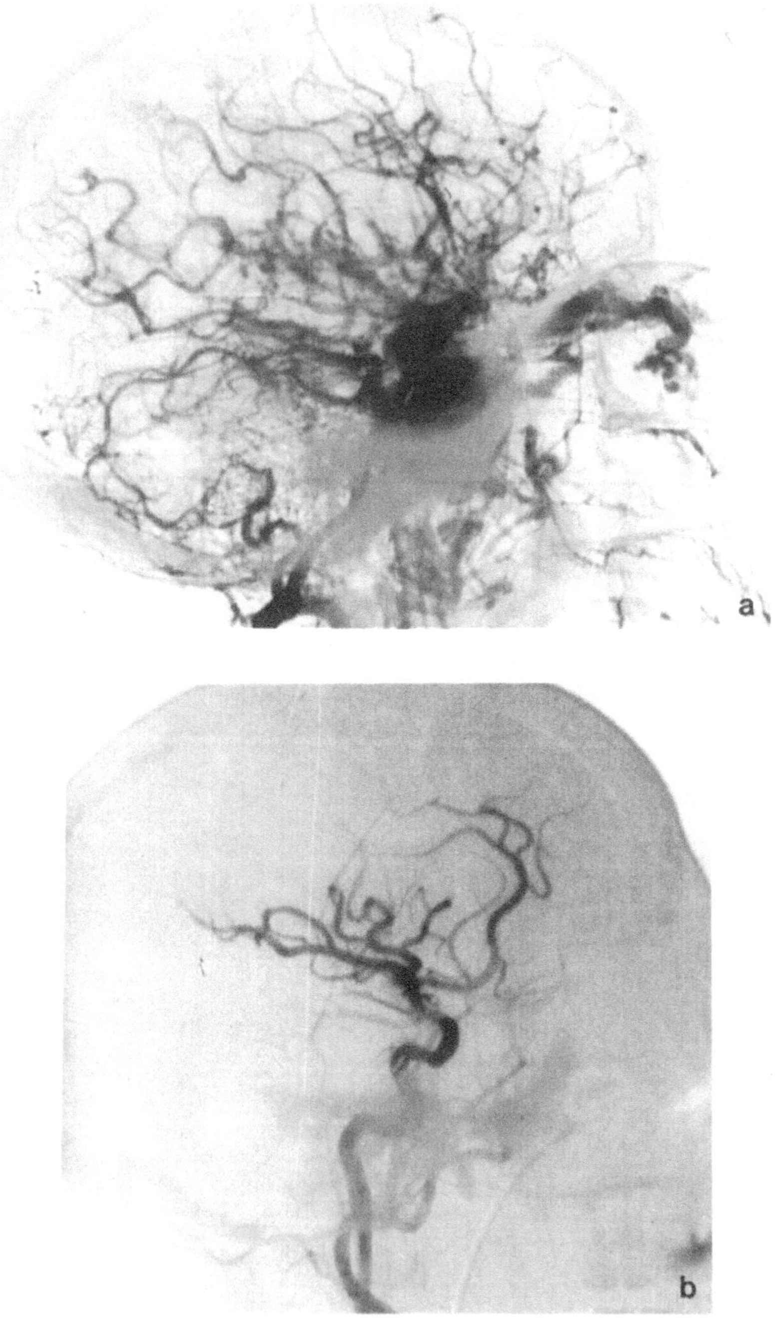

Fig. 4. Moderate-flow CCSF **a** before and **b** after embolization with a DBC

In addition, one also notices a reversal of blood flow within the sphenoparietal sinus. The veins draining the Sylvian fissure are filled retrogradely due to a high pressure. The arterial blood in the Sylvian veins drains through frontal cortical veins, the Rolandic vein and the vein of Trollard into the superior longitudinal sinus. Blood may also pass through the vein of Labbé into the transverse sinus. Thus the increased intravascular pressure may cause even small cerebellar veins to become angiographically visible.

This picture clearly shows the limit of the venous draining capacity of the brain. In the long run this may lead to vascular wall damage, venous insufficiency and congestive edema.

From our angiographic data we can say that large fistulas need to be treated because they seriously disturb the circulation. Considering hemodynamics, it is not absolutely necessary to treat moderate sized fistulas. In the case of small fistulas a spontaneous cure may take place after angiography or an attempt at balloon embolization. In one particular case of the latter a small fistula occluded after a micro-detachable balloon had been positioned in the infundibulum of the fistula for fifteen minutes.

Our experience and results have been derived from 24 cases since 1966. We elaborated nine small, thirteen moderate and two large CCSFs. Up to 1978 eleven CCSFs had been treated with muscle emboli, Fogarty catheters and ligation of the carotid in the neck. After 1978 we used detachable balloon catheters (DBC) [2, 3, 4, 5, 9, 10, 11] in thirteen cases, with preservation of the ICA in six cases, as can be seen in the following example (Fig. 4).

References

1. Barrow DL, Spector RH, Braun IF, Landmann JA, Tindall SC, Tindall GT (1985) Classification and treatment of spontaneous carotid-cavernous sinus fistulas. J Neurosurg 62: 248–256
2. Berenstein A, Kricheff II (1979) Balloon catheters for investigation carotid cavernous fistulas. Radiology 132: 762–764
3. Berenstein A, Kricheff II, Ransohoff J (1980) Carotid cavernous fistulas: intraarterial treatment. AJNR 1: 449–457
4. Brassel F (1983) Hämodynamik und Therapie des Karotis-Kavernosus-Fistel. Dissertation, Bonn, pp 1–89
5. Debrun G, Lacour P, Caron JP, Hurth M, Comoy J, Keravel Y, Loisance D (1976) Technique du ballon gonflable et largable en neurologie. Rev Neurol 132: 23–31
6. Djindjian R, Picard L, Manelfe C (1973) Fistulea artérioveineuses carotide interne-sinus caverneux. Neurochirurgie 19: 75–90

7. Grote W, Schiefer W (1959) Klinik und Behandlung der traumatischen arteriovenösen Aneurysmen. Beitr Neurochir 1: 79–88
8. Huber P (1976) A technical contribution to the exact angiographic localization of carotid-cavernous fistulas. Neuroradiology 10: 239–241
9. Rey A, Cophignon J, Thurel C, Thiebaut JB (1975) Treatment of traumatic cavernous fistulas. In: Krayenbühl H et al (eds) Advances and technical standards in neurosurgery, vol 2. Springer, Wien New York, pp 87–109
10. Serbinenko FA (1974) Balloon catheterization and occlusion of major cerebral vessels. J Neurosurg 41: 125–145
11. White RI, Kaufmann RI, Barth KH, Decaprio V, Strandberg JD (1979) Embolotherapy with detachable silicone balloons. Radiology 131: 619–627
12. Wolff H, Schmidt B (1939) Das Arteriogramm des pulsierenden Exophthalmus. Zentralbl Neurochir 4: 241–250

Closure of carotid-cavernous fistulas by intracavernous surgical insertion of biological materials

F. Isamat

Service of Neurosurgery, Hospital de Bellvitge Princeps d'Espana, University of Barcelona, Barcelona, Spain

Carotid-cavernous fistulas (CCFs) have traditionally been classified into traumatic and spontaneous. Nonetheless the most important implications of a CCF are those related to the anatomical and hemodynamic characteristics of the fistula. Parkinson [21, 22, 23] and, particularly, Barrow et al. [1, 2], have proposed a classification based on these aspects. CCFs belonging to Parkinson's type I or Barrow's type A are direct communications between the internal carotid artery (ICA) and the venous plexus of the cavernous sinus. They are high-pressure high-flow shunts due to a tear in the wall of the intracavernous part of the ICA and are usually of traumatic origin. The clinical manifestations are generally abrupt and severe. They may consist in exophthalmus, chemosis, extraocular palsies, headaches, trigeminal dysesthesias, visual loss and the hearing of a disturbing bruit synchronous with the pulse. Massive epistaxis, although uncommon, can be fatal.

Indications for treatment of high-flow CCFs should be contemplated in the majority of cases since spontaneous resolution is extremely rare. Mandatory indications are intracranial hemorrhage, massive epistaxis, visual deterioration either secondary to the reduction of ocular arterial perfusion or to intraocular venous hypertension and glaucoma, and the neurological deficits due to a steal syndrome of arterial blood from the brain. Nonabsolute indications depend on the severity of the symptoms and they include intolerance of the bruit, the restoration of the orbital contents, the reestablishment of oculomotor functions, the intensity of the headaches and the achievement of a good cosmetic result.

If treatment of a high-flow CCF is indicated this should consist in the obliteration of the fistulous rent while preserving the ICA flow to avoid cerebral ischemia. A selective and complete angiographic study of the internal and external carotid arteries and the vertebral arteries hould be performed to establish the most appropriate treatment, since the definition of a high-flow high-pressure CCF is an angiographic assessment.

Parkinson [21] has shown that it is possible to open the lateral wall of the cavernous sinus and to remain outside the intracavernous arterial and venous components. He described the cavernous sinus as a plexus of veins that incompletely surrounds the ICA, with bare spaces between the artery and the veins.

He concluded that a CCF is a direct pathological connection between the artery and one of the veins in a true Hunterian way, as in arteriovenous shunts of the rest of the body. Therefore he was able to operate on CCFs by opening the cavernous sinus and occluding the fistulous tract without interfering either with the artery or the veins. In this type of high-flow arteriovenous CCFs the arterialized venous blood will leave the cavernous sinus through their distended anatomical exits, particularly via the ophthalmic veins. This originates the well known radiological and clinical pictures of this disorder.

As intracavernous posttraumatic false aneurysm, on the other hand, is a CCF in which the ICA rent flows directly into one of the bare perivascular spaces within the sinus. Radiologically this is shown as a direct ICA rent flowing into a distended cavernous sinus with sparse, if any, venous clearance. This can be present either isolated or in combination with an arteriovenous shunt.

The introduction by Serbinenko [28] of detachable balloon-catheters had changed the treatment of high-flow CCFs. Debrun et al. [7, 8] have obtained total obstruction of CCFs treated with detachable balloons in over 90% of their cases. However, they could not preserve the ICA flow in 41% of the patients. Other published series have similar or even greater morbidity. The appearance of intracavernous pseudoaneurysms following later balloon deflation has been not infrequently observed. Although at present the treatment of choice for a high-flow CCF seems to be the endovascular detachable balloon technique, this is not free of important risks.

Fibrin sealant (Tissucol®, Tisseel®*) consists primarily of fibrinogen and factor XIII with a fibrinolysis inhibitor that in contact with a solution containing thrombin and calcium chloride causes fibrinogen to transform into fibrin, similar to the physiological coagulation process. Rapid solidification takes place in a few seconds after mixing equal volumes of the two components. The intraluminal injection of fibrin sealant has been effective in the occlusion, by thrombosis and later sclerosis, of experimentally created aneurysms, as shown by Moringlane [18].

---

* Tissucol or Tisseel manufactured by Immuno AG, Barcelona, Spain.

Direct muscle plugging of the cavernous sinus with sparing of the ICA flow has been successfully used by Lapras et al. [17] in two patients. None the less the surgical opening of the lateral wall of the cavernous sinus without controlling the hemodynamic conditions leads to a jet of arterialized blood that does not make the introduction of muscle material easy. At the same time it is necessary to suture the lateral wall of the cavernous sinus after the plugging and this can be awkward.

Accordingly a surgical technique to directly obliterate the CCF using biological materials such as muscle and fibrin glue has been developed in my Service and used in a group of patients with high-flow CCFs. The intrasinusal application of this biological fibrin glue will add fast thrombogenic induction as well as support to the fragments of muscle introduced into the cavernous sinus.

Surgical technique

All the patients have been operated on under general anesthesia without hypotension or hypothermia. In addition to the routine intraoperative monitoring a Doppler ultrasound transducer is fixed extracranially to record the bruit. The ICA is first isolated in the neck and surrounded by an elastic band to allow later temporary occlusion. This is followed by a standard pterional craniotomy. The cavernous sinus is exposed by opening the Sylvian fissure and gently elevating the temporal and frontal lobes. The supraclinoid ICA and the free margin of the tentorium are exposed and dissected until identification of the entrance of the cranial nerves III and IV into the cavernous sinus, as described by Parkinson. Due to the distension of the cavernous sinus by the fistulous rent Parkinson's triangular area, formed by cranial nerves III and IV running together within the dural roof of the cavernous sinus towards the superior orbital fissure and the ophthalmic division of cranial nerve V in the inferior lateral dural wall, is spread widely particularly at its posterior base. Therefore it is safe to open the cavernous sinus without injuring these nerves if the incision is done parallel with and beneath the point of entry of the nerve III, as has been shown by Parkinson and others.

At this stage a temporary clip is placed at the supraclinoid ICA proximal to the posterior communicating artery and the cervical ICA is occluded with elastic band. A 10 mm incision is then made in the lateral wall of the cavernous sinus and small elongated and crushed muscular fragments from the temporal muscle are introduced into the sinus. This is done until there is resistance to further introduction and no Doppler signals are received following the removal of the transient ICA occlusions. Prior to the definite withdrawal of the temporal trapping fibrin sealant is injected intracavernously and also spread over the dural incision for a sutureless closure.

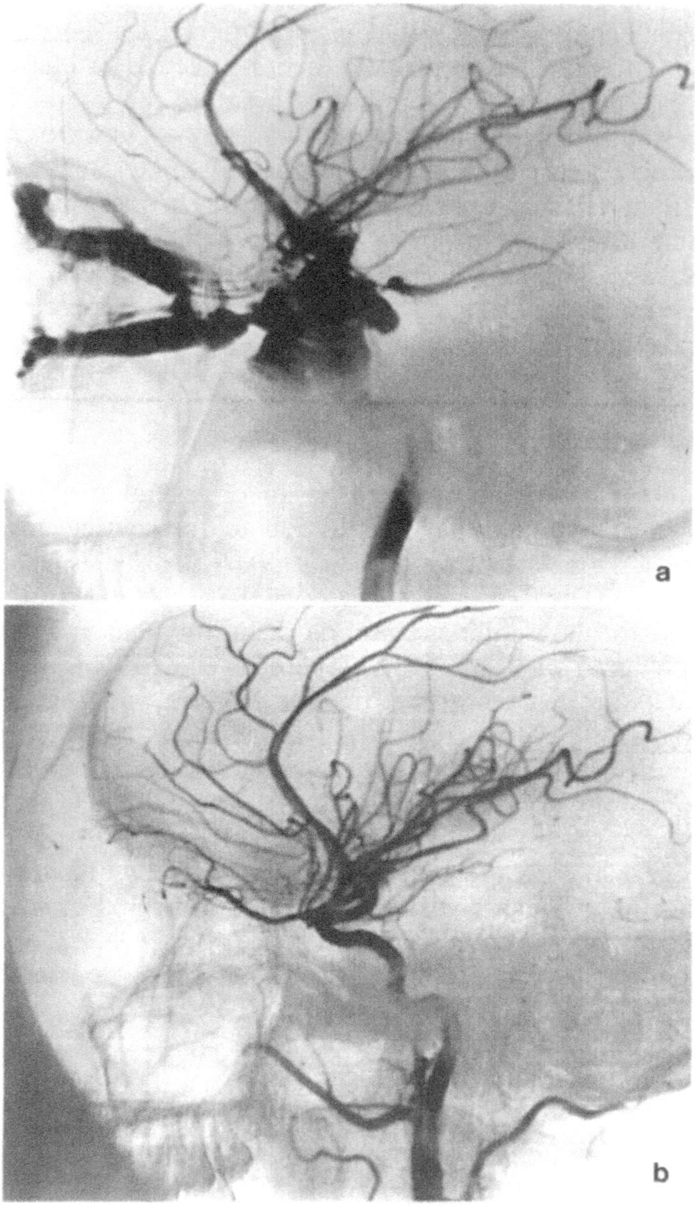

Fig. 1. a CCF of case 1; **b** Postoperative angiography showing the obliteration of the CCF with preservation of the ICA flow

Surgical examples

Case 1

A 32-year-old man was involved in a traffic accident on May 20, 1982. He was admitted to the hospital with severe head and thoracic injuries (Glasgow coma scale score of 4). X-rays of the skull showed large left frontobasal and orbital fractures. Treated conservatively, his neurological condition slowly improved and he was transferred to the Neurosurgical Ward one month after the accident. At that time the patient was completely disoriented and had a left peripheral facial paralysis and a partial left ophthalmoplegia.

Two months after admission he developed left exophthalmus with chemosis, the ophthalmoplegia became complete, and a bruit was noted on the left frontoorbital region. A four vessels angiography demonstrated a left high flow CCF, which was only filled through the left (Fig. 1 a).

On the following week he was operated on by exposing intracranially the left cavernous sinus, which was opened and plugged with small pieces of muscles and Tissucol injected. Surgery resulted in the immediate disappearance of the bruit and in a progressive reduction of the exophthalmus and the ophthalmoplegia, until a complete normalization. Postoperative angiography showed the disappearance of the CCF with preservation of the ICA flow (Fig. 1 b). The patient has remained asymptomatic ever since.

Case 2

A 62-year-old carpenter was admitted to the hospital on December 30, 1983, a few hours following a severe head injury from a casual precipitation. On examination he was unconscious, responding only to painful stimuli and showing as left paresis of the right arm (Glasgow coma scale score of 7). X-ray of the skull documented an extensive fronto-basal fracture with left orbital displacement. Computer tomography (CT) showed bilateral frontotemporal hemorrhagic contusions, intracranial air and proptosis of the left eye which could not be evaluated clinically due to the marked periorbital edema.

With conservative treatment he rapidly improved to a normal neurological condition except for a complete left ophthalmoplegia with exophthalmus and chemosis, and total left eye blindness. He complained of a constant left orbital bruit synchronous with the pulse.

A four-vessel selective angiography showed a high-flow left CCF was only filled by the left ICA. A large false aneurysm was concomitant with the CCF. Clearance was rapidly performed through the enlarged ophthalmic veins and by a striking net of cortical and meningeal veins leading to the sagittal and to the transverse sinuses.

While planning treatment the patient suddenly had a massive epistaxis, which was controlled by emergency nasal tamponade with a double balloon canula. On the following day an occlusion of the fistula using an intra-arterial balloon catheter was unsuccessfully attempted, creating a short lasting dysphasia and right hemiparesis.

This was followed 48 hours later by a direct approach of the cavernous sinus by a left pterional craniotomy. With a transient trapping of the left ICA, at the neck and intracranially, the cavernous sinus was opened, plugged with several fragments of muscle and injected with fibrin sealant.

Postoperatively, he was free of bruit, and the chemosis, the exophthalmus and the ophthalmoplegia improved rapidly. By the third day a very faint bruit could again be occasionally heard by the examiner, but not by the patient himself.

A control carotid angiography showed a complete disappearance of the CCF and the restoration of the intracranial ICA blood flow. The large false aneurysm was still present enclosing the two ends of a completely transected ICA. The cervical ICA had an almost complete stenosis-occlusion at its origin. Due to this the cervical ICA was ligated at the neck. The faint bruit disappaeared. A control digital angiography could not demonstrate filling of the false aneurysm and showed a normal intracranial circulation by crossed-flow.

Since then the patient has maintained a complete regression of the cavernous sinus syndrome.

Case 3

A 33-year-old housewife was admitted to the Neurosurgical Service on February 2, 1984. She had a history of a mild bruit synchronous with pulse on the left ear for four months, and left frontal dysesthesias for three months. In December 1983, and following a short lasting but acute left frontal headache, she developed progressive left exophthalmus and intense left orbital bruit. Forty-eight hours before admission she presented with diplopia, left ophthalmoplegia, enlargement of the exophthalmus and chemosis. There was no previous history of head trauma or of other relevant conditions.

Plain X-ray of the skull were normal. CT showed a large dilatation of the left cavernous sinus and of the opthalmic veins, with proptosis of the left eye.

Selective angiography of both internal and external carotid arteries and of the vertebral artery demonstrated a left high-flow CCF. The fistula was only filled through the left ICA, with clearance by the ophthalmic veins and by a net of corticotemporal veins. There was no evidence of dural arterio-venous malformation or of other vascular anomalies.

By a pterional craniotomy the left cavernous sinus was exposed. While transiently trapping the ICA, intracranially and at the neck, the cavernous sinus was opened, filled with muscle and injected with fibrin sealant.

Posteroperatively the bruit disappeared and she had a complete regression of the exophthalmus, the chemosis and the ophthalmoplegia, with full recovery of the eye movements. A control by digital arterial angiography showed a complete disappearance of the CCF with preservation of the ICA flow. She has remained symptom-free since then.

Case 4

This 55-year-old woman sustained a very severe head injury in a traffic accident in 1957. She had a frontobasal fracture, with immediate right eye blindness and with an acute left pulsating exophthalmus with complete ophthalmoplegia but with preservation of vision. It was reported that a CCF was demonstrated angiographically and treated at that time by a left cervical ICA ligation. Due to the progression of the exophthalmus and to the persistence of a constant bruit she was operated again in 1964 in another hospital, this time by an intracranial ICA clipping, again without success. Two months prior to her referral, she had a massive epistaxis which was controlled by emergency nasal tamponade.

The patient was referred to our Service on July 2, 1984. She had a disfigurating left exophthalmus with huge enlargement of the angular and frontal veins, chemosis and complete opthalmoplegia with preservation of visual acuity in this side. The right eye was blind and internally fixed by retraction. An intense bruit could be heard even from a distance (Fig. 2 a).

CT showed an enormous left cavernous sinus with marked enlargement of the ipsilateral ophthalmic and periorbital extracranial veins (Fig. 3 a, b).

A selective arterial digital angiography demonstrated a high flow left CCF which was only filled through the vertebral circulation by the left posterior communicating artery. The clip at the left ICA was distal to the posterior communicating artery. The left ICA was occluded at the neck (Fig. 4 a).

On July 5, 1984, the left cavernous sinus was approached by a pterional craniotomy. The ICA was exposed and a dilated posterior communicating artery was identified and temporally clipped. The lateral wall of the bulging cavernous sinus was punctured and a total of 12 ml of fibrin sealant was injected intracavernously.

The bruit disappeared immediately. Gradually the exophthalmus, the chemosis, the dilatation of the facial veins and the ophthalmoplegia subsided, while the vision of the left eye was preserved. A control digital arteriography demonstrated a complete disappearance of the CCF (Fig. 4 b).

Since then she has been symptom-free with complete recovery of all the left eye movements and with a remarkable cosmetic result (Fig. 2 b).

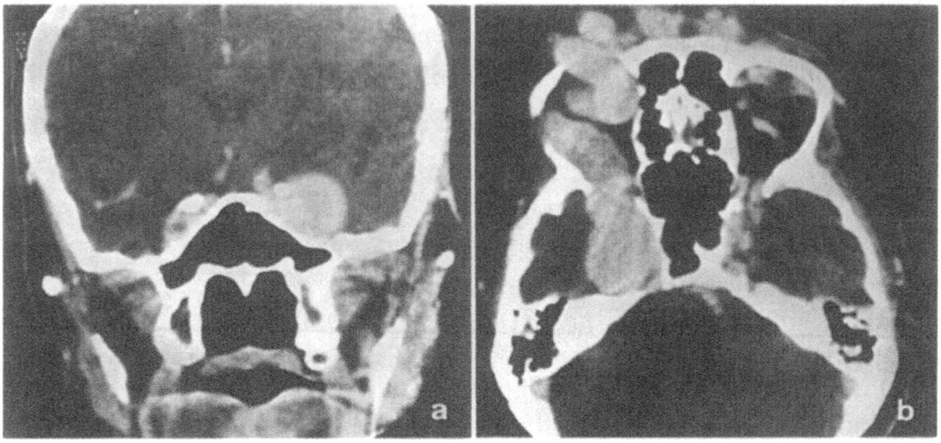

Fig. 2 a and **b.** Computer tomography of case 4

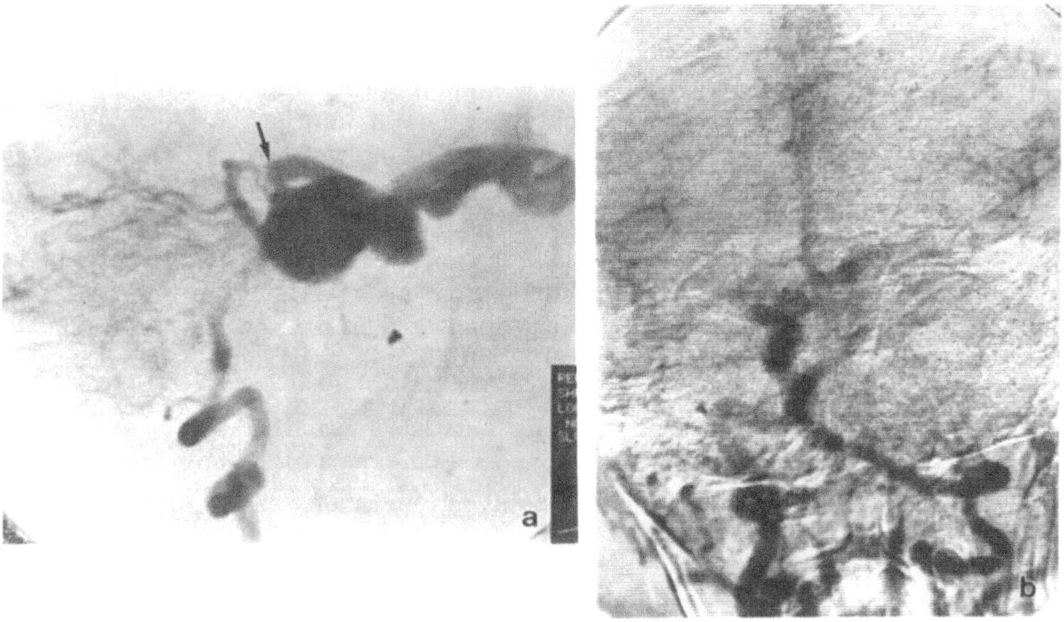

Fig. 3. a Preoperative digital vertebral arteriography. This fistula is filled through the dilated left posterior communicating artery (arrow). The ICA was ligated in the neck and close to the communicating artery; **b** Postoperative digital arteriography showing the resolution of the CCF

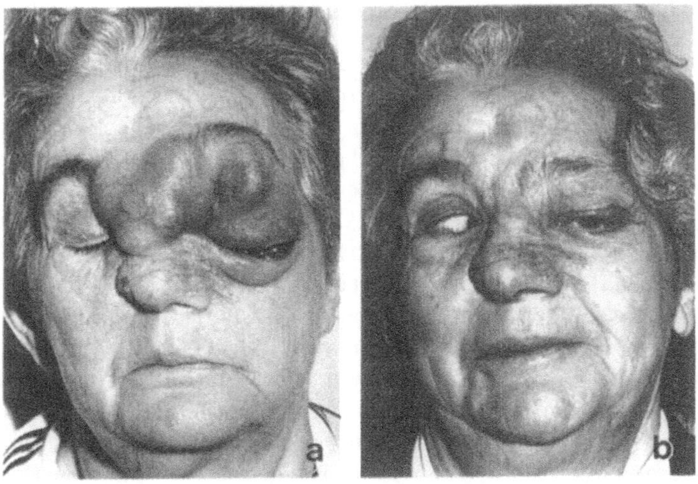

Fig. 4. Preoperative (**a**) and postoperative (**b**) appearance of case 4. The right eye preoperative was blind and internally fixed

Conclusions

In the three cases with a preoperative patent internal carotid artery (ICA) the CCF was occluded while preserving the ICA flow. One of them had a completely concomitant posttraumatic false aneurysm that enclosed the two avulsed ends of a transected intracavernous ICA. A fourth patient to whom an unsuccessful ICA trapping procedure had already been performed elsewhere also obtained a good result. The clinical material and the surgical technique have been presented. Direct intracavernous obliteration with muscle and fibrin sealant fulfills the ideal criteria for treatment of high-flow CCFs: occlusion of the arteriovenous fistula and preservation of the ICA circulation. This surgical technique can be used as a therapeutic option for some cases or as a precise indication for others.

The follow-up period of our patients has been from 18 months to over 3 years, without recurrence. This surgical approach should be considered in the treatment of high-flow CCFs. Unsuccessful and repeated attempts for the introduction of a detachable balloon catheter into a CCF may traumatize the ICA wall producing stenosis or occlusion of the artery. Prior to inducing this morbidity an alternative treatment such as the one presented here should be attempted. CCFs already treated ineffectively by ICA occlusion or ligation are precise indications for a direct intracavernous obliteration with muscle and fibrin sealant, or by fibrin sealant alone if the supraclinoid carotid artery has already been clipped.

References

1. Barrow DL, Fleisher AS, Hoffman JC (1982) Complications of detachable balloon catheter technique in the treatment of traumatic intracranial arteriovenous fistulas. J Neurosurg 56: 396–403
2. Barrow DL, Spector RH, Braun IF et al (1985) Classification and treatment of spontaneous carotid-cavernous sinus fistulas. J Neurosurg 62: 248–256
3. Benati A, Maschio A, Perini S et al (1980) Treatment of posttraumatic carotid-cavernous fistula using a detachable balloon catheter. J Neurosurg 53: 784–786
4. Black P, Umatsu S, Perovic M et al (1973) Carotid-cavernous fistula: a controlled embolus technique for occlusion of fistula with preservation of carotid flow. Technical note. J Neurosurg 38: 113–118
5. Dandy WE, Follis RH Jr (1941) On the pathology of carotid-cavernous aneurysms (pulsating exophthalmos). Am J Opthalmol 24: 356–385
6. Day AL, Rhoton AL Jr (1982) Aneurysms and arterio-venous fistulae in the intracavernous carotid artery and its branches. In: Youmans JR (ed) Neurological surgery, 2nd edn. Saunders, Philadelphia, pp 1764–1785
7. Debrun G, Lacour P, Caron JP et al (1978) Detachable balloon and calibrated techniques in the treatment of cerebral vascular lesions. J Neurosurg 49: 635–349
8. Debrun G, Lacour P, Viñuela F et al (1981) Treatment of 54 traumatic carotid-cavernous fistulas. J Neurosurg 55: 678–692
9. Echols DH, Jackson JD (1959) Carotid-cavernous fistula: a perplexing surgical problem. J Neurosurg 16: 619–627
10. Hamby WB (1964) Carotid-cavernous fistula: report of 32 surgically treated cases and suggestions for definitive operation. J Neurosurg 21: 859–866
11. Handa J, Handa H (1976) Severe epistaxis caused by traumatic aneurysm of cavernous carotid artery. Surg Neurol 5: 241–243
12. Hosobuchi Y (1975) Electrothrombosis of carotid-cavernous fistula. J Neurosurg 42: 76–85
13. Isamat F, Salleras V, Miranda AM (1970) Artificial embolization of carotid-cavernous fistula with postoperative patency of internal carotid artery. J Neurol Neurosurg Psychiatry 33: 674–678
14. Isamat F, Ferrer E, Twose J (1986) Direct intracavernous obliteration of high-flow carotid cavernous fistulas. J Neurosurg 65: 770–775
15. Johnston I (1979) Direct surgical treatment of bilateral intracavernous internal carotid artery aneurysms. Case report. J Neurosurg 51: 98–102
16. Kerber CW, Bank WO, Cromwell LD (1979) Cyanoacrylate occlusion of carotid-cavernous fistula with preservation of carotid artery flow. Neurosurgery 4: 210–215
17. Lapras C, Pierluca P, Taboada F (1983) Direct open surgical approach of the cavernous sinus for the treatment of carotid-cavernous fistula, with preservation of the internal carotid artery, without hypothermia and circulatory arrest. Experience of two cases. Presented at the 7th Eur Congr Neurosurg in Brussels, Aug. 28–Sept. 3, 1983
18. Moringlane JR, Ostertag CB (1985) L'occlusion des anévrismes expérimentaux. Presented at the Annu Meet Soc Neurochir Française in Paris, Dec. 9–12, 1985

19. Morley TP (1976) Appraisal of various forms of management in 41 cases of carotid-cavernous fistulas. In: Morley TP (ed) Current controversies in neurosurgery. Saunders, Philadelphia, pp 223–236
20. Mullan S (1979) Treatment of carotid-cavernous fistulas by cavernous sinus occlusion. J Neurosurg 50: 131–144
21. Parkinson D (1965) A surgical approach to the cavernous portion of the carotid artery. Anatomical studies and case report. J Neurosurg 23: 474–483
22. Parkinson D (1967) Transcavernous repair of carotid cavernous fistula. Case report. J Neurosurg 26: 420–424
23. Parkinson D (1973) Carotid cavernous fistula: direct repair with preservation of the carotid artery. Technical note. J Neurosurg 38: 99–106
24. Peeters FLM, van der Werf AJM (1980) Detachable balloon technique in the treatment of direct carotid-cavernous fistulas. Surg Neurol 14: 11–19
25. Prolo DJ, Burres KP, Hanbery JW (1977) Balloon occlusion of carotid cavernous fistula: introduction of a new catheter. Surg Neurol 7: 209–214
26. Samson D, Ditmore QM, Bayer CW Jr (1981) Intravascular use of isobotyl-2-cyanocrylate: 2. Treatment of carotid-cavernous fistulas. Neurosurgery 8: 52–55
27. Sbeih IA, O'Laoire SA (1984) Traumatic carotid-cavernous fistula due to transection of the intracavernous carotid artery. Case report. J Neurosurg 60: 1080–1084
28. Serbinenko FA (1974) Balloon catheterization and occlusion of major cerebral vessels. J Neurosurg 41: 125–145
29. Viñuela F, Fox AJ, Debrun G et al (1984) Spontaneous carotid-cavernous fistulas: clinical, radiological and therapeutic considerations. Experience with 20 cases. J Neurosurg 60: 976–984

Surgery of vascular lesions

Carotid cavernous aneurysms and fistulae

S. Mullan

Neurological Surgery, University of Chicago Medical Center,
Chicago, Illinois, U.S.A.

Aneurysms

Our experience in treatment includes conservative management, internal carotid occlusion, and thrombosis by wire, by needles, and by balloon.

Conservative management

We do not have enough information on the natural history of the accidentally discovered small aneurysm to evaluate its spontaneous risks. At the moment our policy is to control blood pressure and evaluate by serial angiography. We have followed one such patient for twenty years. A few symptomatic older patients (65+) who cannot tolerate carotid occlusion have accepted unilateral extraocular palsy rather than any surgical risk. We have only known of two patients with an intracavernous aneurysm who have had an intracranial hemorrhage. A confirmatory autopsy was obtained in one but not in the other. (It might have been an intracerebral hemorrhage.)

Internal carotid occlusion

This is a perfectly safe procedure for any patient who can tolerate manual carotid compression. The key of safety is to carry out the occlusion under full heparinization (as taught by Rasmussen T, in the early fifties).

Step 1
The Selverstone clamp is applied (open), under local or general anesthesia.

Step 2
When the patient is fully awake, the clamp is totally closed to verify ischemic

tolerance. If the patient tolerates occlusion for one minute, the clamp is set with 5/8 of one turn open, *i.e.*, almost totally closed. If not tolerated for a full minute, we have on two occasions successfully slowly occluded the clamp over a period of two to three weeks. We have not had any others in whom this slow attempt failed. If the total occlusion produces ischemic symptoms very rapidly, we have not attempted a slow occlusion.

Step 3
Over a two-day period, subtotal occlusion is continued for the patient who tolerates the initial trial occlusion. This interval permits the distal carotid to shrink in proportion to the new volume it transmits, so that eventually when a clot is allowed to develop within it, there will be no further elasticity, and therefore, no force to extrude the clot intracerebrally. The clamp is adjusted each day since it sometimes opens slightly under the continued pulsation.

Step 4
The patient is totally heparinized. Heparinization is not started earlier because of the risk of wound hematoma immediately after surgery. The clamp is fully occluded. Heparinization is maintained for two days. If symptoms occur, the clamp is opened.

Step 5
The stem of the clamp is removed.

We have twice observed hemispheric signs and symptoms. One patient developed these suddenly, associated with a slight fall in systemic blood pressure. The clip was opened, and he made an immediate recovery. It was then successfully occluded over a two-week period. It was never certain whether the problem was ischemic or embolic. Another patient had a slow decrease in higher intellectual function, beginning about three hours after total occlusion, noted by his family but not observable by the medical and nursing staff, over a period of a few hours. It was finally recognized as dysphasia appeared. All symptoms and signs completely reversed over a few hours upon opening the clamp. It was not reapplied.

We have had several patients subjected to a week or more of subtotal clamp. This demonstrated that these large aneurysms close down by internal thrombosis and virtually or completely disappear. Upon opening the clamp, the aneurysm became fully patent again within a few weeks without any trace of embolization. One patient, subsequent to a permanent subtotal clamp, showed disappearance of the aneurysm at the days. At two years, angiography was carried out. The carotid was totally occluded, and the patient was asymptomatic.

A limitation to the carotid occlusion method is that giant aneurysms are not infrequently bilateral.

We have some experience with initial carotid occlusion using balloons. They have the advantage over a Selverstone clamp in that being inflated high up, they eliminate the long "sump" in which clot forms and from which emboli exited. This problem has been solved by the combined Selverstone and heparin technique; and with thirty years of virtuality trouble-free occlusion, we have elected no change merely for the sake of simplicity. The single problem has been a fatal postoperative pneumonia in a patient with a recent aplastic anemia.

Thrombosis of carotid cavernous aneurysms

We have attempted to occlude the aneurysms while preserving carotid flow by three methods.

Wire thrombosis

This has been described in detail [1]. It is suitable for small aneurysms of about 1 cm diameter with small necks. It is not suitable for giant aneurysms, most of which have broad necks, which permit the thrombus to extend into the carotid. In one patient with a very small aneurysm, the wire itself, finding inadequate room within the aneurysm, extended into the carotid and thrombosed it asymptomatically.

Needle thrombosis

This method is suitable for relatively small aneurysms with a well defined neck. Copper clad steel needles of 0.2 mm diameter inserted transdurally across the neck will effectively thrombose it. These are so small that they have not injured the extraocular nerves in any instance.

Balloon thrombosis

This is our current area of interest. It is indicated for patients with giant symptomatic aneurysms who may not tolerate carotid occlusion, in whom carotid occlusion is inadvisable because of bilateral aneurysms, or in whom there is contralateral atherosclerosis. The experience has been with the use of Debrun balloons and Fogerty Balloon catheters (no. 4). Neither is ideal. The Debrun balloon catheter is too flexible and cannot be forced against the neck. It floats freely within the blood stream. The Fogerty catheter (cut off short) can be pushed against the neck, but the volume of each balloon (0.75–1.0 ml) is too small. Three to six such balloons must be used. It is, however, preferable to the Debrun. One balloon is positioned against the neck and held there by subsequently positioned balloons.

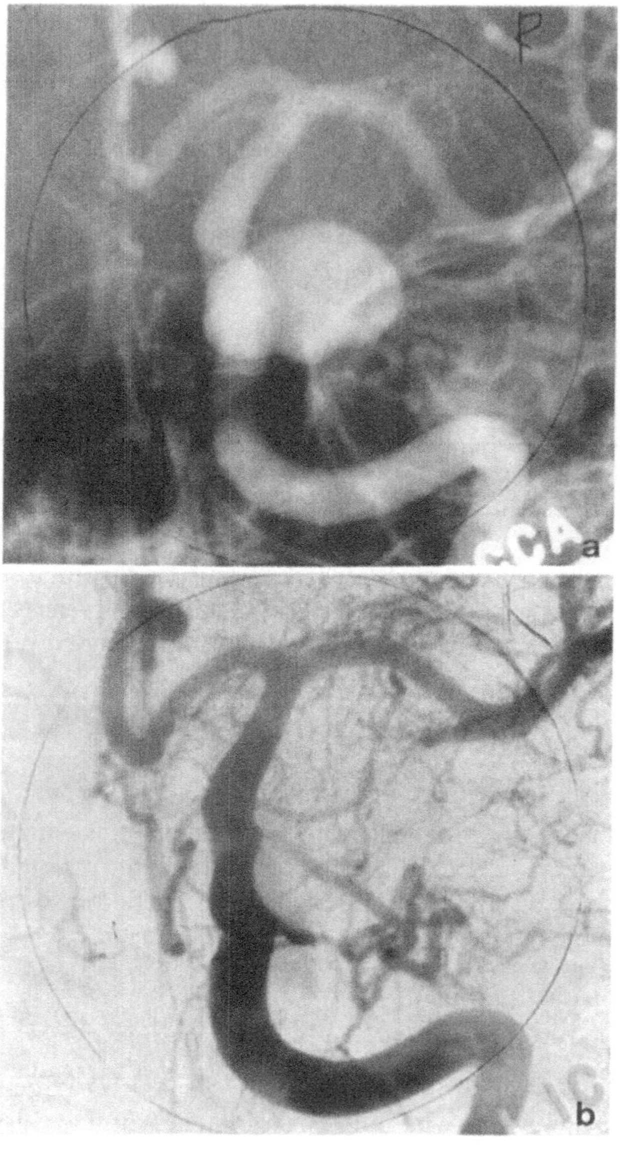

Fig. 1. Size of neck cannot be determined, therefore a balloon is preferable to wire (**a**), the postoperative appearance suggests a large neck (**b**)

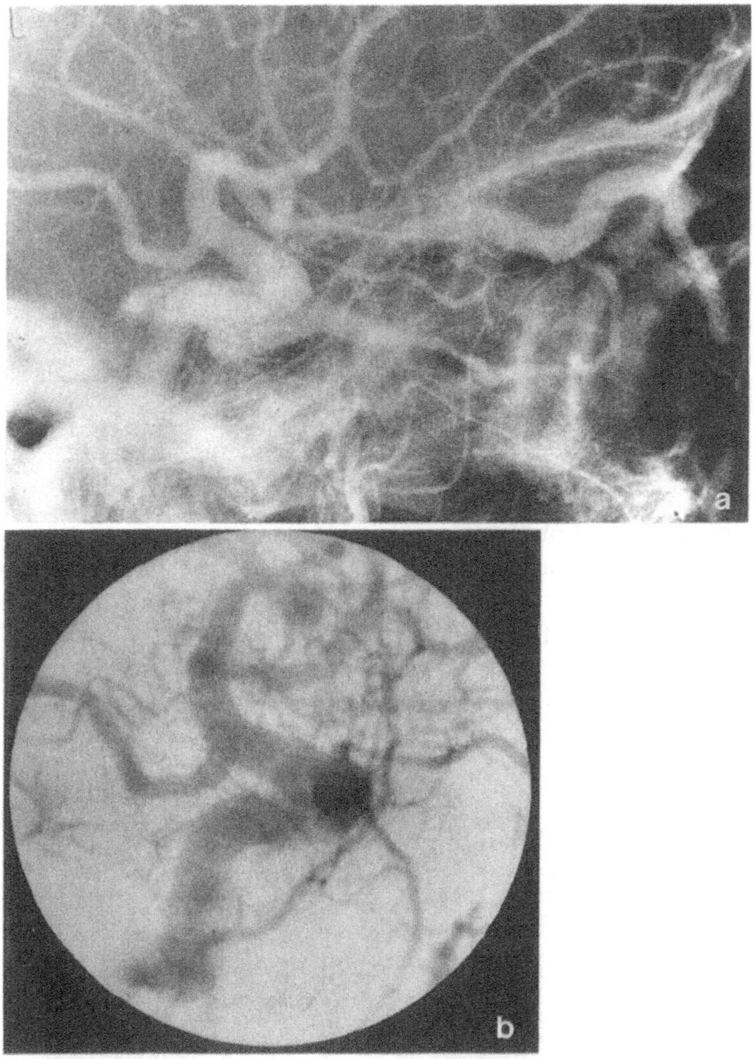

Fig. 2. Note that superior and inferior ophthalmic veins join in orbit and enter skull through inferior orbital fissure (**a**), obliteration achieved by packing vein in retrograde fashion at its entrance into dura (**b**)

The balloon catheters are inserted by craniotomy with exposure of the cavernous dura. They are inserted through separate needles which are withdrawn, leaving the balloon catheter in place. Hemorrhage from the needle tract is stopped by "surgical" and slight pressure. The balloons are inflated by saline, one at a time, and occlusion is monitored by serial angiography (usually performed through a retrograde superficial temporal artery catheter). When the exact degree of occlusion has been achieved, the balloons are deflated and then filled sequentially by silastic. The end point is close to the volume of saline previously used but may not be identical and must, again, be arrived at by serial angiography. We have used continuous corticography to monitor cerebral function during occlusion [2] (Fig. 1).

Carotid cavernous fistulae

The technique employed has varied somewhat since that previously described [3]. In that publication we advocated insertion of thrombogenic material in a retrograde manner through the ophthalmic vein and the superior petrosal sinus. We also used wire inserted into any cavernous areas not radiographically filled by artery and needles in to the fistulous communication.

As experience progressed, we continued to utilize the ophthalmic vein and the superior petrosal sinus as the approaches of choice, but have become more familiar with direct incision and packing into the sinus immediately above the foramen rotundum and into the posterior superior bulge lateral to the third and fourth nerves (Parkinson's triangle). We have used wire infrequently, not because it is not effective, but because its insertion is somewhat tedious (Fig. 2).

Complications

Judgements and delay

The major problem was in delay in initiating treatment due to either the patient, the referring physician, or our own judgement.

Case 1
A young man, psychologically disturbed, probably the victim of an attempted homicide rather than an accident, delayed closure until vision in the affected eye had irreversibly disappeared.

Case 2
An alcoholic woman sustained a severe head injury, was in coma about two weeks, and had extensive open infected gluteal wounds. She was blind in her

left eye from direct optic nerve compression and had a right fistula. Because we planned to insert "foreign material", we spent some days trying to minimize her infection. In this interval, the vision of the right eye, which because of her confused state, could not be examined "objectively", disappeared. There was no recovery following the technically simple closure of the fistula.

Case 3
A schizophrenic youth shot himself through the left ear, sustaining a cerebrospinal fluid fistula and a carotid cavernous fistula. While awaiting stabilization of his mental state, he developed a refractory meningitis and died before either fistula was closed.

Case 4
An elderly lady developed a fistula after a head injury received during a burglary. Her physician and neurosurgeon did not advise treatment because there was no diplopia and no loss of vision. She suffered an extensive subarachnoid hemorrhage and was in coma for three weeks when she came under our care. Closure of the fistula was carried out in the hope that it might improve cerebral blood flow and permit her to waken up. A technically successful closure was carried out, but she did not improve and died several weeks later.

Technical problems

Case 5
An elderly lady with colon carcinoma had extreme pain from her fistula. She could not tolerate carotid compression. A lumbar drain was inserted after anesthesia was induced, as was our custom. The initially clear CSF became blood tinged before the craniotomy was started. A massive acute subdural hematoma was present extending medially as well as laterally over the hemisphere. The fistula was closed easily, but she did not survive.

Case 6
Following the report of the use of a direct cyanoacrylate occlusion of the sinus [4], we placed a small catheter (craniotomy) in the sinus of a middle-aged man. Two injections of contrast showed no reflux into the carotid, but subsequent to the injection of the thrombogenic liquid, he sustained a carotid occlusion and expired.

These experiences have taught us that delay in treatment, whether caused by the patient or by those in charge of his management, can have serious consequences, that fatal spontaneous subarachnoid hemorrhage can occur, that subdural drainage can precipitate a fatal subdural hemorrhage, and that a liquid thrombogenic agent should not be used in the cavernous sinus.

There have been no ischemic complications and no permanent extra-ocular and motor palsies. One patient completely recovered from a sixth nerve palsy at the end of a year.

Balloon occlusion of fistulae

This is now the method of choice for the acute traumatic fistula if the patient can tolerate unilateral manual carotid compression. It is recognized that in a large number of cases, occlusion is affected by occluding the carotid rather than the fistula itself. For all patients who cannot tolerate manual occlusion, for those with contralateral cavernous fistulae or aneurysms, and for those with evidence of atherosclerosis, we prefer to maximize the possibility of saving the carotid by using the craniotomy and direct packing method. For those in whom balloon embolization has failed or for those in whom symptoms recur despite a previous trapping operation, there seems to be no good alternative to direct occlusion in most instances. A very occasional recurrence after direct trapping might be subject ot arterial embolization if only one external arterial branch was involved.

References

1. Mullan S (1974) Experiences with surgical thrombosis of intracranial berry aneurysms and carotid venous fistulas. J Neurosurg 41: 657–670
2. Mullan S, Duda EE, Patronas NJ (1980) Some examples of balloon technology in neurosurgery. J Neurosurg 52: 321–329
3. Mullan S (1979) Treatment of carotid cavernous fistulas by cavernous sinus occlusion. J Neurosurg 50: 131–144
4. Sampson D, Ditmore QM, Beyer CW (1981) Intravascular use of isobutyl 2-cyanoacrylate: 2. Treatment of carotid cavernous fistulas. Neurosurgery 8: 52–55

Traumatic carotid aneurysms of the cavernous sinus

J. R. van Dellen

Department of Neurosurgery, Faculty of Medicine, University of Natal and Wentworth Hospital, Durban, Natal, South Africa*

In general, traumatic aneurysms of the intracavernous carotid artery can be regarded as rare complications of a head injury. Injury to the carotid artery in this situation may occur directly or indirectly. The reason for an aneurysm forming, rather than a fistula, can be deduced from the modern anatomical concept of the cavernous sinus. Provided the walls of the venous vessels of the sinus are not breached when the carotid artery is damaged, compression by the extravasating blood would create a stronger venous vessel wall and lead to the development of a false aneurysm.

The classical triad of loss of vision, a fracture in the vicinity of the cavernous sinus of the base of the skull and a massive arterial epistaxis, however, are common presenting features. These may, however, not all be present.

A large series, since 1974, of seven cases of this rare complication, is presented highlighting the problems of diagnosis, management and subsequent complications. All were treated surgically—one by extracranial carotid ligation, four by a carotid trapping procedure and in two cases by a direct approach. One case was associated with a carotico-cavernous fistula on the opposite side, necessitating a direct attack on the carotico-cavernous fistula.

In two cases total circulatory arrest utilizing profound hypothermia was used as an adjunct to the direct approach. Two of the seven patients died, only one for reasons related to the surgical management. The surgical treatment of choice appears to be a trapping procedure (probably associated with an anastomotic bypass procedure when indicated), since the extensively damaged wall of the carotid artery in the confined space of the cavernous sinus does not easily allow repair.

* Present address: Division of Neurosurgery, Harbor/UCLA Medical Center, Los Angeles, Torrance, California, U.S.A.

Patients and treatment methods

Traumatic aneurysms of the intracavernous carotid artery are rare complications of a head injury. The world literature comprises just over one hundred reports. In a recent report by Wang et al. a comprehensive list of the reported cases is provided [8, 13, 14, 15].

They may be caused by direct or indirect trauma. Sharp objects or bone spicules may damage the vessel or a shear stress may be applied to the artery or its intracavernous branches as a result of this segment being mobile between the two points of firm dural fixation, as it enters and leaves the cavernous sinus. A carotico-cavernous fistula is a more common complication of this type of trauma. The reason that an aneurysm rather than a fistula forms is probably best explained by the more recently described microanatomy of the cavernous sinus [4, 6, 9, 10, 11]. If the walls of the veins present in the sinus are not breached and if these canals are compressed by the blood extravasating from the damaged adjacent carotid artery, it is likely that they will be less friable and that a false aneurysm can develop rather than a fistulous connection.

A classical triad, originally reported by Maurer [7], has been described in the majority of these aneurysms [1, 2]:

a) a fracture of the skull base in the vicinity of the cavernous sinus;
b) loss of vision;
c) often an arterial epistaxis.

Although the clinical presentation of the sequelae usually occurs up to 1–3 months after the initial injury, it may occur much later. The symptoms and clinical findings are in keeping with an enlarging space-occupying lesion, of any cause, in the cavernous sinus, with effects on the adjacent vascular nervous and bony structures. The progressive loss of vision is interesting and in the case of an intracavernous aneurysm it cannot be explained by an ischemic process as would occur in a fistula [12]. In a recent book edited by Wilson and Stein on "Intracranial Arteriovenous Malformations", Hosobuchi [15] describes the development of a glaucomatous condition due to chronic venous stasis, which may be a reason for the progressive visual loss. Immediate loss of vision is from damage to the optic nerve at the time of injury. The arterial epistaxis presumably occurs from rupture of the aneurysm when the normal or damaged walls of the adjacent nasal sinus, usually the sphenoid, are eroded. The epistaxis may be mild and repetitive, or massive and exsanguinating. Some patients have a warning of the epistaxis in the form of a strange sensation or feeling of fullness in the surrounding facial and forehead area. The delayed complication of intracerebral hemorrhage is rare, although Shallat et al. [13] have reported a case with this complication. This could obviously only take place if the dura of the cavernous sinus is breached on its intracranial aspect.

Six proven cases and one likely case of a posttraumatic intracavernous carotid artery aneurysm are presented to highlight the diagnosis, management and subsequent complications of the condition.

The first, a 62-year-old male, had been stabbed 3 years previously and lost vision as a result of the right orbital injury. He presented with pulsatile proptosis of the right eye and an obvious arterial thrill on palpation of the eye. He also had a partial nerve IV palsy. Angiography demonstrated a carotid aneurysm in the cavernous sinus on the right and no evidence of any angiographic cross-circulation. After discussion with the patient a direct approach on the aneurysm was carried out using the technique of profound hypothermia and total circulatory arrest [14] for 46 minutes in an attempt to preserve the damaged carotid artery. At surgery the aneurysm and the carotid walls were extremely friable and surrounded by dense adhesions, believed to be the result of previous hemorrhage. The extent of these may also have been due to the late presentation after the initial injury. It was not possible to repair the carotid artery or deal directly with the aneurysm, and the separated proximal and distal portions of the damaged artery were clipped and occluded within the sinus. Postoperatively the patient had a left upper limb monoparesis but was otherwise neurologically intact. On the 7th postoperative day his level of consciousness deteriorated and he developed a right hemiplegia. A CT scan demonstrated an infarct of the right middle cerebral territory. He deteriorated further and died on the 12th postoperative day. The outcome on this patient may have been different had a bypass procedure been used extensively at that time.

The second patient sustained a stab injury to the right eye which was then enucleated. Eight months later this 22-year-old woman presented with failing vision, ptosis and a complete ophthalmoplegia of the left eye. A massive aneurysm extending well beyond the normal confines of the cavernous sinus infratemporally was demonstrated by angiography. After considering the alternative possibilities and in consultation with the patient, a direct approach to the aneurysm was decided upon in an attempt to reduce the bulk of the lesion rapidly. Profound hypothermia in association with total circulatory arrest was again utilized for 41 minutes. In this case, as with the previous patient, due to grossly damaged and distorted carotid arterial wall at the origin of the aneurysm, the carotid lumen could not be reconstituted. Postoperatively she was well but no obvious improvement in vision or in the degree of ptosis was detected. She discharged herself on the 22nd postoperative day, did not return for follow-up visits and could not be traced.

The third patient was a 20-year-old male who had sustained a head injury, had been admitted to an outlying hospital for 2 days and then discharged. He returned 12 days later with a right hemiplegia and facial palsy. He also had an expressive aphasia, a total left nerve III palsy and proptosis. There was not bruit present. Prior to transfer to the neurosurgical department he had a severe arterial epistaxis. Unfortunately we were not able to obtain further history regarding the clinical sequence of events which occurred from his initial discharge from the outlying hospital until his representation to the same hospital. An angiogram demonstrated an intracavernous carotid aneurysm and a Hamby-type trapping procedure was carried out. He did well and at his last visit had only a right upper limb monoplasia and was able to speak, but still had a severe expressive dysphasia. The reason for the right middle cerebral infarct in this patient was probably embolic to clot formation in the large traumatic aneurysm which has been well described.

The next case was an 11-year-old boy who had collided with a tree whilst riding his bicycle. On admission he had bruising of the nose and right side of the face and was found to be blind in the rigt eye. X-ray of the skull showed an opaque ethmoid paranasal sinus and a fracture of the base of the skull also involving the ethmoid bone. He was observed and discharged. Two weeks later, after 5 episodes of severe epistaxis, he was readmitted. The otolaryngologists who had seen the boy for the epistaxis, after repeated attempts at nasal packing, eventually obliterated both the right anterior and posterior ethmoidal arteries on this admission. Despite the surgical procedure, further severe bouts of epistaxis followed and 8 weeks later an external carotid ligation was carried out, but this surgical intervention also did not reduce the nasal bleeding. A CT scan was done but was not helpful in making a diagnosis. Twelve weeks later, after a neurosurgical consultation, an angiogram was carried out which showed the intracavernous carotid aneurysm. After discussion with the parents, with regard to the alternatives of management, a common carotid ligation was carried out. The patient made a full recovery with no further bouts of epistaxis but remained blind probably due to an initial direct optic nerve injury.

The fifth case was a 19-year-old girl involved in a motor vehicle accident who suffered severe facial and frontal injuries. The CT scan on admission demonstrated blood in the right ethmoid sinus and extensive fracturing of the base of the skull. A debridgement of the wounds was carried out. Twelve days later, after being fully conscious she developed confusion and a left hemiparesis. A CT scan showed a delayed frontal intracerebral hematoma which was evacuated and she returned to her previous state. A few days later she had a severe epistaxis which responded to plugging and the junior staff felt it too "minor" an episode to report to a senior member of staff. On day 21 she had another extremely severe epistaxis and became deeply unconscious with a fixed, dilated right pupil and a left hemiplegia. Angiography done at this stage showed rupture of an intracavernous aneurysm into the cerebral hemisphere. She was taken to the operation room and a Hamby-type trapping procedure immediately carried out and the intracerebral hematoma evacuated. She improved to a state where she was moving all her limbs to painful stimuli but not to commands. She then developed a Klebsiella septicemia and died from a coagulopathy 42 days after admission. The patient is almost identical to the patient reported on by Shallat et al. in 1981 [13].

These two cases highlight the need for special care to be taken in evaluating the parasellar nasal sinuses both on straight radiology and on CT scanning, since the latter investigation has superseded the use of angiography in the management and diagnosis of head trauma. Information gained from these two investigations may well provide valuable additional guides to the diagnosis and the need for angiography to identify or confirm vascular pathology.

The sixth case, a 47-year-old male, also sustained a stab wound of the forehead. He also had a swollen left eye and complained of retroorbital pain. He was transferred to the neurosurgical department two weeks later with a markedly proptotic and chemotic left eye, limitation of movement, a nerve VI palsy and hypoanesthesia of the first division of the cranial nerve V. He also had a systolic bruit on auscultation over the eye. He was tentatively diagnosed as a carotico-cavernous fistula and angiography booked. Prior to this being done, he had a severe epistaxis which terminated spontaneously, but he required a blood transfusion. Whilst the transfusion was in progress he had a second exsanguinating hemorrhage which could not be controlled despite the use of a Foley catheter in the nasopharyngeal space [8]. He was immediately taken to the operating room and a Hamby-trap carried out. He made a full recovery apart from some minor visual loss and a palsy of nerve VI.

This case, who did not have angiography, raises the question of whether this was an aneurysm or a fistula. Sattler reported on 6 cases with carotico-cavernous fistula who had died as a result of epistaxis and three cases who had bled intracranially. It appears therefore that both an aneurysm and a fistula in this situation, when posttraumatic, may have dire and often fatal complications from hemorrhage.

The final case is a 36-year-old male who sustained a compression fracture of the skull. He had severe comminuted fracturing of the skull base with bilateral petrous bone dislocations and a CSF leak from both ears which, fortunately, resolved spontaneously. However, he remained with bilateral VI and lower motor neuron nerve VII palsies. He returned 3 months later with bilateral visual deterioration which, in the left eye, had led to total blindness and on the right a severe loss of acuity and a field loss. There was also proptosis and chemosis of the right eye and a bruit was heard over the left eye. The CT scan suggested a carotico-cavernous fistula on the right. A Doppler study showed abnormal signals from the right carotid artery. Angiography was then carried out which showed an unexpected typical carotico-cavernous fistula on the left and a traumatic aneurysm on the right side. In view of our previous experience with traumatic aneurysms, it was decided to carry out a direct approach on the left carotico-cavernous fistula to preserve the carotid artery. The use of a detachable balloon was believed to be too risky. The cavernous sinus was opened and the fistula occluded with muscle. The carotid artery was preserved with an intact lumen. Seven days later the patient had a Hamby-trap of the traumatic carotid aneurysm on the right. He did extremely well and there was improvement of vision on the right, which would tend to support the view of Hosobuchi regarding the mechnism of visual loss.

From this experience, it appears that traumatic intracavernous carotid aneurysms may have typical clinical features which allow for diagnosis, are not amenable to direct repair and that the best option would appear to be a Hamby trapping procedure with possibly a bypass procedure e.g. STA-MCA or saphenous vein carotico-carotid anastomosis where indicated. The use of detachable balloons is an alternate form of treatment of achieve trapping by placing balloons above and below the cavernous aneurysm (Fox et al. comment to Ming-Ying) [8].

In conclusion, direct attack on a carotico-cavernous fistula under standard operative conditions with muscle packing of the cavernous sinus and preservation of the carotid artery, is eminently feasible and rewarding.

References

1. Araki C, Handa S, Handa J, Yoshida K (1965) Traumatic aneurysm of the intracranial portion of the internal carotid artery. J Neurosurg 23: 64–67
2. Benoit BG, Wortzman G (1973) Traumatic cerebral aneurysms clinical features and natural history. J Neurol Neurosurg Psychiatry 36: 127–138
3. Chadduck WM (1969) Traumatic cerebral aneurysms due to speargun injury. Case report. J Neurosurg 31: 77–79
4. Harris FS, Rhoton AL (1968) Anatomy of the cavernous sinus. J Neurosurg 45: 169–180
5. Hosobuchi Y (1984) Carotid cavernous fistulas. In: Wilson CB, Stein BM (eds) Intracranial arteriovenous malformations. Williams and Wilkins, Baltimore, p 250
6. Kaplan HA, Browder J, Krieger AJ (1976) Intracavernous connections of the cavernous sinus. J Neurosurg 45: 166–168
7. Maurer JJ, Mills M, German WJ (1961) Triad of unilateral blindness, orbital fracture and massive epistaxis after head injury. J Neurosurg 18: 837–840
8. Ming-Ying L, Chun-Jen S, Yeon-Chih W, Shin Han T (1985) Traumatic intracavernous carotid aneurysm with massive epistaxis. Neurosurgery 17: 569–573
9. Parkinson D (1973) Carotid cavernous fistula: Direct repair with preservation of the carotid artery. J Neurosurg 38: 99–106

10. Parkinson D, Shields CB (1974) Persistent trigeminal artery, its relationship to the normal branches of the cavernous carotid. J Neurosurg 39: 244–248
11. Penn WH, Rhoton AL (1975) Microsurgical anatomy of the sellar region. J Neurosurg 43: 288–298
12. Sanders MD, Hoyt WF (1969) Hypoxic ocular sequelae of carotid-cavernous fistulae. Study of the cause of visual failure before and after neurosurgical treatment in a series of 25 cases. Br J Ophthalmol: 5382
13. Shallat RF, Tackman MS, Nagle RC (1981) Delayed complications of craniocerebral trauma. Case report. Neurosurgery 8: 569–573
14. Van Dellen JR (1980) Intracavernous traumatic aneurysms. Surg Neurol 13: 203–207
15. Wang AN, Winfield JA, Gucer G (1986) Traumatic internal carotid artery aneurysm with rupture into the sphenoid sinus. Surg Neurol 25: 77–81

Strategies in intracavernous saccular aneurysms

G. PENDL, P. VORKAPIC, B. RICHLING, and W. T. KOOS

Department of Neurosurgery, University of Vienna Medical School, Vienna, Austria

Since the introduction of EC-IC bypass surgery in 1975 an additional method in the management of infraclinoid aneurysms has been available, as well as balloon catheter techniques in recent years and in addition to clipping, rhaphy, wrapping of the aneurysm and ligation of the internal carotid artery or trapping. We encountered 28 cases of infraclinoid aneurysms up until the end of 1985. Five patients were seen in severe condition on admission; they had no treatment and one of them eventually died. Direct clipping was possible in only 7 aneurysms regardless of their size, since dissection within the cavernous sinus even in large aneurysms was possible. Wrapping in broad-based large aneurysms was performed in 4 cases, since the clinical signs and symptoms as well as topographic anatomy did not lead us to expect an encroachment onto the cranial nerves. Endovascular techniques with a detachable balloon catheter were executed in 3 cases with an additional EC-IC bypass in two of these cases. Ligation of the internal carotid artery combined with an EC-IC bypass was achieved in 3 cases and in a further 2 cases only an EC-IC bypass was performed. In 2 cases trapping of the giant aneurysm by ligation of the internal carotid artery at the neck as well as distal to the aneurysms was performed. The results were satisfactory since the clinical signs and symptoms improved in most cases and no further deficits were encountered. Four patients died postoperatively. The various indications for the strategies applied are further discussed.

Introduction

Although a direct surgical approach with clipping of the neck is the treatment of choice for intracranial aneurysms this might not be possible in some locations especially for aneurysms arising from the infraclinoid portion of the internal carotid artery. The proximity of the cavernous sinus with its close relationship to the optic nerve and nerve III makes the direct approach hazardous and clipping of the neck is technically impossible in many of these cases. Therefore various concepts of surgical strategies have been developed (Fig. 1):

1. The direct approach with neck clipping or rhaphy of the aneurysm.
2. Internal carotid ligation or trapping of the aneurysm with or without EC-IC bypass.
3. EC-IC bypass only.
4. Endovascular occlusion by detachable balloon catheter with or without EC-IC bypass.
5. Common carotid ligation.

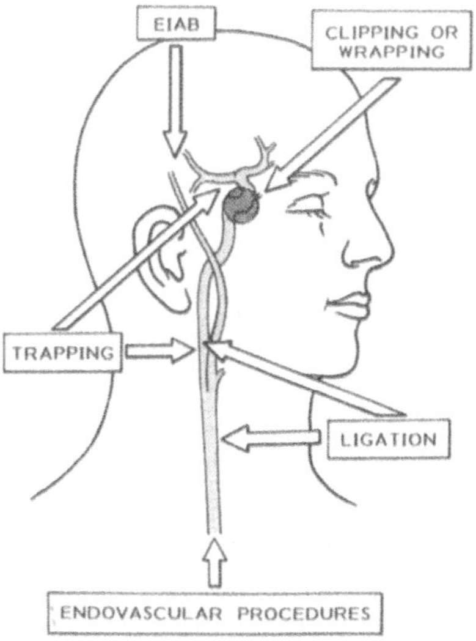

Fig. 1. Various surgical strategies for infraclinoid intracavernous saccular aneurysms

Clinical material and methods

During the years from 1964 to 1985, 1,120 intracranial aneurysms were encountered and 28 of these patients were diagnosed as having intracavernous aneurysms (Table 1). The size of these aneurysms was mostly less than 1 cm. Eleven were less than 2.5 cm and 14 from 2.5 up to 6 cm and in one case of bilateral appearance the left was 4 cm, the right 1 cm in diameter. Therefore more than half of these cases should be called giant aneurysms (Fig. 2).

Table 1. Treatment of intracavernous saccular aneurysms

		Good	Fair	Poor	Died
Direct approach with clipping	7	4	—	—	3*
Direct approach with wrapping	4	3	—	—	1*
Trapping	2	2	—	—	—
Internal carotid ligation	1	1	—	—	—
EIAB	2	2	—	—	—
Direct balloon occlusion of siphon	2	2	—	—	—
Internal carotid ligation with EIAB	3	3	—	—	—
Detachable balloon occlusion with EIAB	2	1	1	—	—
No treatment	5	1	3	—	1*
Total	28	19	4	—	5

* See Table 2

The sex ratio was 23 female to only 3 male patients, with the age distribution showing 9 patients younger than 50, the youngest 15 years of age, and 17 patients older than 50, the oldest 80 years old.

The direct surgical approach was chosen in 11 cases, but direct clipping was achieved only in 7 cases as the small size as well as the narrow neck enabled a good enough exposure by a standard pterional approach on the ipsilateral side with resection of the anterior clinoid process (Fig. 3). In 4 of the other cases of wrapping and rhaphy the size as well as the wide neck prevented a save dissection or clipping of the neck. Wrapping was performed with muscle and fibrin glue. Postoperative complications were severe with a lethal outcome in 4 of these 11 cases with the direct approach: one case was lost because of a myocardial infarction, another patient died due to an extensive ischemic lesion in the territory of the middle cerebral artery on the side of the aneurysm, the third patient died by hemorrhage of an accompanying cerebellar angioma, and the fourth case was lost due to the poor condition following a severe subarachnoid hemorrhage by a concomitant anterior communicating artery aneurysm (Table 2).

Internal carotid ligation after securing an effective cross flow and perfusion after temporary occlusion with EC-IC bypass was performed in 3 cases of the giant type with satisfactory results (Fig. 4).

Endovascular occlusion of the internal carotid artery at the site of the aneurysm with occlusion of the aneurysm itself with a detachable balloon

Table 2. Mortality rate in 28 cases of treatment of intracavernous saccular aneurysms

		Age	Treatment
Myocardial infarction	1	78	direct clipping
Cerebellar angioma with hemorrhage	1	64	direct clipping
Cerebral infarction	1	80	direct approach
Fatal subarachnoid hemorrhage by concomittant aneurysms	1	68	wrapping
Fatal recurrent subarachnoid hemorrhage	1	53	No treatment
Total	5		

was performed in 2 cases. In a further case with balloon occlusion an additional EC-IC bypass was necessary to establish sufficient perfusion of the according hemisphere (Fig. 5). All these 3 patients did very well.

In 2 symptomatic cases in elderly patients with trigeminal pain, ophthalmoplegia and giant aneurysms, a trapping maneuver with good results was performed.

Five elderly patients with SAH and in very poor condition were not treated, since the operative risk was too high even after recovery from the hemorrhage; one of them eventually died (Table 3).

Discussion

Aneurysms arising from the internal carotid artery proximal to the posterior communicating artery are rare. If they arise even proximal to the origin of the ophthalmic artery, they are extradural and therefore unlikely to be the source of SAH [14], as we have lost a patient with SAH and an unrecognized anterior communicating aneurysm associated with a large infraclinoid aneurysm treated with wrapping. They are less likely to bleed, because they are covered by the clinoid process, the optic apparatus and the basal dura [6]. In cases of the giant type these infraclinoid aneurysms may partly extend into the intracranial subarachnoid space and are therefore more likely be associated with SAH. Also small infraclinoid aneurysms, even at the site of the origin of the ophthalmic artery, are not expected to be intradural.

Another characteristic of these aneurysms is that they occur much more frequently in females than in males [5, 6, 9, 12].

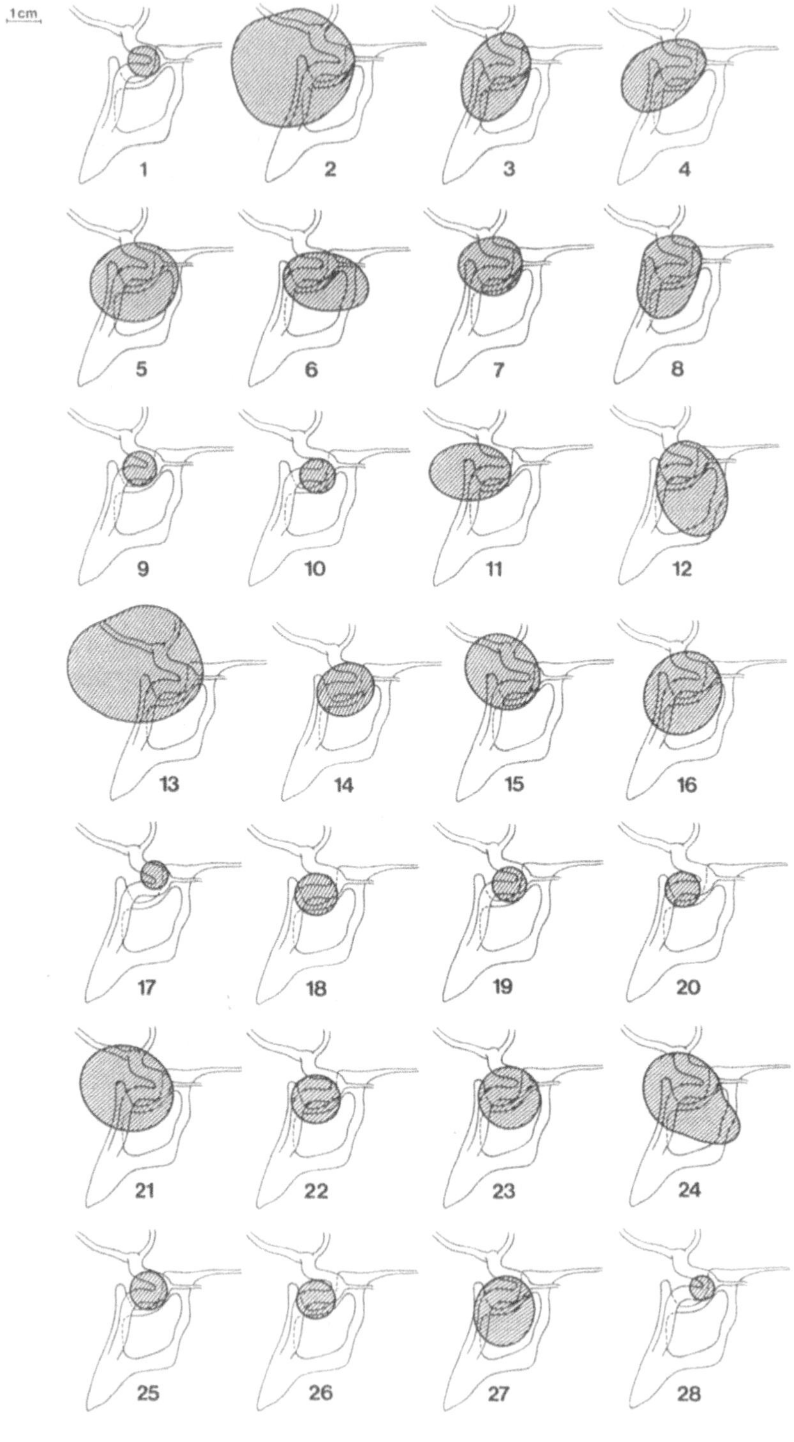

Fig. 2. The size and shape of 28 observed cases of infraclinoid partly intracavernous saccular aneurysms

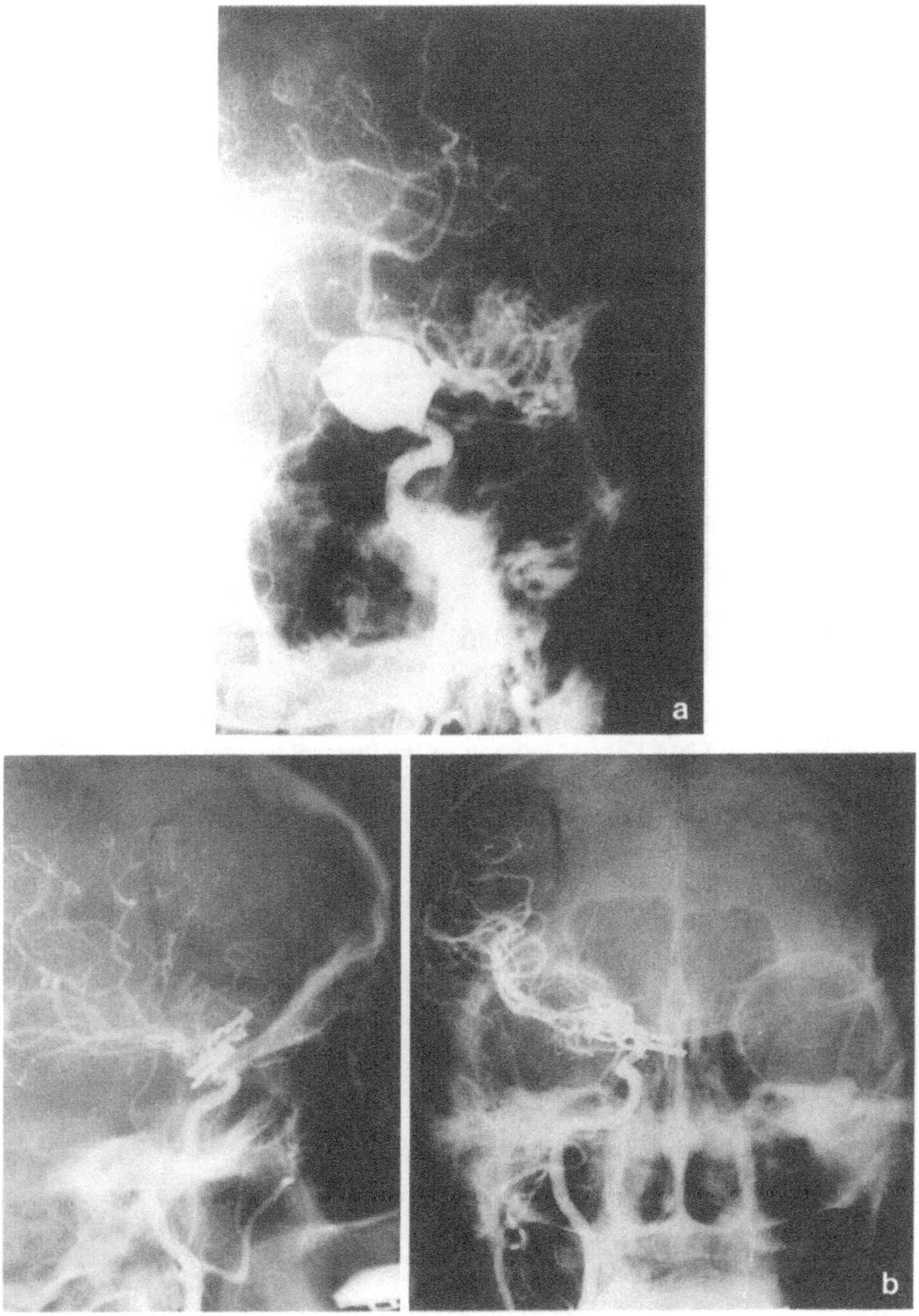

Fig. 3. a Arteriogram of a saccular infraclinoid aneurysm with rather narrow neck in an oblique projection (Case 11); **b** Arteriogram of Case 11 after clipping of the neck of the infraclinoid intracavernous aneurysms with several Sugita clips

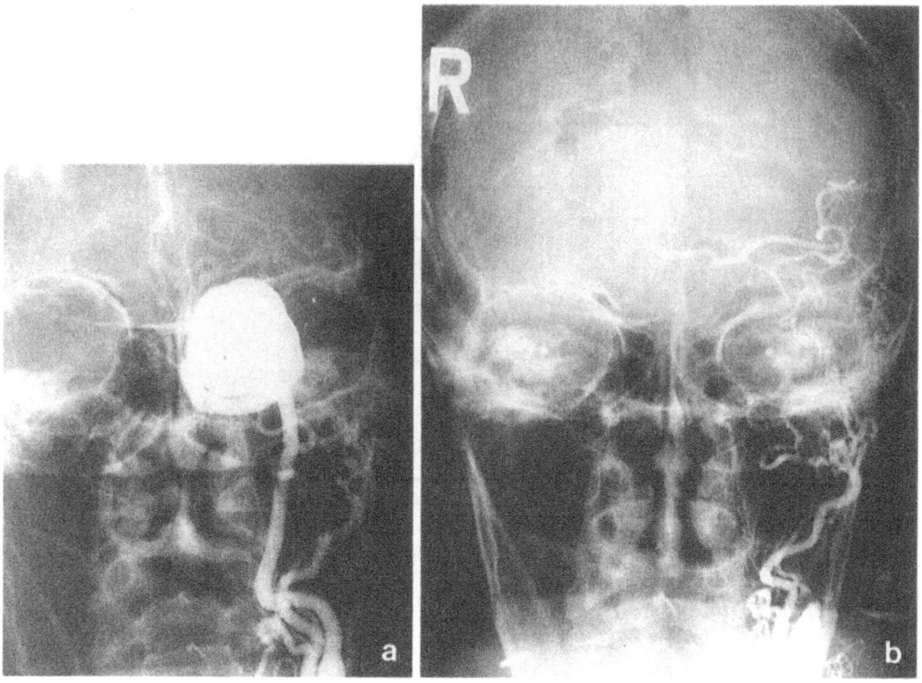

Fig. 4. a Giant infraclinoid saccular aneurysm in the arteriogram (Case 13); **b** Arteriogram of Case 13 after ligation of the internal carotid artery and EC-IC bypass

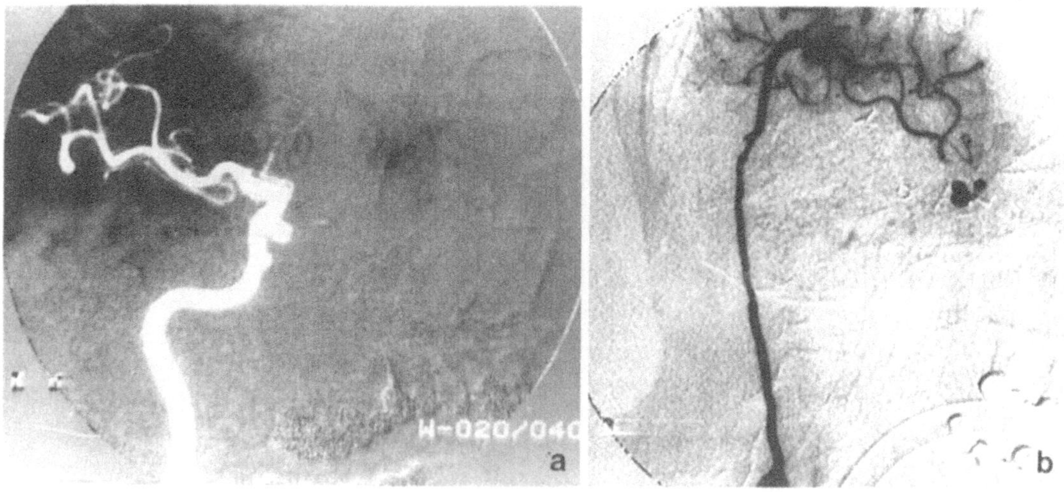

Fig. 5. a Infracavernous berry aneurysm in the digital substraction angiogram (Case 28); **b** DSA of Case 28 after endovascular balloon occlusion and EC-IC bypass with vein graft

The clinical symptoms associated with intracavernous aneurysms and giant carotid-ophthalmic aneurysms are various dysfunctions of the nerves III, IV and VI with pain mainly in the first branch of the nerve V. Visual impairment and visual field defects will be present if the aneurysm extends towards the optic nerve, chiasm, or tract in cases of giant aneurysms.

Since the advent of microsurgery and microvascular surgery in association with endovascular techniques, sole carotid artery ligation has become problematic, as has common artery ligation, which proved to be safer, but internal carotid artery ligation has been more effective in producing a permanent reduction in distal blood pressure and in preventing recurrent SAH [6, 7, 11, 13]. Finally, with primary ligature of the internal carotid or common carotid artery, endovascular techniques became impossible. The additional possibility of EC-IC bypass with internal carotid occlusion has improved the tolerance for this maneuver as well as gradual occlusion of the vessel [5, 6, 19]. In our series we had no ischemic complications using this method.

Lowered morbidity with microsurgery had made the direct intracranial approach the procedure of choice for most aneurysms and even infraclinoid and giant aneurysms should be explored directly, when there is evidence from arteriography that there is a suitable neck for clipping [4, 6, 7, 9] with a pterional approach with preservation of the main branches of the temporal artery for possible EC-IC bypass later. The anterior clinoid process has to be removed extradurally and occasionally the roof of the optic canal as well. Then the dura is further opened, if necessary, to expose the neck of the aneurysm. If a clip has been applied it might be necessary to reinforce the clip by applying a second clip parallel to the first or across it and secure the clips with fibrin glue; fenestrated clips are very useful here [9, 10]. Temporary clamping of the internal carotid in the neck or temporary occlusion by an intraoperatively managed nondetachable balloon, is helpful during surgery to reduce the blood flow and soften the aneurysm for clipping.

Since the introduction of detachable balloons for carotid-cavernous sinus fistulas, this endovascular technique has also been introduced for intracavernous internal carotid aneurysms [4, 9, 17]. As in infraclinoid aneurysms with distinct neck selective aneurysm, occlusion with detachable balloons is reported [15] (while preserving the internal carotid artery), and there generally exists the opinion that the risk of thrombo-embolic complications during manipulations there is relatively high [2]. When no neck exists, the manipulation of several balloons into the sac of the aneurysm might achieve thrombosis of the aneurysm.

Generally, ligature of the internal carotid artery by a detachable balloon, placed at the site of the aneurysm, is preferred [2]. Crossflow-studies before detaching the blown-up balloon indicates the necessity of an EC-IC bypass,

Table 3.

Case no.	Age	Sex	Clinical presentation	Size	Treatment	Result	Remarks
1	68	F	SAH	1 cm	wrapping	died	concomitant ACoA-aneurysm with SAH, clipped
2	72	F	orbital pain, IIIrd nerve palsy	5 cm	EC-IC	good	concomitant stenosis of ICA
3	71	F	trigeminal pain V/1	3 cm	trapping	good	
4	74	F	orbital pain, IIIrd nerve palsy	4 cm	none	died	poor condition
5	15	M	trigeminal pain V/1, 2; ophthalmoplegia amaurosis left	3 cm	trapping	excellent	amaurosis left unchanged
6	43	F	none	4 cm	balloon occlusion with ligation of ICA	good	accidental diagnosis after postoperative CT and transnasal hypophysectomy
7	80	F	SAH	2.5 cm	direct clipping	died	ischemic lesion MCA right
8	68	F	left trigeminal pain V/1, 2, IIIrd nerve palsy	4 cm	balloon occlusion with ligation of ICA	excellent	trigeminal pain V/1, 2, resolved, IIIrd nerve palsy improved, 2nd ICA aneurysm right (1 cm) unchanged
9	64	F	SAH	1 cm	direct clipping	died	1. postop. transient meningitis—recovered 2. died after 6 weeks from cerebellar hemorrhage (A-V malformation)
10	54	F	headache, trigeminal pain	1 cm	wrapping	good	
11	52	F	loss of visual field	3 cm	direct clipping	excellent	
12	34	M	loss of visual field bilateral, pituitary dysfunction	6 cm	ICA ligation with EC-IC	good	
13	63	F	IIIrd and VIth nerve palsy, exophthalmos	6 cm	ICA ligation with EC-IC	excellent	IIIrd nerve palsy improved
14	78	F	loss of visual field	3 cm	direct clipping	died	1. patient already fully mobilized, no deficit

							2. died 4th day postop., myocardial infarction
15	65	F	IIIrd nerve palsy, headache	1.5 cm	ICA ligation with EC-IC	good	
16	31	F	SAH	2.5 cm	direct clipping	excellent working	
17	35	M	SAH	6 mm	rhaphy and wrapping	excellent	
18	53	F	SAH	1.5 cm	no treatment	died	1. patient did not tolerate ligation, no treatment 2. died 1 month after SAH
19	38	F	stroke like onset with hemiparessis left, trigeminal pain	1 cm	exploration, EC-IC	good	
20	54	F	SAH	1 cm	direct clipping	excellent	concomitant ACoA-aneurysm
21	50	F	VIth nerve palsy, trigeminal pain, exophthalmos	4 cm	partial rhaphy balloon occlusion with EC-IC	good	broad neck, enlargement again after rhaphy
22	72	F	trigeminal pain V/1, 2	2 cm	none	no follow-up	
23	47	F	SAH	1.5 cm	wrapping	excellent	concomitant A-V angioma left frontal lobe
24	71	F	IIIrd nerve palsy	3.5 cm	none	no follow-up	
25	25	F	SAH	1 cm	direct clipping	excellent	
26	38	F	SAH	1 cm	none	excellent	2nd aneurysm of ICA, clipped
27	72	F	complete ophthalmoplegia left, trigeminal pain V/1	2.5 cm	ICA ligation	*no* trigeminal pain, ophthalmoplegia *not* improved	
28	58	M	epistaxis	0.5 cm	balloon occlusion with EC-IC	excellent	

which might be performed during the same operation. This technique is similar to the intramural thrombosing induced with varius metallic material [8].

Conclusion

The management of infraclinoid and intracavernous internal carotid aneurysms should follow these strategies:

1. The direct approach in symptomatic cases if the patient is in good general condition and there is radiological evidence of a suitable neck for clipping;

2. If no direct approach for clipping is possible internal carotid ligation or, much preferable occlusion with a detachable balloon should be performed when there is evidence of good collateral circulation;

3. With insufficient collateral circulation an EC-IC bypass with an occlusion of the internal carotid artery to follow might be performed;

4. Asymptomatic small intracavernous aneurysm cases should be followed by periodic neuroimaging, since they have a tendency to enlarge [2, 6, 9, 18].

References

1. Berenstein A, Ransohoff J, Kupersmith M, Flamm E, Graeb D (1984) Transvascular treatment of giant aneurysms of the cavernous carotid and vertebral arteries. Surg Neurol 21: 3–12
2. Debrun G, Fox A, Drake C (1981) Giant unclippable aneurysms: treatment with detachable balloons. AJNR 2: 167–173
3. Diaz FG, Ausman JI, Pearce EP (1982) Ischemic complications after combined internal carotid artery occlusion and extracranial-intracranial anastomosis. Neurosurgery 10: 563–570
4. Dolenc V (1983) Direct microsurgical repair of intracavernous vascular lesions. J Neurosurg 58: 824–831
5. Gelber BR, Sundt TM Jr (1980) Treatment of intracranial and giant carotid aneurysms by combined internal carotid ligation and extra- to intracranial bypass. J Neurosurg 52: 1–10
6. Heros RC (1983) Surgical management of large paraclinoid aneurysms. Contemp Neurosurg 5: 1–6
7. Hopkins LN, Grand W (1979) Extracranial-intracranial arterial bypass in the treatment of aneurysms of the carotid and middle cerebral arteries. Neurosurgery 5: 21–31
8. Hosobuchi Y (1985) Giant intracranial aneurysms. In: Wilkins RH, Rengachary SS (eds) Neurosurgery. McGraw-Hill, New York, pp 1404–1414
9. Kodama N, Mineura K, Fujiwara S, Suzuki J (1979) Surgical treatment of carotid-ophthalmic aneurysms. In: Suzuki J (ed) Cerebral aneurysms. Neuron Publ, Tokyo, pp 268–274

10. Koos WT, Perneczky A, Schuster H, Vorkapic P (1985) Zerebrale Riesenaneurysmen. In: Schürmann K (ed) Der zerebrale Notfall. Urban & Schwarzenberg, Munich, pp 163–176
11. Nishioka H (1966) Results of the treatment of intracranial aneurysms by occlusion of the carotid artery in the neck. J Neurosurg 25: 660–682
12. Parkinson D (1982) Surgical management of internal carotid artery aneurysms within the cavernous sinus. In: Schmidek H, Sweet WH (eds) Operative neurosurgical techniques. Grune & Stratton, New York, pp 815–828
13. Pilcher C, Thuss C (1934) Current blood flow: III cerebral effects of occlusion of the common or internal carotid arteries. Arch Surg 29: 1024–1035
14. Punt J (1979) Some observations on aneurysms of the proximal internal carotid artery. J Neurosurg 51: 151–154
15. Romodanov AP, Shcheglov VI (1982) Intravascular occlusion of saccular aneurysms of the cerebral arterized by means of detachable balloon catheter. In: Krayenbühl H et al (eds) Advances and technical standards in neurosurgery, vol 9. Springer, Wien New York, pp 25–49
16. Roski RA, Spetzler RF (1985) Carotid ligation. In: Wilkins RH, Rengachary SS (eds) Neurosurgery. McGraw-Hill, New York, pp 1414–1422
17. Scialfa G, Vaghi A, Valsecchi F, Bernardi L, Tonon C (1982) Neuroradiological treatment of carotid and vertebral fistulas and intracavernous aneurysms. Neuroradiology 24: 13–25
18. Spetzler RF, Schuster H, Roski RA (1980) Elective extracranial-intracranial arterial bypass in the treatment of inoperable giant aneurysms of the internal carotid artery. J Neurosurg 53: 22–27
19. Vorkapic P, Schuster H, Koos WTh, Perneczky A (1984) Die Bedeutung der extra-intrakraniellen Anastomose in der Behandlung von intrakraniellen Aneurysmen. Angio Arch 6: 117–119

Para- and infraclinoidal aneurysms. Anatomy, surgical technique and report on 22 cases

A. Perneczky, E. Knosp, and Th. Czech

Department of Neurosurgery, University of Vienna Medical School, Vienna, Austria

The internal carotid artery in its intracavernous portion is covered by a soft connective tissue layer. At the entrance of the artery into the subarachnoid space there is a very dense fibrous ring fixing the artery wall at the roof of the cavernous sinus. After cutting the fibrous ring it is possible to dissect along the artery wall without opening the cavernous sinus. The anatomical details are described.

22 patients with aneurysms situated para- and infraclinoidally were treated by the direct surgical approach. In 10 cases the aneurysm was clipped. In 10 patients clipping and resection of the aneurysm sack was performed, while in 2 cases the aneurysm was occluded by sutures. The aneurysm was attacked by the fronto-temporo-basal approach in all cases. In one case the infraclinoidal aneurysm was dissected by a contralateral exposure. In 20 cases the anterior siphon knee of the internal carotid artery was dissected by opening the fibrous ring at the level of the roof of the cavernous sinus. In one case the approach to the lateral sinus wall was performed. Postoperatively 2 patients died because of epidural hematoma and edema, one patient died following myocardiac infarction and one patient died of pneumonia. The ipsilateral and contralateral approaches are anatomically and surgically described.

Introduction

In cases with aneurysms located in the area of the anterior siphon knee, subarachnoid hemorrhage occurs despite their intracavernous location, since part of the aneurysm sack may bulge into the subarachnoid space superiorly. In such cases direct surgical management with the possibilities of partial resection of the aneurysm sack is preferable to interventional

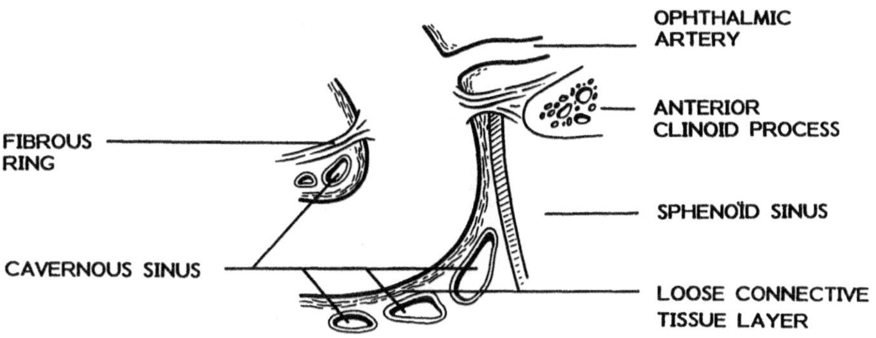

Fig. 1. Sagittal section through the clinoid region demonstrating the dural attachment of the carotid artery wall (fibrous ring)

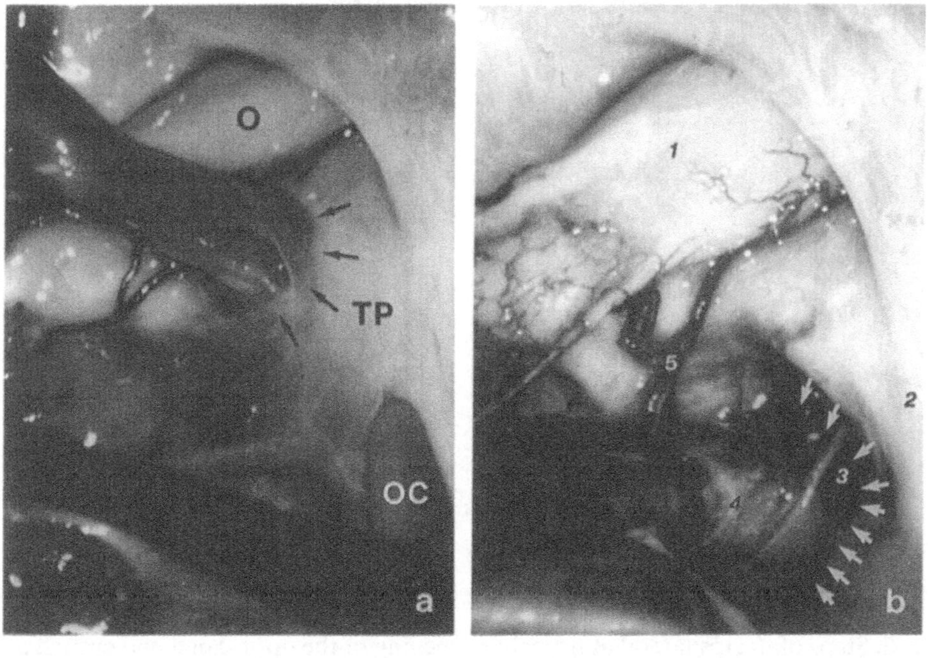

Fig. 2. Anatomical specimen demonstrates the fibrous ring before (**a**) and after (**b**) cutting. Observe the space between carotid artery and cavernous sinus approached by opening the fibrous ring (white arrows). Fibrous ring (arrows), right optic nerve (*O, 1*), transversal plate (*TP*), oculomotor nerve (*OC*), anterior clinoid process (*2*), space with soft connective tissue (*3*), internal carotid artery (*4*), ophthalmic artery (*5*)

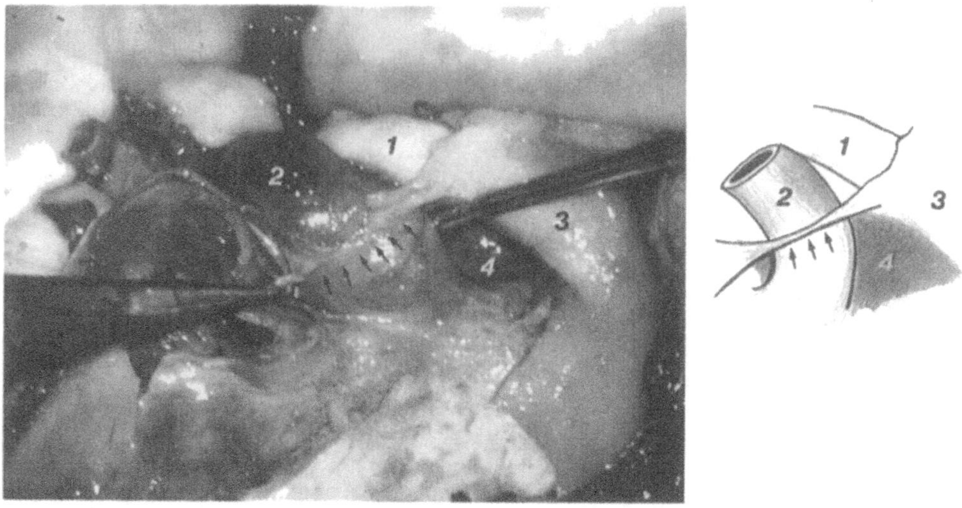

Fig. 3. Anatomical dissection of the fibrous ring with correlation to the optic canal. Lateral view. Right optic nerve (*1*), internal carotid artery, subarachnoidal portion (*2*), optic canal after removal of the bony structures (*3*), region anteriorly of the anterior siphon knee where very rarely venous canals of the cavernous sinus can be found (*4*), fibrous ring (arrows)

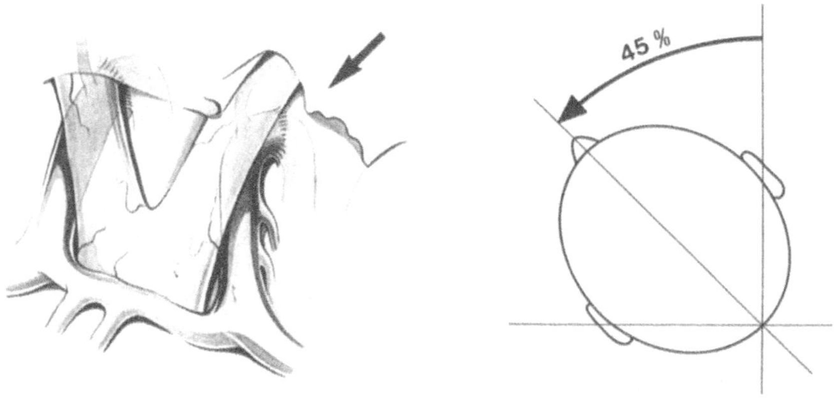

Fig. 4. Scheme of the ipsilateral approach

Fig. 5. Steps of the ipsilateral approach: **a** Opening of the optic canal and cutting a triangle-like dura flap over the anterior clinoid process; **b** Drilling off the clinoid process. Note the dura flap (*df*) protecting the carotid artery and optic nerve during the bone removal; **c** After removal of the anterior clinoid the transversal plate is demonstrated. Subarachnoid bulging of the infraclinoidal aneurysm (arrows); **d** Visualization of the aneurysm dome (arrow) by the use of a mirror; **e** Dissection of the fibrous ring (arrows) by a crystal knife; **f** Slipping of the dissector along the carotid artery wall infraclinoidally after opening of the fibrous ring (arrows). Right optic nerve (*1*), internal carotid artery (*2*), removed anterior clinoid process (*3*), crystal knife (*4*)

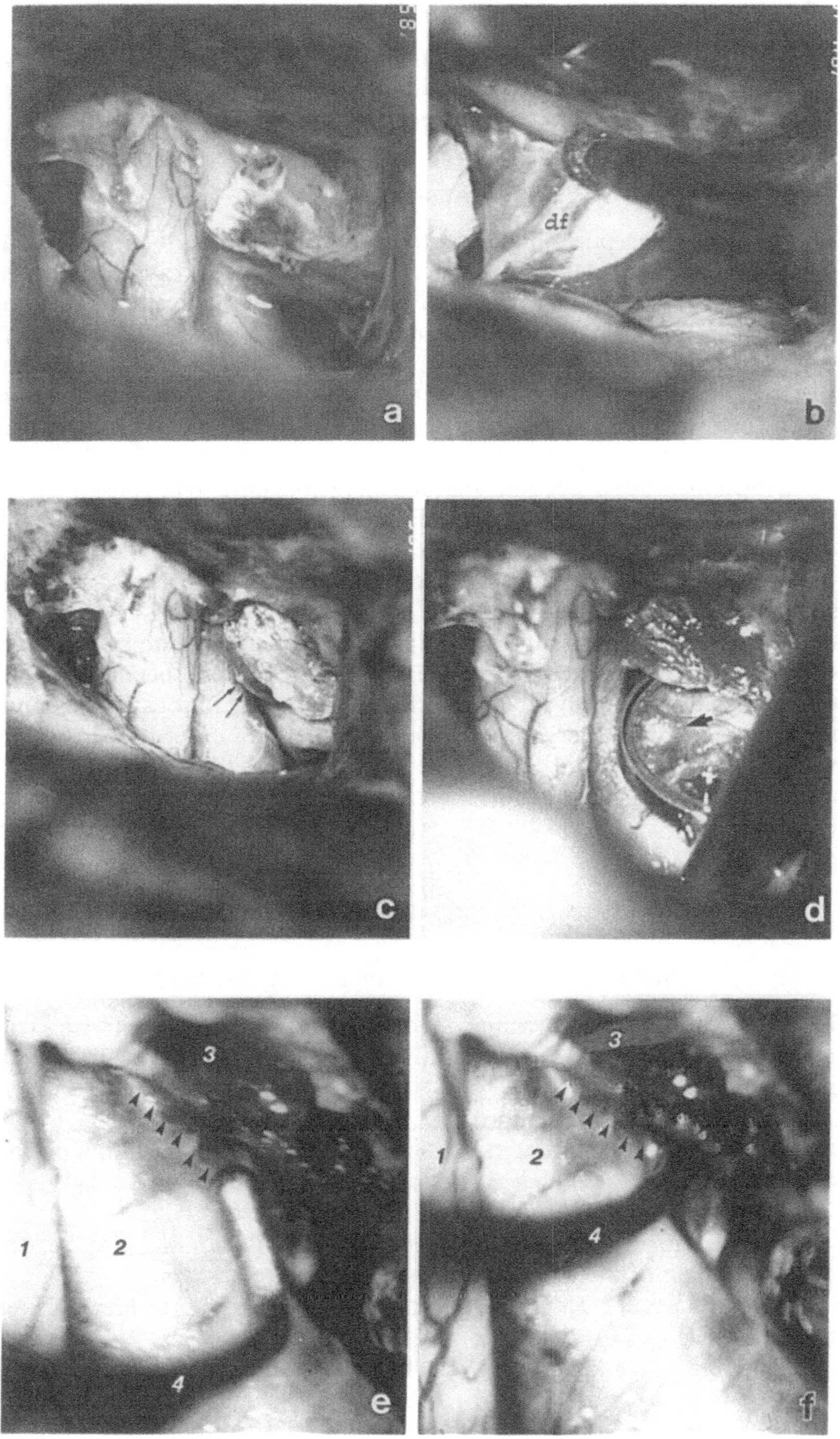
a
df
b
c
d
3
1
2
4
e
3
1
2
4
f

neuroradiological techniques. The microsurgical approach to the anterior siphon knee of the internal carotid artery is discussed by means of anatomical studies [8, 9] and clinical cases.

Anatomy

The intracavernous portion of the internal carotid artery is loosely covered by connective tissue. Only at the level of the roof of the cavernous sinus (transversal plate), a solid radial attachment of the carotid wall to the dura can be seen (Fig. 1). If this attachment is sharply dissected, a loose layer of connective tissue is reached, where blunt exposure of the anatomical structures can be undertaken along the entire wall of the intracavernous carotid artery without opening the sinus. This dissection is easier in younger post-mortem cases (Fig. 2).

In intraoperative dissection, anatomical factors have to be considered as well. On the one hand, the anterior siphon knee is very rarely surrounded by venous canals of the cavernous sinus. On the other hand, the level of the transversal plate is located deeper than the anterior clinoid process, planum sphenoidale and tuberculum sellae.

Thus, in the ipsilateral approach, the anterior clinoid has to be resected. Equally, in the contralateral approach a part of the planum sphenoidale and the tuberculum sellae have to be resected to expose the fibrous ring around the internal carotid artery in the transversal plate. In order to gain better visibility, the appropriate canal of the optic nerve has to be opened in both cases in order to make gentle mobilization of the optic nerve possible (Fig. 3).

Surgery

Ipsilateral approach to the anterior siphon knee

In cases with para- and infraclinoidal aneurysms, where the aneurysm sack points antero-laterally, posterolaterally or laterally, we choose an ipsilateral pterional approach (Fig. 4).

Steps of the ipsilateral approach:

a) unroofing of the ispilateral optic canal for gentle mobilization of the nerve (Fig. 5 a);

b) removal of the anterior clinoid process (Fig. 5 b);

c) identification of the transversal plate and the fibrous ring (Fig. 5 c, d);

d) dissection of the fibrous ring sharply (Fig. 5 e);

e) blunt dissection along the internal carotid artery up to the anterior siphon knee (Fig. 5 f);

f) clipping of the aneurysm neck (Fig. 6).

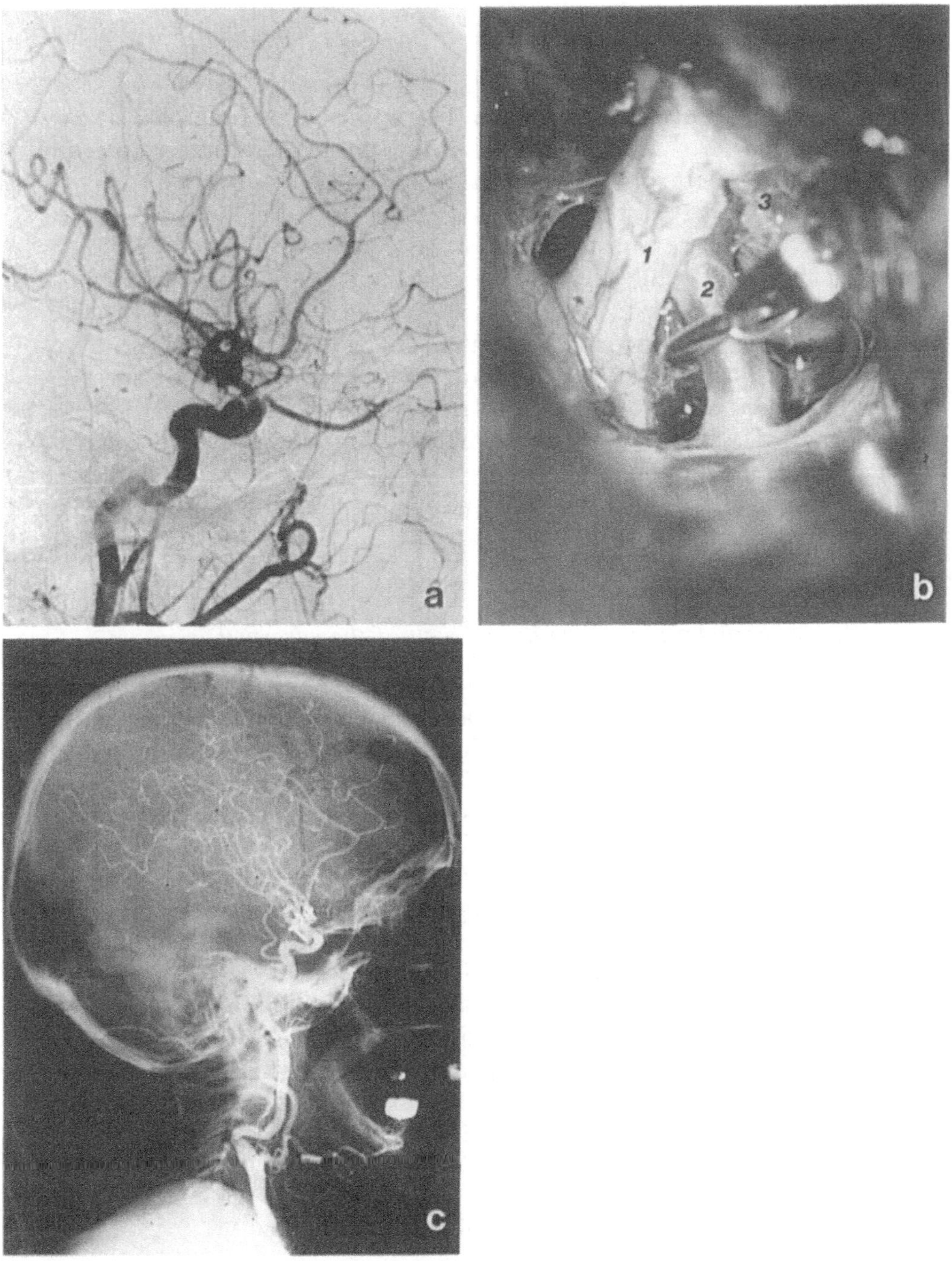

Fig. 6. Angiograms and clipping in the case demonstrated in Fig. 5. **a** Preoperative angiogram with small infraclinoidal aneurysm located posteriorly to the carotid artery. **b** Clipping of the aneurysm by an angled fenestrated Sugita-clip. Right optic nerve (*1*), carotid artery (*2*), removed anterior clinoid process (*3*). **c** Postoperative angiogram

Contralateral approach to the anterior siphon knee

In cases where the aneurysm points from infraclinoidal to medial the contralateral approach is appropriate. This approach obliquely leads below the optic chiasm to the medial wall of the contralateral internal carotid artery. The craniotomy is performed fronto-latero-basaly (Fig. 7).

The steps of the dissection are:

a) opening of the chiasmatic cistern (Fig. 8 a);

b) removal of the tuberculum sellae: the mucosa of the sphenoid sinus is left intact and retracted (Fig. 8 b);

c) removal of the medial wall of the contralateral optic canal;

d) identification of the contralateral transversal plate and fibrous ring;

e) sharp dissection of the fibrous ring (Fig. 8 c);

f) blunt dissection along the medial and anterior wall of the carotid artery up to the anterior siphon knee;

g) clipping of the aneurysm neck: the opened sphenoid sinus is closed by muscle and fibrin glue (Fig. 8 d).

Approach through the lateral wall of the cavernous sinus

If the lesion is located more proximally along the intracavernous carotid artery portion and direct surgery has been chosen, we use a modified approach through the lateral wall of the cavernous sinus. The craniotomy is orbito-pterional (Fig 10 a, b).

Since the lateral sinus wall consists of two layers, between them nerves III, IV and V are located, it is possible to open the outer layer like a flap without tearing the venous space (Fig. 10 c, d). So the Gasserian ganglion and the peripheral divisions of the trigeminal nerve can be visualized. The fibers of the nerve can be held away and the medial layer of the sinus wall is demonstrated. In cases of vascular lesions it is necessary to use plugging of the venous space after opening of the lateral wall (tabotamp, cotton pieces). In tumor cases the sinus is occluded by the tumor mass: therefore in such cases there is no risk of bleeding by opening the lateral wall (Fig. 11, case 16).

At the end of the dissection the lateral sinus wall can be closed by suturing of the flap. The only nerve which hardly can be saved this way is the abducent nerve.

Cases and results

22 cases of para- and infraclinoidal aneurysms were operated on by the surgical approach described above. There were 18 women and 4 men. Thirteen patients had subarachnoid hemorrhage and 5 of them underwent acute surgery. In 10 cases the aneurysm had a diameter of more than 2.5 cm and two other patients had an aneurysm larger than 1.5 cm (Table 1).

In all 22 cases presented the anterior portion of the intracavernous internal carotid artery was dissected. There were no intraoperative complications. Eighteen patients had carotido-ophthalmic aneurysms with partial extradural extension of the aneurysm neck. Four other patients had an extradural aneurysm with intradural bulging of the aneurysm dome. In 10 cases the aneurysm was clipped by one or more clips. In 10 patients the aneurysm sack was evacuated, resected and the neck clipped. In two cases the sack was occluded by sutures.

One patient died on the first postoperative day following epidural hemorrhage. Another patient died on the second day because of brain edema and vasospasm. Three patients had fatal late complications. One died on the sixth day following myocardiac infarction, one on the 21st day because of cerebellar hemorrhage caused by an intracerebellar AVM and one patient died on the 42nd day following pneumonia. All other patients showed good or excellent results.

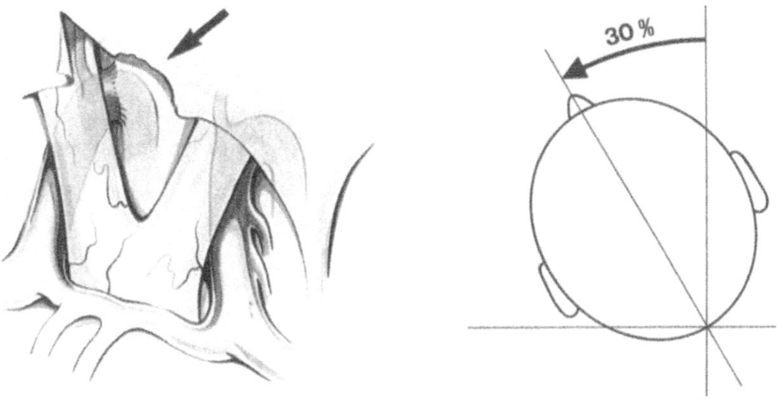

Fig. 7. Scheme of the contralateral approach

Discussion

Aneurysm originating in the area of the anterior siphon knee may partly reach into the subarachnoid space and thus cause subarachnoid hemor-

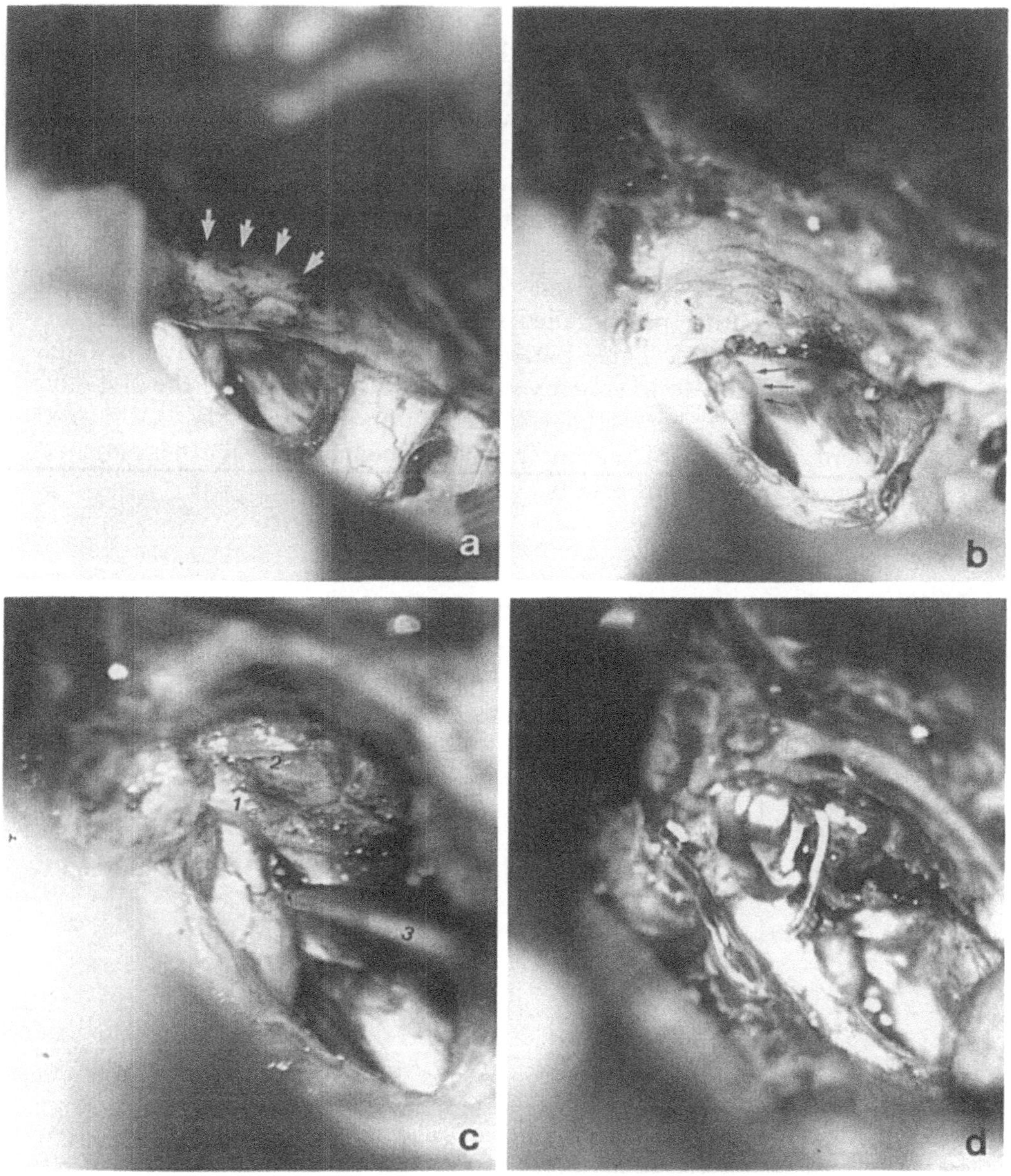

Fig. 8. Steps of the contralateral approach: **a** After opening of the chiasmatic cistern the dura will be removed (arrows) above the tuberculum sellae; **b** Drilling of the tuberculum sellae. The transversal plate and the fibrous ring (arrows) of the opposite side can be seen; **c** Sharp dissection of the fibrous ring by a crystal knife. Aneurysm dome (*1*), intact mucosa of the sphenoid sinus (*2*), crystal knife (*3*); **d** Clipping procedure

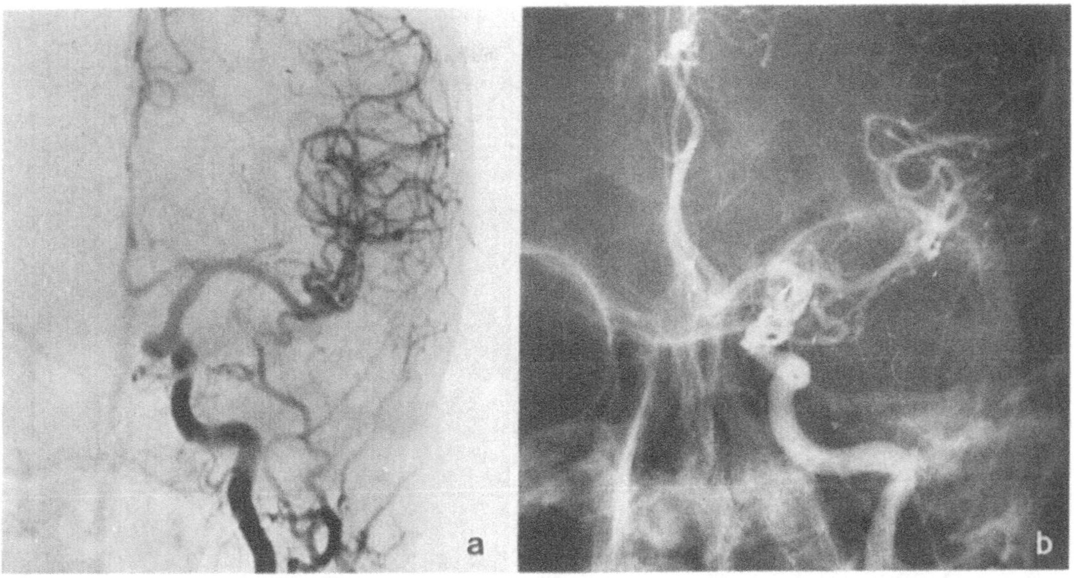

Fig. 9. Angiograms of the case demonstrated in Fig. 8 with an aneurysm arising medially from the internal carotid artery. Preoperative (**a**), postoperative (**b**)

rhage. Very few publications, however, indicate direct surgical management of such aneurysms by a transcavernous approach [1, 7]. This approach presents considerable risks. It requires a major amount of anaesthesiological attention and is inferior to the interventional neuroradiological methods. This is particularly the case with occlusion of carotid cavernous fistulas. Indirect methods such as carotid artery ligation and trapping do not lead to a satisfying result, since often ischemic complications and amaurosis occur ipsilaterally [4, 6, 13].

The anatomical investigations we performed [8, 9, 10] have shown that it is possible to expose the anterior siphon knee without opening the cavernous sinus in a way as to provide good visibility of the adjacent structures and to permit constant control. This approach makes the direct surgical management of infraclinoidal aneurysms in the anterior C3 segment of the internal carotid artery possible.

The loose layer of connective tissue along the wall of the intracavernous carotid artery, which has already been described, represents a good guide layer for preservation of the artery when dissecting tumors [9].

Even in many cases with carotido-ophthalmic aneurysm the fibrous ring has to be divided for making possible the closure of the whole aneurysm neck with patency of the internal carotid and ophthalmic arteries (Figs. 12, 13).

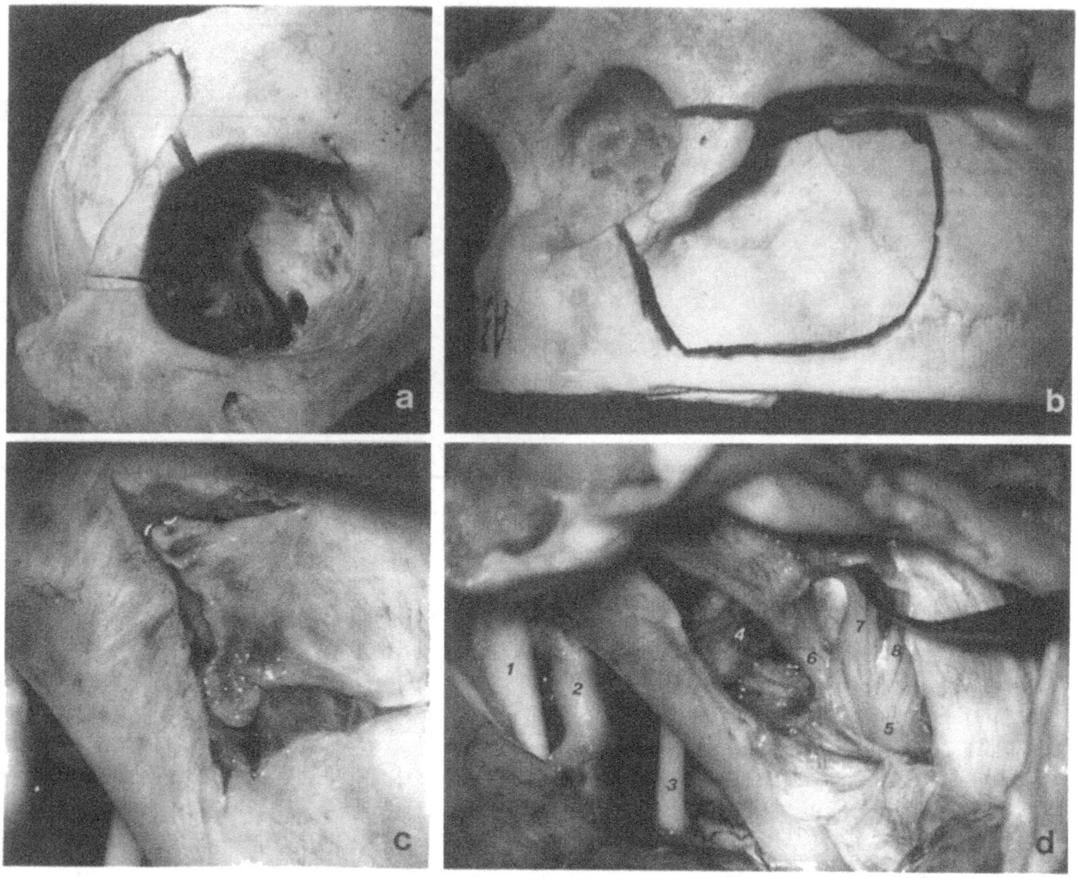

Fig. 10. Anatomical demonstration of the approach to the lateral cavernous sinus wall: **a** Frontal view of the combined orbito-pterional approach demonstrating the line of the craniotomy; **b** Surgeons view of the craniotomy; **c** Flap-like dissection of the superficial layer of the dura in the lateral cavernous sinus wall; **d** Demonstration of the different divisions of the trigeminal nerve between them a save approaching to the posterior siphon knee is possible. Right optic nerve (*1*), right internal carotid artery, subarachnoid portion (*2*), right oculomotor nerve (*3*), posterior siphon knee (*4*), Gasserian ganglion (*5*), ophthalmic nerve (*6*), maxillary nerve (*7*), mandibular nerve (*8*)

Fig. 11. Giant infraclinoid aneurysm of the right internal carotid artery treated by direct surgery through the lateral wall of the cavernous sinus as described in Fig. 10 (case 16). **a** Intraoperative view of the approach. Right optic nerve (*1*), right internal carotid artery, subarachnoid portion (*2*), right temporal lobe (uncus) (*3*), bulging of the lateral sinus wall by the large intracavernous aneurysm (*4*); **b** Intraoperative situation after flap-like opening (*df*) of the lateral sinus wall. Maxillary nerve (*5*); **c** Intraoperative angiography before occlusion of the aneurysm; **d** Intraoperative angiography demonstrating the closure of the aneurysm and patency of the internal carotid artery

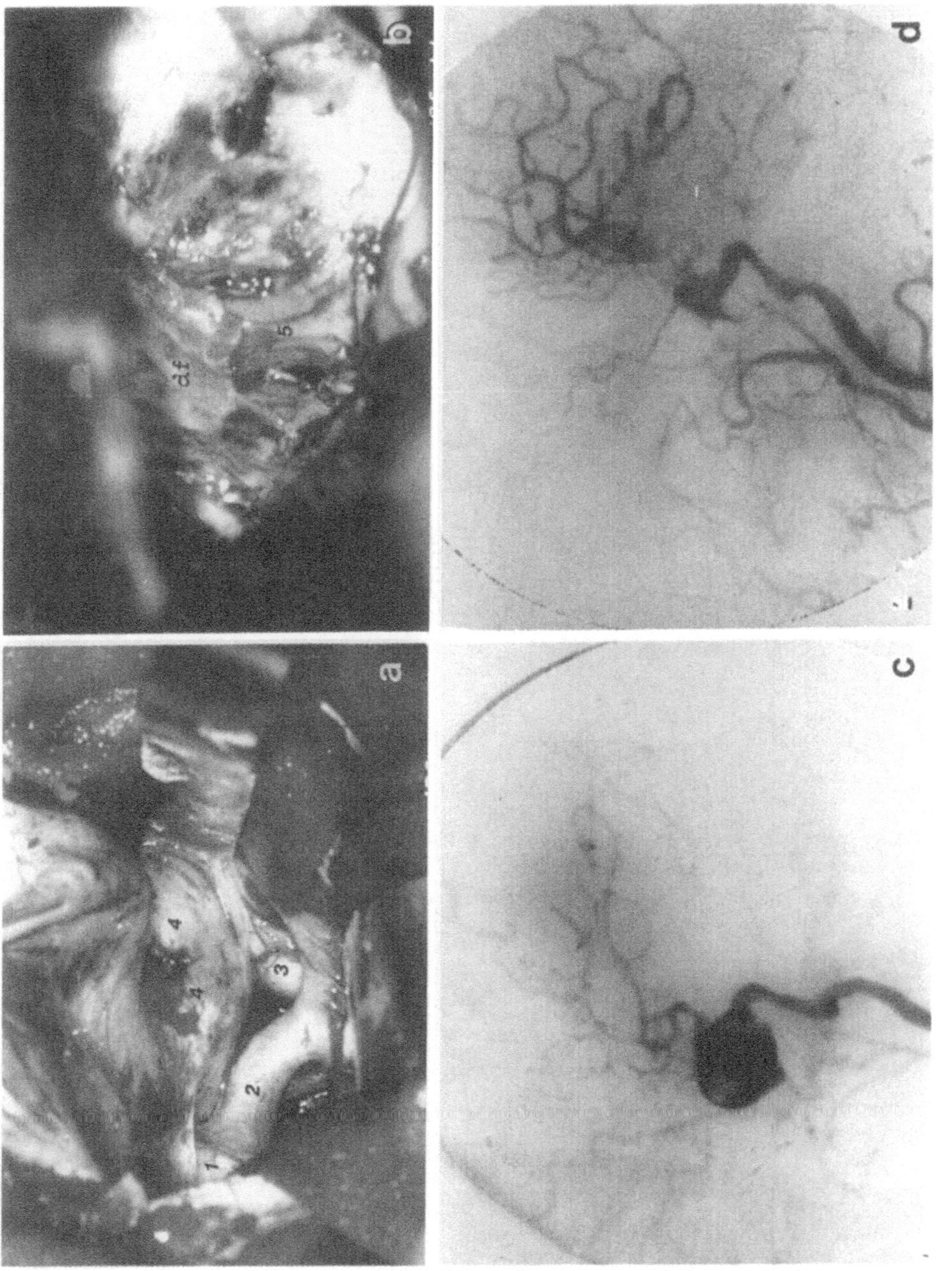
a
b
c
d
1
2
3
4
5
df

Table 1. The description of cases and their results (para- and infraclinoidal aneurysms)

Case	Name	Sex	Location	∅	SAH	Surgery	Result	Remarks
1	S. E.	F	right ophth.	1 cm	+	clipping (1 clip)	excellent	
2	M. G.	F	right ophth.	3 cm	—	clipping (3 clips) resection	excellent	
3	B. M.	F	left ophth.	2.5 cm	+ a.	clipping (2 clips) resection	excellent	
4	L. E.	F	right ophth.	3 cm	—	clipping (3 clips) resection suture	excellent	post-traumatic aneurysm
5	Sch. A.	M	left ophth.	2.5 cm	—	clipping (4 clips) resection	excellent	post-traumatic aneurysm
6	Sch. M.	F	right ophth.	5 cm	—	clipping (3 clips)	died	on 6th postop. day, myocard. infarction

7	S. H.	F	left ophth.	2.5 cm	+ a.	clipping (2 clips) resection	excellent	vasospasm
8	J. M.	F	left ophth.	1 cm	+ a.	clipping (1 clip) resection	excellent	intraop. rupture
9	H. H.	F	left ophth.	1.5 cm	—	clipping (1 clip)	excellent	
10	M. O.	F	right carot.	1 cm	+	clipping (1 clip)	excellent	
			right ophth.	3 mm		clipping (1 clip)		
11	W. E.	F	comm. ant.	3 mm	+	clipping (1 clip)	excellent	
			left ophth.	3 mm		clipping (1 clip)		
12	L. R	M	right ophth.	1 cm	+	clipping (1 clip)	good	
13	F. M.	F	right ophth.	2.5 cm	+	clipping (2 clips) resection	on 42th day stage III, pulm. died	temp. clipping of internal carotid, 4.5 min.

Table 1. (continued)

Case	Name	Sex	Location	∅	SAH	Surgery	Result	Remarks
14	S. W.	F	left ophth.	2.5 cm	died	clipping (2 clips)	excellent	
15	R. J.	F	left ophth.	5 cm	—	clipping (3 clips)	on 2nd day edema died	intraop. rupture, temp. clip. of carotid 10 min.
16	Z. M.	F	extradural right	3.5 cm	—	direct surg., (lat. sinus wall) balloon occlus., suture	no change	2nd stage balloon embolization
17	Z. R.	F	partial intradural right	5 mm	+	clipping (1 clip)	died	

18	T. R.	M	partial intra-dural right	4 mm	+	suture	excellent	
19	J. St.	F	partial intra-dural left	5 mm	+	contra-lateral approach clipping (1 clip)	excellent	after 3 weeks, cerebel. he-morrh. AVM
20	A. M.	F	left ophth.	8 mm	—	clipping (1 clip) resection	excellent	tuberculum sel-lae meningioma
21	W. Ch.	M	partial intra-dural left	8 mm	+ a.	clipping (1 clip)	excellent	two more aneu-rysms, all clip-ped
22	I. R.	F	right ophth.	20 mm	+ a.	clipping (2 clips) resection	excellent	pregnancy 4th month

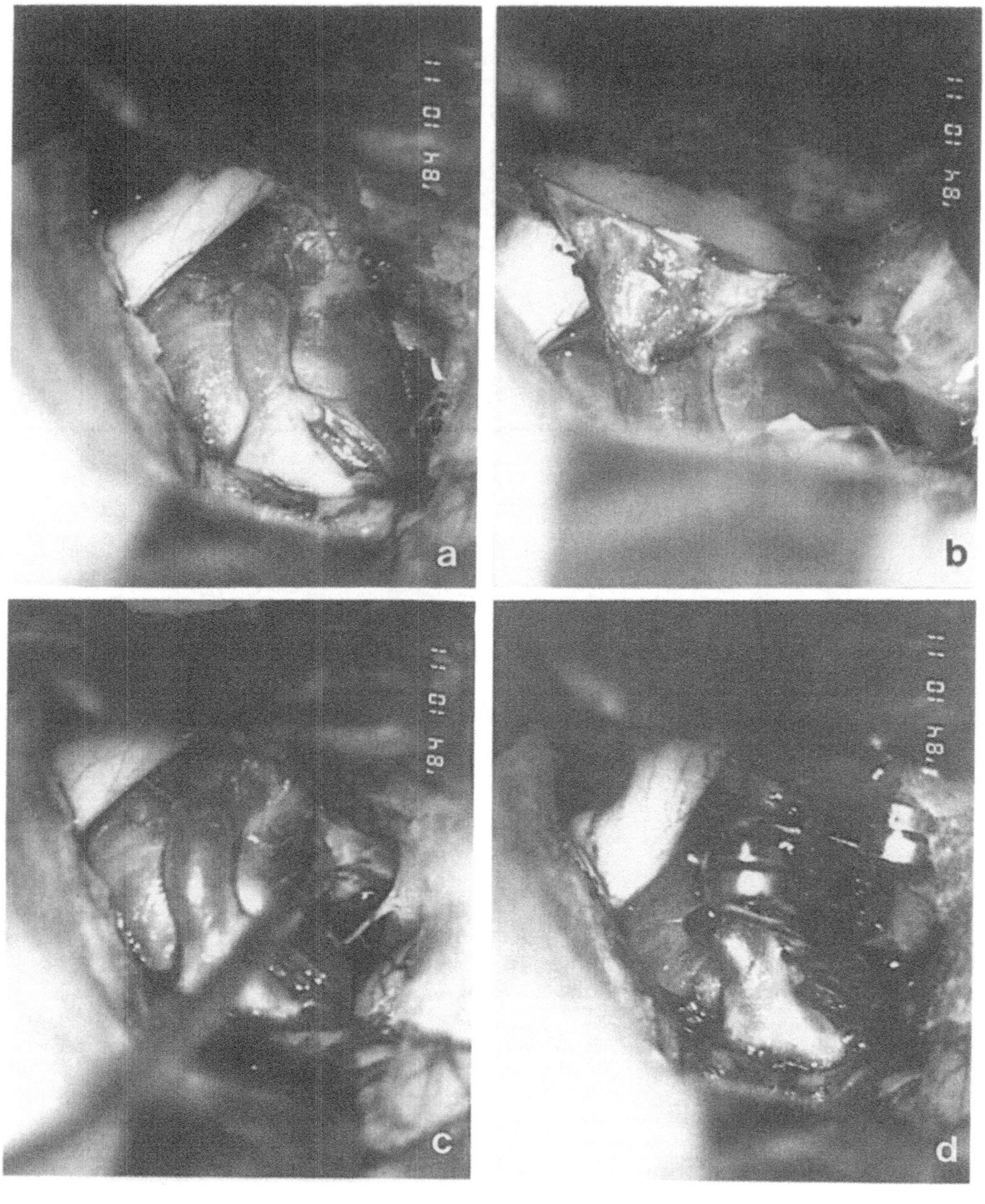

Fig. 12. Giant para- and supraclinoidal aneurysm of the right carotid artery (case 2). The extension of the fusiform aneurysm neck made the infraclinoidal dissection necessary. **a** Intraoperative survey. **b** Dura flap protecting the aneurysm, carotid artery and optic nerve during the removal of the anterior clinoid process and surrounding bony structures. **c** The fusiform paraclinoidal portion of the aneurysm neck after the bone removal. **d** Clipping procedure with 3 fenestrated Sugita-clips

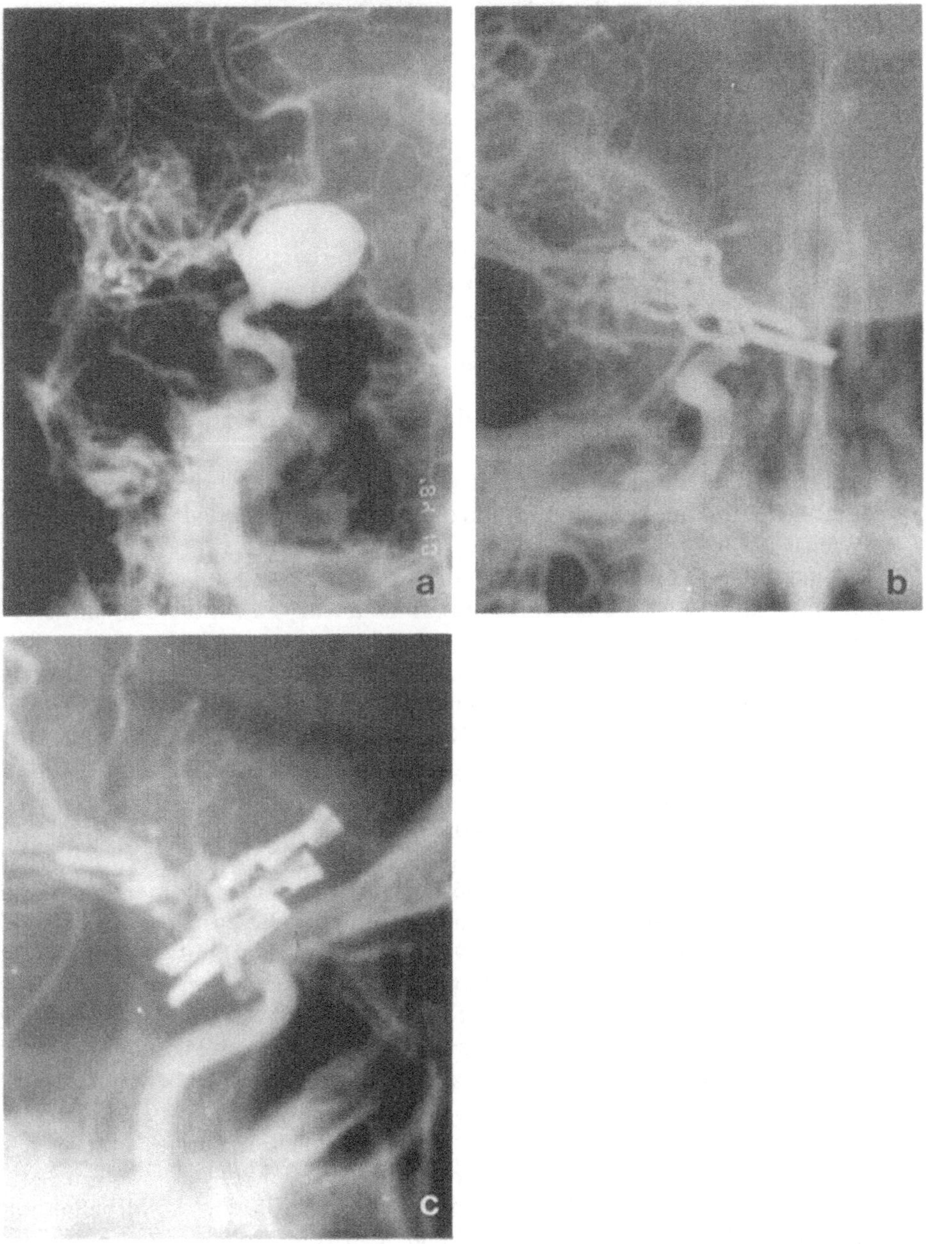

Fig. 13. Angiograms of the case (case 2) demonstrated in Fig. 12. Preoperative angiogram (**a**), postoperative angiograms (**b, c**)

With regard to the aneurysm it has been demonstrated that for those originating antero-laterally and postero-laterally, an ispilateral approach is preferred.

In cases of smaller aneurysm (diameter < 1 cm) originating anteromedially or posteromedially the best approach is from the contralateral side. In the latter case, the first part of the exposure is similar to the description provided by other authors [5, 3, 14].

References

1. Dolenc V (1983) Direct microsurgical repair of intracavernous vascular lesions. J Neurosurgery 58: 824–831
2. Iwabuchi T, Suzuki Sh, Sobata E (1978) Intracranial direct operation for carotid-ophthalmic aneurysm by unroofing of the optic canal. Acta Neurochir (Wien) 43: 163–169
3. Milenkovic Z, Gopic H, Antovic P, Jovicic V, Petrovic B (1982) Contralateral pterional approach to a carotid-ophthalmic aneurysm ruptured at surgery. J Neurosurg 57: 823–825
4. Mitsugi T, Kikuchi H, Karasawa J, Itoh K, Takahashi N (1981) Surgical treatment of carotid-siphon aneurysms. Neurol Med Chir (Tokyo) 22: 513–520
5. Nakao S, Kikuchi H, Takahashi N (1981) Successful clipping of carotid-ophthalmic aneurysms through a contralateral pterional approach. J Neurosurg 54: 532–536
6. Nutik S (1978) Carotid paraclinoid aneurysms with intradural origin and intracavernous location. J Neurosurg 48: 526–533
7. Parkinson D (1965) A surgical approach to the cavernous portion of the carotid artery. Anatomical studies and case report. J Neurosurg 23: 474–483
8. Perneczky A, Knosp E, March (1982) The intracavernous portion of the internal carotid artery. Presented at the am eur neurosurg winter conf on cerebrovascular diseases and posterior fossa pathology in Obergurgl (Austria)
9. Perneczky A, Knosp E (1986) The intracavernous connective tissue cover of the internal carotid artery. Anatomy and surgery. In: Scheunemann H (ed) Tumors of the skull base. de Gruyter, Berlin New York, pp 177–177
10. Perneczky A, Knosp E, Vorkapic P, Czech T (1985) Direct surgical approach to infraclinoidal aneurysms. Acta Neurochir (Wien) 76: 36–44
11. Perneczky A, Knosp E, July (1985) direct surgical approach to infraclinoidal aneurysms. Presented at the world congr neurosurg in Toronto
12. Perneczky A, Knosp E (1985) Direct surgical approach to infraclinoidal aneurysms. In: Auer LM (ed) Timing of aneurysm surgery. de Gruyter, Berlin New York, pp 323–329
13. Tesal JS, Bergeron R Th, Rumbaugh CL, Segall HD (1973) Aneurysms of the petrous or cavernous portions of the internal carotid artery associated with nonpenetrating head trauma. J Neurosurg 38: 568–574

14. Yamada K, Hayakawa T, Oku Y, Maeda Y, Ushio Y, Yoshimine T, Kawai R (1984) Contralateral pterional approach for carotid-ophthalmic aneurysm: usefulness of high resolution metrizamide or blood computed tomographic cisternography. Neurosurgery 15: 5–8

Direct approaches to vascular lesions in the cavernous sinus via the medial triangle

A. Hakuba, Y. Matsuoka, T. Suzuki, M. Komiyama, T. B. Jin, and Y. Inoue

Department of Neurosurgery and Radiology,
City University Medical School, Osaka, Japan

Vascular lesions in the cavernous sinus were radically operated on under normal body temperature in a semi-sitting position which reduced pressure in the sinus. In this series of 17 cases of various kinds of vascular lesions in the cavernous sinus, the approach leads by a fronto-latero-basal craniotomy to the superior and lateral walls of the cavernous sinus. Via an ispilateral approach, the medial triangle in the superior wall was opened for repair of the vascular lesions of the C 3 and C 4 portions of the internal carotid artery, and Parkinson's triangle in the lateral wall was opened for lesions of the C 5 portion. Via a contralateral approach, the medial side of the medial triangle was opened for clipping of the aneurysm originating from the medial wall of the C 3 portion. Both the ipsilateral and the contralateral approaches to the vascular lesions in the cavernous sinus are presented in this paper.

Introduction

From the anatomical point of view, the medial triangle [3, 4] is a part of the superior wall of the cavernous sinus (CS); it forms the roof of both the medial part of the posterior superior cavity and the medial cavity of the CS, in which there are no important neural structures. Therefore it is very safe and easy to open the medial triangle in order to explore the C 3 and C 4 portions of the internal carotid artery (ICA). The medial triangle is hidden antero-laterally by the anterior clinoid process, anteriorly by both the optic canal and the optic nerve and medially both the planum sphenoidale and the tuberculum sellae. Hence in the ipsilateral approach, the anterior clinoid process, and, in the contralateral approach the planum sphenoidale and tuberculum sellae, have to be resected, and also in both approaches the optic canal and its dural sheath must be opened [3, 4, 5, 8, 12].

The purpose of this paper is to describe the detailed surgical techniques for radical operation on the vascular lesions under normal body temperature and their operative results.

Anatomy of the cavernous sinus

The CS is a kind of pentahedron (Fig. 1). The lateral wall of the CS is a dural fold consisting of an outer layer of dense connective tissue and an inner layer of loose connective tissue, in which the third, fourth and fifth cranial nerves are enveloped and Parkinson's triangle is present. The posterior wall of the CS is bounded by the plica petroclinoidea posterior above and the lateral part of the upper end of the clival dura mater below. The medial wall is bordered by the lateral wall of the pituitary gland. And the superior wall is a triangular shape which is bordered laterally by Parkinson's triangle, posteriorly by the plica petroclinoidea posterior and medially by the diaphragma sellae. In the superior wall, the medial triangle [3, 4] is bounded by the line connecting between the dural entrance of the oculomotor nerve and the anterior rim of the origin of the C 2 portion of the ICA laterally, by the line between the anterior rim of the origin of the C 2 portion of the ICA and the lateral edge of the posterior clinoid process medially and by the line between the lateral edge of the posterior clinoid process and the dural entrance of the oculomotor nerve posteriorly (Figs. 1, 4 d). When the ICA is freely present within the CS, the CS can be divided into four cavities instead of three as reported by Harris et al. [6] with respect to the cavernous portion

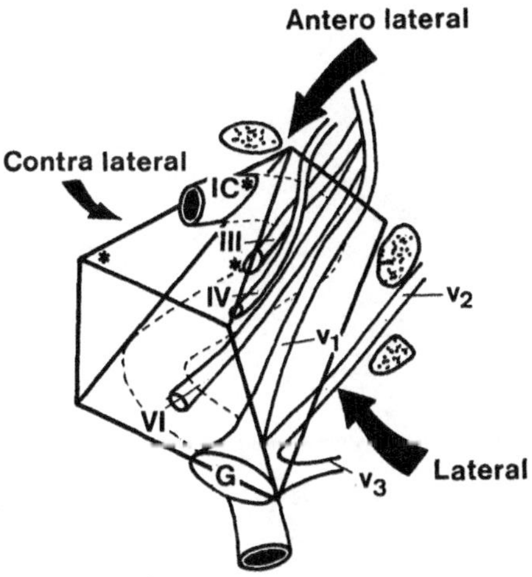

Fig. 1. Schematic diagram of the cavernous sinus. The medial triangle is formed by connecting three points (*) in the superior wall of the cavernous sinus. Arrows indicate the respective approaches. *G* Gasserian ganglion; *III* oculomotor nerve; *IV* trochlear nerve; *V*/1, V/2, and *V*/3 first, second and third divisions of trigeminal nerve; *VI* abducens nerve

of the ICA; the anterior inferior cavity, posterior superior cavity, lateral cavity and medial cavity. This was confirmed by the explorations of the sinuses in our cases.

Operative techniques

There are two principal approaches according to the location of the lesions in the cavernous portion of the ICA: ipsilateral approach and contralateral approach.

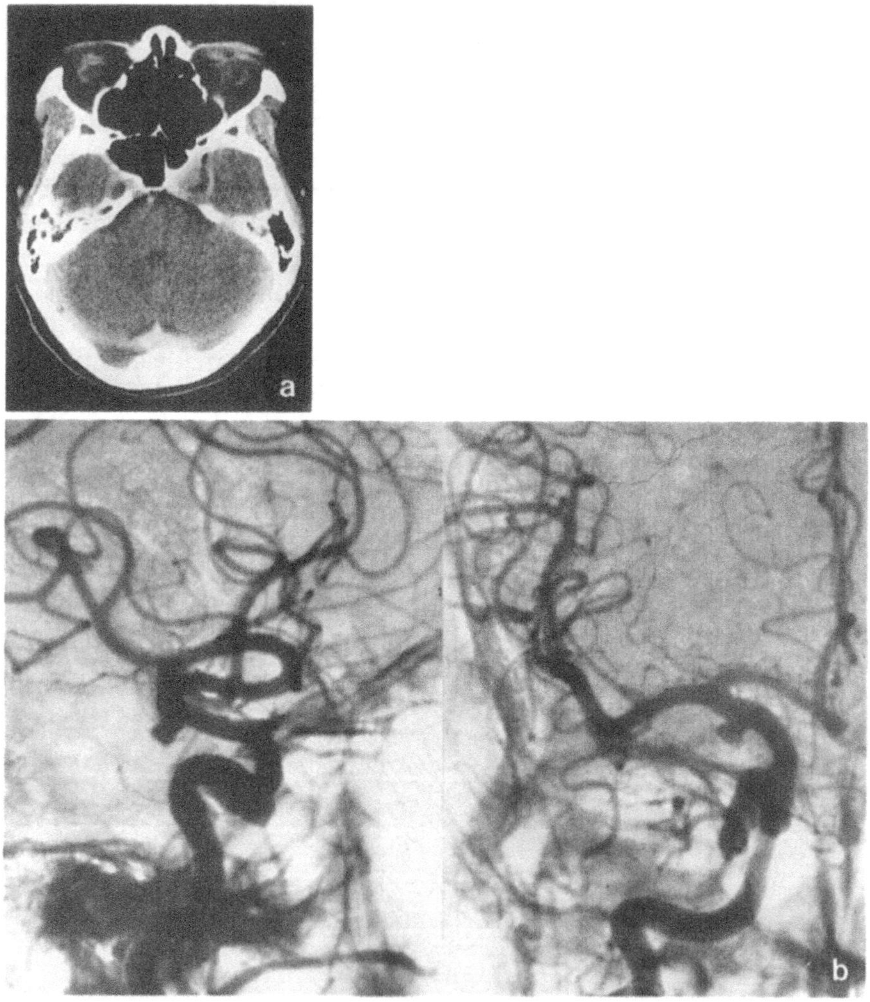

Fig. 2. A 54-year-old woman with an aneurysm originating in the lateral wall of the C4–C5 portion of the internal carotid artery. **a** Enhancement CT scan showing a cystic mass in the right cavernous sinus, of which the lateral wall and the medial half are enhanced. **b** Carotid arteriogram. Left: lateral view, right: A-P view. A small aneurysm at the bifurcation of the anterior choroidal artery and a large partially thrombosed aneurysm at the C4–C5 junction

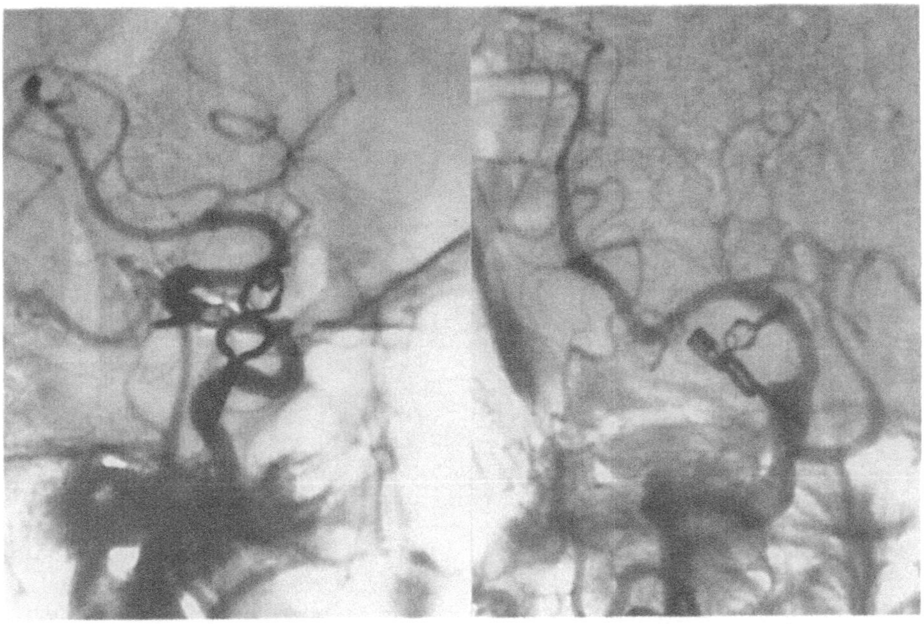

Fig. 3. The same case. Postoperative right carotid arteriogram showing no aneurysm and Yaşargil's clips applied successfully to the neck of the aneurysms

Ipsilateral approach

Via the ipsilateral subfronto-pterional transsylvian approach, the vascular lesions of the lateral parts of the C 3 and C 4 portions, and the C 5 portion can be managed.

The surgical technique for clipping a large aneurysm originating at the lateral wall of the C 4–C 5 junction is described as follows (Figs. 2a, b, and 3).

Positioning and skin incision

The patient is placed on the healthy side in a semi-sitting position (Fig. 4 a). By using a Mayfield's three-pin headholder, the head is elevated and kept in an extended position at the craniovertebral junction and then rotated about 15 degrees toward the healthy side. The skin flap is reflected forward. A unilateral fronto-lateral-basal craniotomy is performed.

Exposure of the medial trangle

Via a subfronto-pterional transsylvian approach, the dura mater along the limbus sphenoidalis, the posterior rims of the anterior clinoid process and the medial part of the sphenoid wing is divided, which are exposed

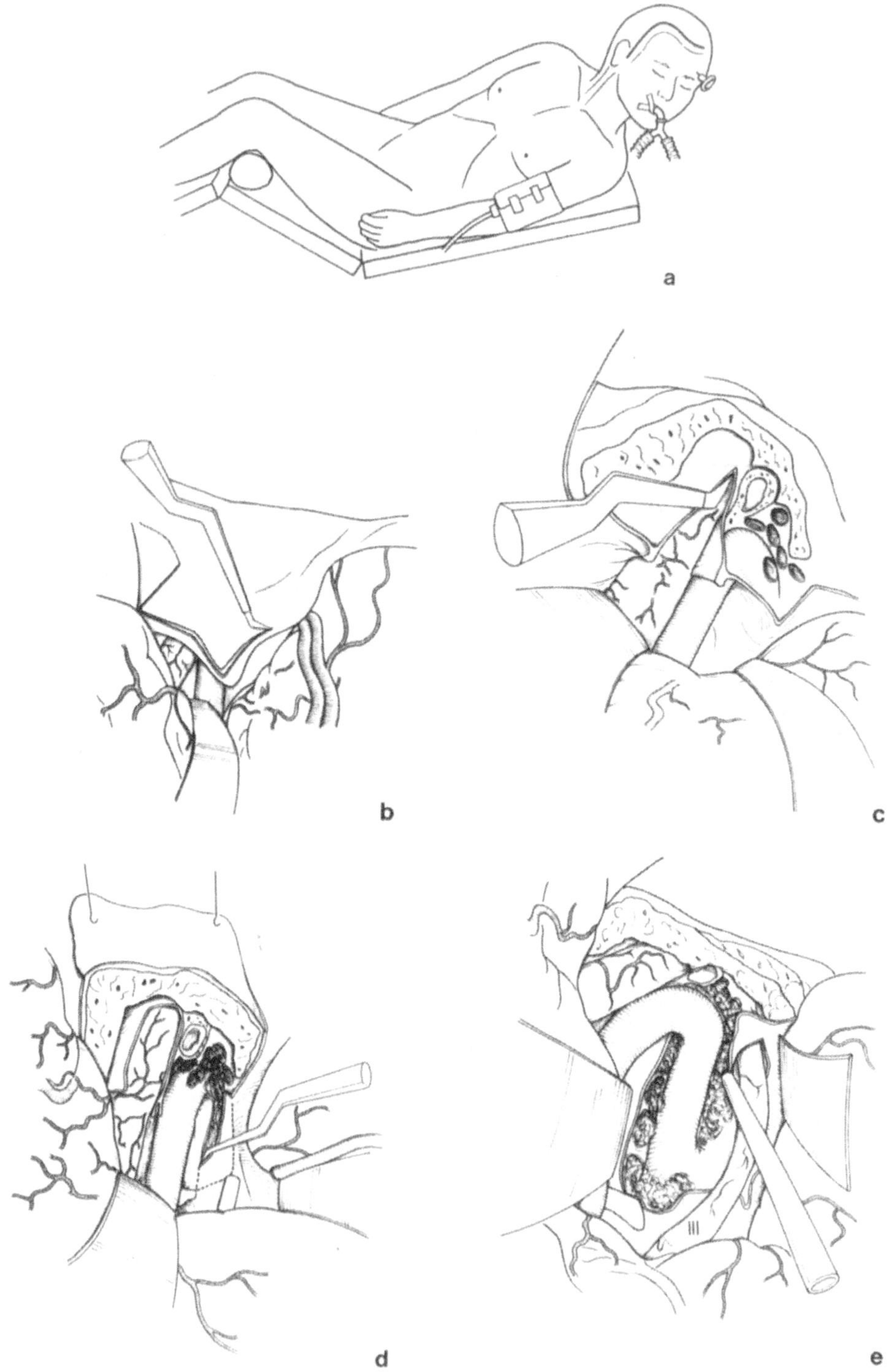

Fig. 4. a–e

subperiosteally with the dural fringe retracted forward by suture ligations to the more anterior dura mater. The anterior clinoid process and the superior, lateral and inferior walls of the optic canal are drilled out by using a high speed air drill. The dura propria and the falciform dural fold covering the optic nerve are opened forward (Fig. 4c). The lateral leaf of the opened optic sheath along the anterior margin of the origin of the C 2 portion is divided, and the medial triangle is now well exposed.

The exposure of the C 3 and C 4 portions of the ICA through opening of the superior wall of the CS via the medial triangle

In order to expose the lateral part of the C 3 portion, the anterior part of the medial triangle is opened along the lateral rim of the origin of the ICA and the antero-lateral part of the anterior inferior cavity of the CS is plugged by either insertion of * Biobond-soaked Oxycel [3] or insertion of Fibrinogen-soaked Gelfoam and Thrombin-soaked Gelfoam [4].

The medial side of the medial triangle is opened while plugging the medial cavity with multiple pieces of the same material as described above (Fig. 4 d), and the C 4 portion is exposed. The oculomotor nerve is denuded by opening the dorsal wall of its dural sheath in the lateral wall of the CS in order to bring about gentle mobilization of the nerve and then the remaining posterior part of the lateral side of the medial triangle to the dural entrance of the nerve is opened while plugging the posterior superior cavity. The dural fringe of the opened medial triangle is elevated and retracted backwards, and the C 4 portion is exposed while dividing the trabeculae and plugging the medial and lateral cavities. An additional opening of the posterior side of the medial triangle between the dural entrance of the oculomotor nerve and the lateral margin of the posterior clinoid process is made while plugging the remaining posterior part of the posterior-superior and lateral cavities.

The distal part of the C 5 portion and the neck of the aneurysm are exposed from their medial side by this means (Fig. 4 e) and a clip is applied to it (Fig. 3).

Fig. 4. a Positioning of the patient and a half coronal incision along the hairline. **b** Via the subfronto-pterional-transsylvian approach, the dura mater along the posterior margins of the medial part of the sphenoid wing, the anterior clinoid process is divided. **c** The dura propria of the optic nerve is opened along the lateral margin of the nerve. The medial triangle is exposed. **d** The medial triangle is about to be opened. Dotted lines indicate the medial triangle. **e** The medial triangle has been opened and the neck of the aneurysm is exposed. The oculomotor nerve (*III*) has been well exposed

Contralateral approach

The contralateral subfronto-pterional transsylvian approach is suitable for clipping aneurysms originating from the medial wall of the C 3 portion of the ICA (Fig. 5 a, b).

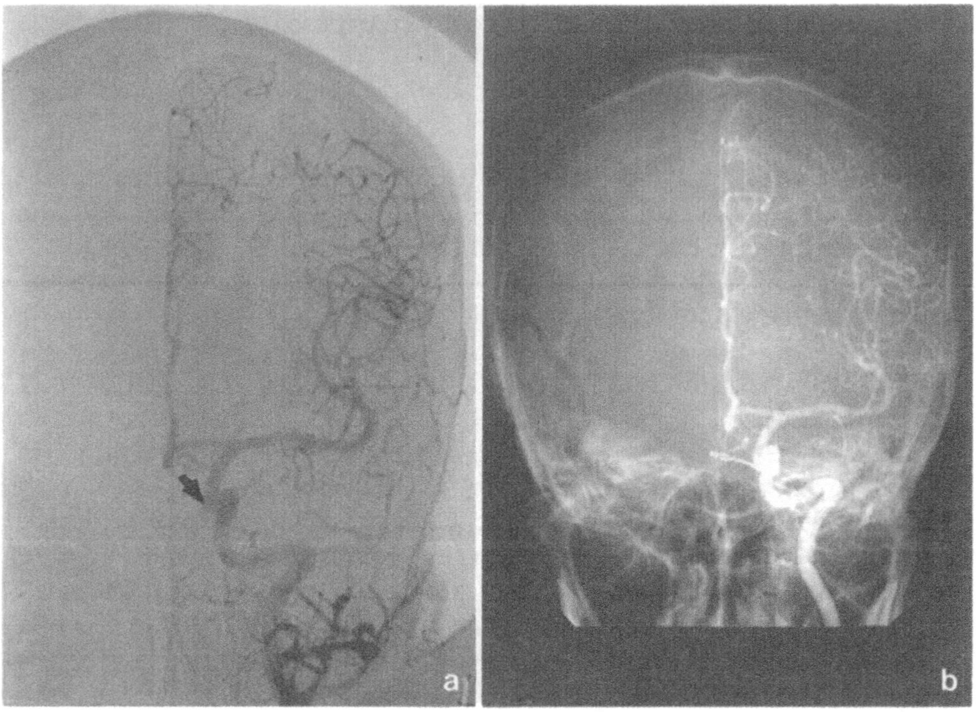

Fig. 5 a. Preoperative left carotid arteriogram of a 52-year-old woman with an aneurysm (arrow) originating from the medial part of the C 3 portion of the left internal carotid artery. **b** The postoperative left carotid arteriogram of the same patient

Positioning and craniotomy

The positioning is the same as described above, but the head is turned toward the side of the lesion about 15 degrees and a contralateral frontotemporal craniotomy with removal of the lateral part of the sphenoid wing is performed.

Exposure of the medial side of the medial triangle

Via the contralateral fronto-pterional transsylvian approach, the dura mater on the planum sphenoidale is divided in the midline toward the limbus sphenoidalis and then the dural incision is made along it extending into the posterior margin of the anterior clinoid process on either side (Fig. 6 a). The dural fringes are elevated and retracted forward by suture ligations. The planum sphenoidale and the superior, medial and inferior walls of the optic canal on the side of the lesion as well as the tuberculum sellae and the anterior wall of the sella turcica more on the side of the lesion are drilled away with preservation of the mucosa of the sphenoïd sinus. The dura propria and falciform dural fold covering the optic nerve are opened forwards (Fig. 6 b). The dura mater of the tuberculum sellae and anterior wall of the sella turcica are divided obliquely from the midline to the medial rim of the origin of the C 2 portion and the medial side of the medial triangle is exposed (Fig. 6 c).

Dividing the medial site of the medial triangle for exposure of the medial anterior, medial and medial posterior walls of the C 3 portion of the ICA.

The dura mater along the medial and anterior rims of the origin of the C 2 portion is opened and the medial part of the anterior inferior cavity is opened while plugging it in the same manner (Fig. 6 d). The medial anterior part of the C 3 portion can be exposed by this means. The dura mater in the lateral part of the diaphragma sellae is opened along the medial side of the medial triangle, and the roof of the medial cavity is opened by this means (Fig. 6e). The medial posterior wall of the C 3 portion is well exposed. The neck of the aneurysm is dissected out and a clip is applied to it.

The opened paranasal sinuses and the defects of the dura mater are closed and made watertight by using muscle pieces and a fascia lata graft taken from the patient's thigh.

Materials and results

Since 1974, the authors have operated on 17 patients with vascular lesions in the CS. Thirteen of them were operated upon via an ipsilateral approach; 6 aneurysms originating in the lateral wall of the C 3 portion of the ICA, one carotid-cavernous fistula (CCF) originating in the antero-medial wall of the C 3 portion, two aneuryms, one traumatic aneurysm and one CCF originating in the lateral wall of the C 4 portion, and one CCF and one tentorial arteriovenous malformation originating in the antero-lateral wall of the C 5 portion. A contralateral approach was applied to the remaining four patients for clipping of the aneurysms originating from the medial wall of the C 3 portion (Table 1). Out of 17 patients, one with an aneurysm of the lateral wall of the C 3 portion complicated by a malignant glioma died of a recurrent tumor 6 months after the surgery. Oculomotor palsy developed as an operative complication in 8 cases in whom exploration of the lateral wall of the CS was performed. This dysfunction was improved within three to four months after the interventions in 6 cases. And the remaining 2 cases (one CCF and one aneurysm originated at the C 4 portion) had double

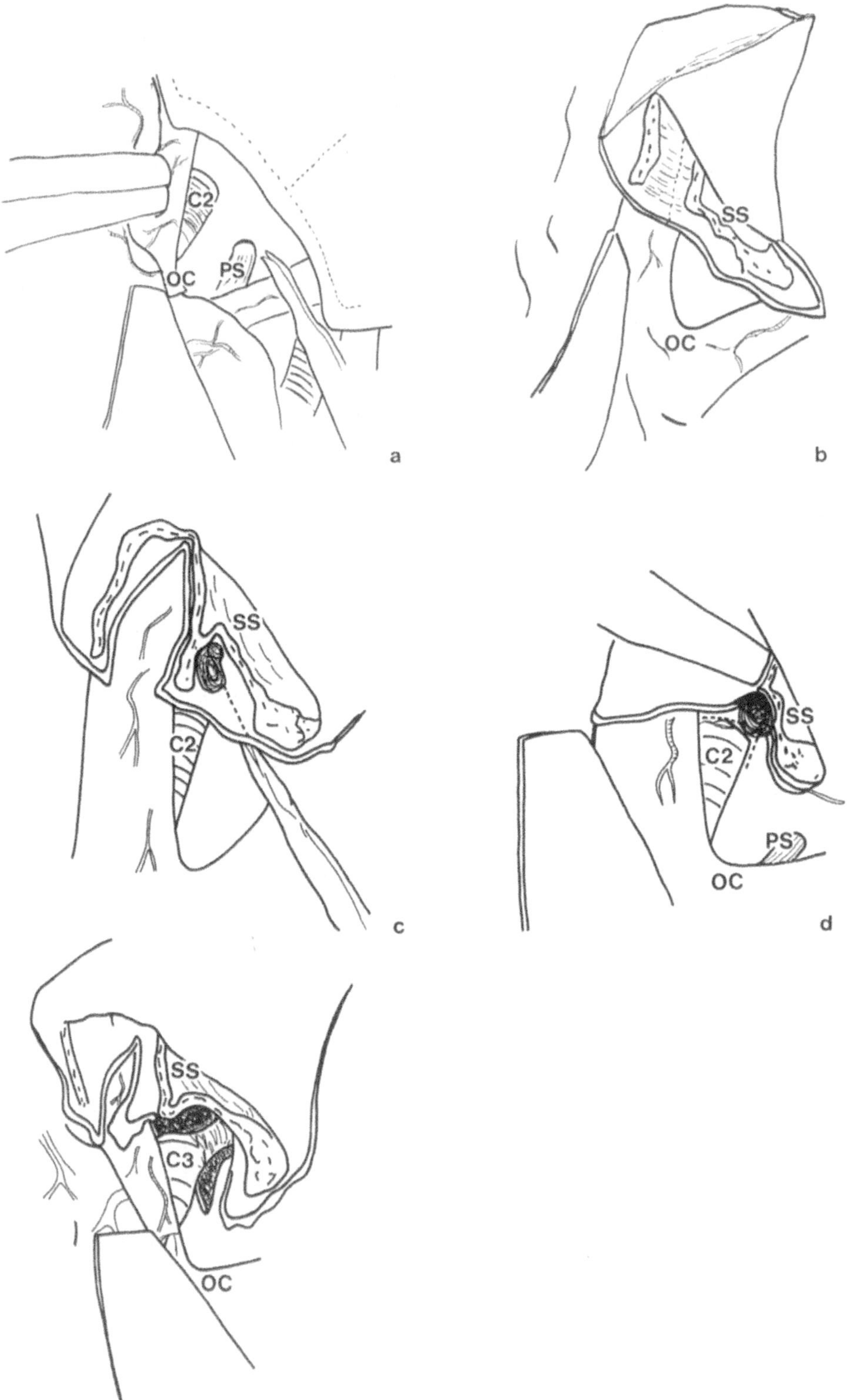

e

Fig. 6 a.–e.

vision due to permanent partial oculomotor palsy. Two cases of giant aneurysms originated at the medial part of the C 3 portion developed blindness on the side of the operation. One with a large traumatic aneurysm, who was blind O.U. with diabetes insipidus and whose carotid arteriograms showed complete obstruction of the C 3 portions of both the internal carotid arteries, remained blind but diabetes incipidus was improved and both the internal carotid arteries became patent after the repair of the lacerated C 5 portion of the left ICA via the medial triangular approach.

Eleven patients (9 aneurysms, one AVM of the tentorium and one CCF originating in the C 3 portion) recovered completely and returned to their work within three to four months after surgery.

Discussion

The approach to the lateral cavity and the posterior superior cavity is done through Parkinson's triangle, via which a direct surgical approach to the cavernous sinus was successfully performed by Parkinson [10, 11] more than 20 years ago. His technique was conducted under hypothermia and a CCF was successfully operated upon.

However, this technique was soon replaced by introduction of the balloon catheter technique and the successful treatment of the CCF and aneurysm in the CS has been accomplished in increasing numbers [1].

Recently after the introduction of the microsurgical technique, the direct approach to the cavernous sinus became feasible under normal body temperature. The anterior part of the anterior inferior cavity was approached by Mullan [9] who successfully treated a CCF with a large

---

Fig. 6. a Via the antero-lateral approach, the dura mater along the posterior margins of the anterior clinoid process and the planum sphenoidale (*PS*) is about to be opened; **b** The full length of the medial half of the optic nerve inside the optic canal has been exposed, and the dura propria of the optic nerve is about to be opened along the medial margin of the optic nerve; **c** The dura mater of the tuberculum sellae and the anterior wall of the sella turcica are about to be divided obliquely from the midline to the medial rim of the origin of the C 2 portion; **d** The medial and anterior margins of the dura mater of the origin of the C 2 portion of the ICA and the dura mater of the lateral part of the diaphragma sellae which is divided in the line of the medial side of the medial triangle under the C 2 portion are about to be opened (dotted line); **e** The anterior inferior cavity and the medial cavity have been opened and the neck of the aneurysm has been exposed. *C 2, C 3* C 2 and C 3 portions of the left ICA; *OC* Optic chiasma; *SS* Sphenoid mucosa

Table 1. Approaches to vascular lesions in the cavernous sinus

	Aneurysm	Traumatic aneurysm	CCF	Tentorial AVM	Total
1. Approach to the lateral part of the C 3 portion: fronto-temporal craniotomy, transsylvian approach, removal of the anterior clinoid process and the superior, lateral and inferior walls of the optic canal and opening of the anterior part of the medial triangle in order to explore the lateral part of the anterior inferior cavity and the anterior part of the posterior superior cavity	6		1		7
2. Approach to the lateral part of the C 4 portion: includes all steps under 1. and is followed by opening the medial triangle in order to explore the medial cavity and the medial part of the posterior superior cavity	2	1	1		4
3. Approach to the C 5 portion: includes all steps under 2. and is followed by opening Parkinson's triangle			1	1	2
4. Approach to the medial part of the C 3 portion: contralateral-frontotemporal craniotomy, transsylvian approach, removal of the superior, medial and inferior walls of the optic canal and opening the medial site of the medial triangle in order to explore the medial part of the anterior inferior cavity and the anterior part of the medial cavity	4				4
					17

anterior inferior cavity via an anterior extradural approach to the triangular portion between the superior and inferior orbital fissures above the foramen rotundum. The medial cavity was approached successfully through the transethmoidal-transsphenoidal approach by Laws [7]. Dolenc [2] reported a successful direct approach to the cavernous sinus via a lateral approach with exposure of the C 6 portion. Perneczky et al. [12] performed successful clippings of infraclinoidal aneurysms without opening the sinus, especially in cases with extradural extension of the aneurysmal neck.

The authors reported 17 cases of vascular lesions in the CS which were operated upon directly under normal body temperature. Good results were obtained in all cases without mortality directly related to the operations. A semi-sitting position was used in all cases in order to reduce the venous pressure nearly to 0 except for the cases of CCF [3, 4, 5, 8], and bleeding at the CS opening is very easily controlled by insertion of multiple pieces of glue-soaked Oxycel [3, 4] or Gelfoam [4, 5]. The opening of the CS via the medial triangle in its superior wall is a relatively easy and safe procedure because there are no important anatomical structures except for the ICA and with such precautions as described above we can perform relatively safe operations for vascular lesions under normal body temperature.

References

1. Debrun G, Lacour P, Caron JP (1977) Balloon arterial catheter techniques in the treatment of arterial intracranial disease. In: Krayenbühl H et al (eds) Advances and technical standards in neurosurgery, vol 4. Springer, Wien New York, pp 131–145
2. Dolenc VV (1983) Direct microsurgical repair of intracavernous vascular lesions. J Neurosurg 58: 824–831
3. Hakuba A, Nishimura S, Shirakata S, Tsukamoto M (1982) Surgical approaches to the cavernous sinus; report of 19 cases. Neurol Med Chir (Tokyo) 22: 295–308
4. Hakuba A (1985) Surgical approaches to the cavernous sinus via the medial triangles: report of an aneurysm at the C 4–C 5 junction of the internal carotid artery. Geka Shinryo 26. 1385–1390
5. Hakuba A (1986) Surgical approaches to the cavernous sinus: repair of a C-C fistula at the C 5 portion of the internal carotid artery. Neurol Surg (Tokyo) 14: 601–607
6. Harris FS, Rhoton AL (1976) Anatomy of the cavernous sinus. A microsurgical study. J Neurosurg 45: 169–180
7. Laws ER Jr, Onofrio BM, Pearson BW, Mc Donald TJ, Dirrenberger RA (1979) Successful management of bilateral carotid-cavernous fistulae with a trans-sphenoïdal approach. Neurosurgery 4: 162–167

8. Matsuoka Y, Hakuba A, Kishi H, Nishimura S (1986) Direct surgical treatment of intracavernous internal carotid artery aneurysms; report of four cases. Surg Neurol 26: 360–364
9. Mullan S (1979) Treatment of carotid-cavernous fistulas by cavernous sinus occlusion. J Neurosurg 50: 131–144
10. Parkinson D (1965) A surgical approach to the cavernous portion of the carotid artery. Anatomical studies and case report. J Neurosurg 23: 474–483
11. Parkinson D (1967) Transcavernous repair of carotid cavernous fistula. Case report. J Neurosurg 26: 420–424
12. Perneczky A, Knosp E, Vorkapic P, Czech TH (1985) Direct surgical approach to infraclinoidal aneurysms. Acta Neurochir (Wien) 76: 36–44

Treatment of internal carotid infraclinoid aneurysms

H. Sano, V. K. Jain, Y. Kato, M. Hoshino, M. Shoda, H. Tanji, Y. Kamei, K. Katada, and T. Kanno

Department of Neurosurgery, Fujita-Gakuen Health University, Toyoake, Aichi, Japan

Operation on aneurysms has become safe and easy because of the development of microsurgery and many instruments. However, some kinds of surgery are still difficult due to the aneurysm's location or size. The carotid cavernous or ophthalmic aneurysm is one of the most difficult aneurysms. Therefore this paper reports our operative results on carotid ophthalmic and intracavernous aneurysms.

Patients

660 cases of aneurysm surgery were performed personally in several institutes until May 1986, including 16 cases of carotid ophthalmic and 5 cases of intracavernous carotid aneurysms. Five cases of carotid ophthalmic aneurysms and 4 cases of intracavernous carotid aneurysms were giant.

Table 1. Patients

Total number of personal cases of aneurysm operation until May 1986		660
IC ophthalmic aneurysm		16
Giant aneurysm	5	
Small aneurysm	11	
IC cavernous aneurysm		5
Giant aneurysm	4	
Large aneurysm	1	

Method

Carotid ligation or trapping with SAT-MCA anastomosis were performed in 7 cases. Two of them developed ophthalmoplegia and visual disturbance 1–2 weeks after surgery. Coating was done in one case of aneurysm situated in the sella turcica who has been living normally now for over 7 years. Clipping of the aneurysm neck was done in 13 cases. A curved fenestrated clip was the most useful for giant ophthalmic aneurysms. Two cases of small carotid ophthalmic aneurysms directed inferiomedially were operated on using the contralateral approach. In two cases of intracavernous carotid aneurysm the neck was exposed after drilling of the anterior clinoid process and the sphenoid wing. As regards the giant aneurysm the cavernous sinus was open after trapping the aneurysm completely. The aneurysm was opened to examine its cavity internally. Reconstruction of the internal carotid artery was done.

Table 2. Method

Clipping	13 cases
IC ligation + STA–MCA anastomosis	7 cases
Coating	1 case*

* Aneurysm situated in the sella turcica

Results

Two cases of ophthalmic aneurysm were operated on in the early stage. Both cases died because of severity at the onset in a grade V case, and severe vasospasm in a grade III case which was operated on 4 days after SAH. There were 19 cases who were operated on in the chronic stage. Fifteen cases were excellent without any neurological deficit. One case of intracavernous giant aneurysm developed postoperative ophthalmoplegia which disappeared after about 6 months. Three cases developed a permanent neurological deficit postoperatively. Two cases of ophthalmic giant aneurysm in whom IC ligation and STA-MCA anastomosis was done developed ophthalmoplegia and visual disturbance 1–2 weeks after operation. Angiography showed the aneurysm as having disappeared completely at this time. Hemiparesis and aphasia remained after postoperative convulsion in a case of clipping of IC ophthalmic giant aneurysm. Postoperative angiogram revealed the internal carotid artery was occluded at the site of the temporary clipping at the neck.

Table 3. Results

Early operation			2
Dead	2 <	Gr. III (vasospasm) Gr. V	
Delayed operation			19
Excellent (no deficit)	15		16
Good (temporary deficit)	1		
Poor (permanent deficit)	3		

Discussion

Recently ligation of internal carotid artery with EC-IC bypass surgery was recommended on intracavernous or ophthalmic IC aneurysm. However, in the case of a giant aneurysm a mass effect causes the patient's neurological deficit. So aneurysm size must be reduced. Therefore direct clipping should be a better procedure. If the aneurysm can be trapped permanently, it should be possible to tap and reduce the size of the aneurysm. Then aneurysm can be easily clipped. Usually a carotid ophthalmic aneurysm is located inferiorly and medially. In the case of a giant aneurysm a fenestrated clip is the most useful because an operation on a giant aneurysm is not really clipping but reconstruction of the internal carotid artery with clips. In case of a small carotid ophthalmic aneurysm directed inferiomedially the contralateral pterional approach should be selected because the anterior clinoid process, sphenoid wing and orbital roof must be drilled for the ipsilateral pterional approach. However, clipping is easy on the contralateral approach to see the aneurysm directly through the optic chiasma except for the prefixed type of chiasma. A thin sliced amipaque CT scan may help to make a diagnosis of chiasma type. Intracavernous aneurysm is the most difficult operation because of control of bleeding, preservation of nerves and prevention of cerebral ischemia while using temporary clips. As regards control of bleeding, a giant aneurysm is easier than a small aneurysm because a giant aneurysm blocks cavernous sinus by itself. As regards preservation of nerves, an aneurysm is much simple than a tumor. The nerves can be preserved between the aneurysm wall and the sinus dural wall. Therefore we try to prepare the aneurysm just around the entrance of the internal carotid artery. The most important problem is to prevent cerebral ischemia during the temporal trapping of the internal carotid artery. Before and during the operation monitoring is essential, for example angiographical findings and especially cross circulation. The balloon Matas test with EEG, CBF should be applied. If one of these monitors suggests no maintenance of CBF during temporary clipping, simultaneous EC-IC bypass surgery is necessary.

Direct operation on intracavernous giant aneurysm

H. Sano, V. K. Jain, Y. Kato, M. Shoda, H. Tanji, K. Katada, and T. Kanno

Department of Neurosurgery, Fujita-Gakuen Health University, Toyoake, Aichi, Japan

Operation on an intracranial giant aneurysm is one of the most difficult types of surgery. On the other hand operation of the cavernous sinus poses a challenge to neurosurgeons. We had a case of bilateral intracavernous giant aneurysms clipped by direct surgery. This woman developed bilateral abducens palsy, CT showed round contrast enhanced masses situated in both cavernous sinuses. Angiography showed bilateral intracavernous giant aneurysms. The patient was followed up in the outpatient clinic. She started complaining of a headache 2 years afterward. Repeat angiography showed the aneurysm increasing in size. An operation was scheduled following a balloon Matas test monitored by EEG, SEP and clinical symptoms. Frontotemporal craniotomy was done by the usual method. The anterior clinoid process and sphenoid wing were drilled. The cavernous sinus was opened after temporary trapping of the internal carotid artery. The aneurysm was opened and cut to make a carotid artery by clipping. The embolus and air was flushed out before opening and temporary clips. Patient had developed ophthalmoplegia which was improving 3 months after the operation.

Operation on cerebral aneurysms has become easier and safer after the introduction of the operating microscope. However, it is still difficult to operate upon some aneurysms because of their location and size. Giant aneurysms, posterior fossa and intracavernous aneurysms are some of the most difficult aneurysms to operate on [1–11]. We report a case of bilateral intracavernous giant aneurysms one of which was successfully clipped.

Case report

A 73-year-old woman had been suffering from hypertension for 14 years. Four years ago her right eye ball deviated inwards. Three years ago, the left eye also deviated inwards. CT scan and angiography showed bilateral intracavernous giant aneurysms (Figs. 1, 2, 3). She was being followed up in the out-patient clinic. She started having headaches in December 1985. Therefore she was admitted to the neurosurgical ward on May 7, 1986.

Neurological examination on admission revealed nothing except bilateral abducens palsy and right trigeminal neuralgia. CT and angiography were performed again which showed that the right aneurysm had become larger than before (5.7 cm in maximum diameter) (Fig. 4). Collateral circulation came from vertebrobasilar artery to the right internal carotid artery through the posterior communicating artery and from the ophthalmic artery to the right carotid artery. Manual Matas test with EEG monitoring showed δ-activity within 1 minute after compression of the left internal carotid artery, however, there was no clinical manifestation. EEG and clinical status remained unchanged on compression of the right internal carotid artery. The balloon Matas test was repeated monitoring EEG, SEP and clinical status on May 23, which showed the same results.

Surgery was carried out on May 29, 1986. The patient was placed in the supine position with flexion of the head to 30 degrees and rotation of the face to 60 degrees (Fig. 5). A frontotemporal craniotomy was done. The anterior clinoid process and sphenoid wing were drilled. We could see the cavernous sinus under the sphenoid ridge. On opening the dura, the cavernous sinus was found to be swollen with a giant aneurysm (Fig. 6). The internal carotid artery was clipped temporarily in the neck and between the ophthalmic and posterior communicating artery.

The ophthalmic artery was also clipped to trap the aneurysm completely. The aneurysm was punctured through the dura of the cavernous sinus after trapping the aneurysm. The cavernous sinus was opened in the Parkinson's triangle and the aneurysm wall was also opened. The aneurysmal cavity was examined. The aneurysm wall was dissected free and was cut near the internal carotid artery. The aneurysm wall was thin and partly calcified. Reconstruction of the internal carotid artery was done using Sugita clips. Air was flushed out before finally closing the aneurysm (Fig. 7). Then temporary clips were removed and pulsations of the internal carotid artery were recognized. The cavernous sinus was closed with interrupted sutures. The dura and craniotomy wound were closed as usual. Postoperatively the patient was well except for right ophthalmoplegia which gradually recovered in three months (Fig. 8). Postoperative angiogram showed an almost normal internal carotid artery without aneurysm (Fig. 9).

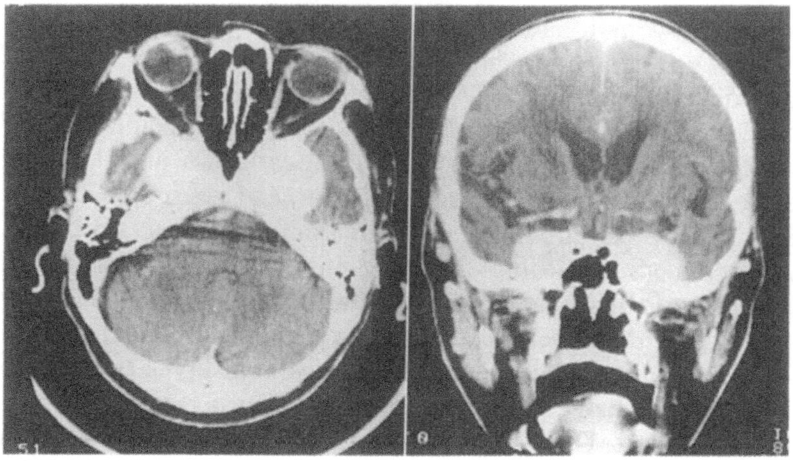

Fig. 1. Preoperative CECT showed a bilateral symmetric contrast enhanced mass at parasellar lesion

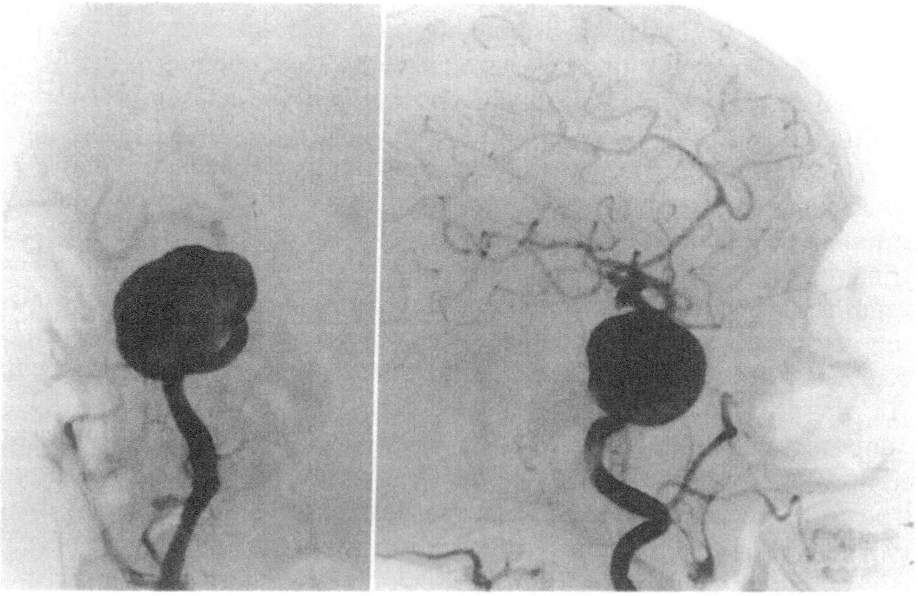

Fig. 2. Right carotid angiogram in 1982 showed an intracavernous giant aneurysm

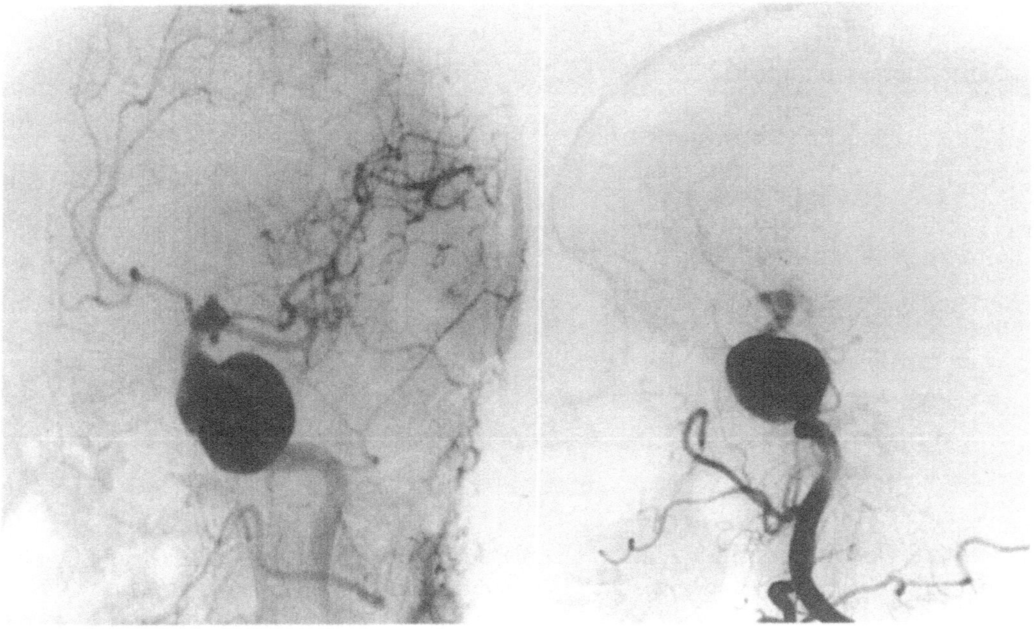

Fig. 3. Left carotid angiogram in 1982 showed intracavernous giant aneurysm, which is smaller than the right

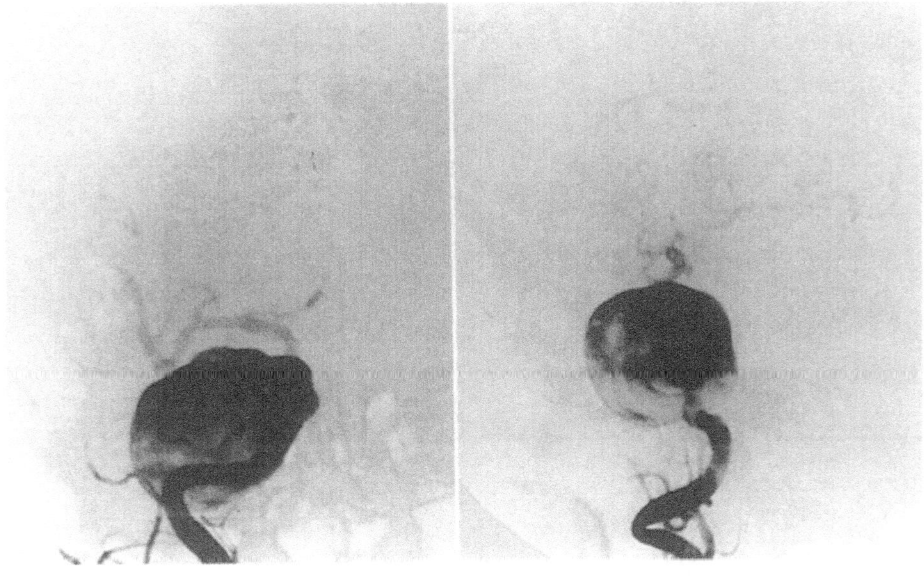

Fig. 4. Right carotid angiogram in 1986 showed aneurysm size increased to 5.7 cm in maximum diameter

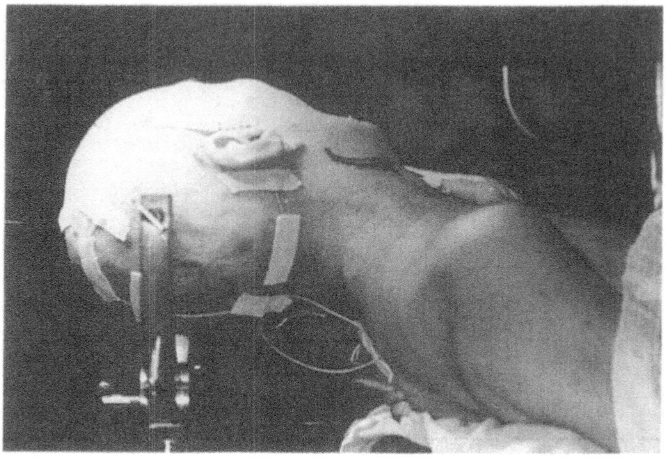

Fig. 5. Operating position. Patient was placed in supine position with the head tilted to 30 degrees and the face rotated to 60 degrees

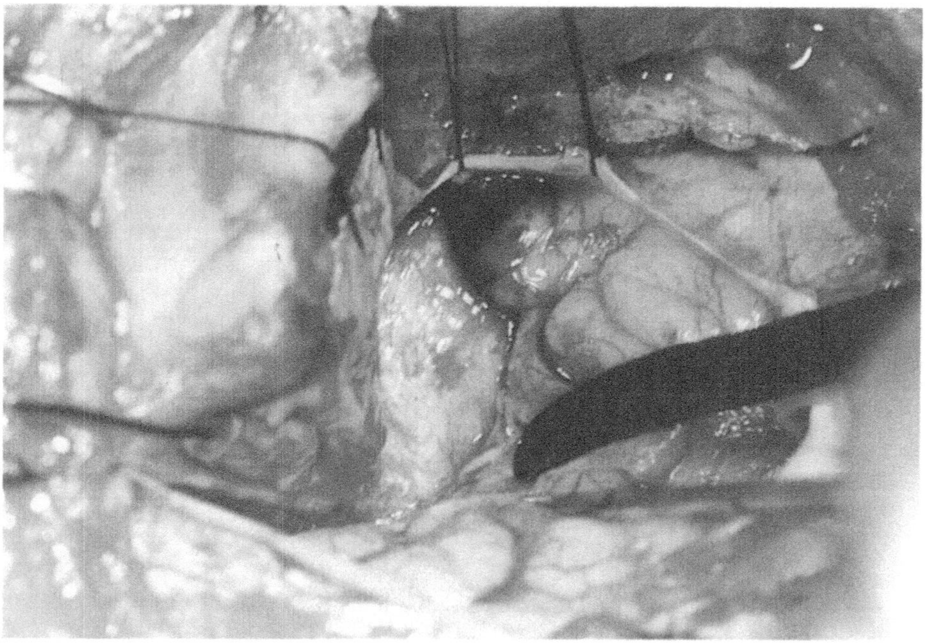

Fig. 6. On opening the dura, the cavernous sinus was swollen by a giant aneurysm

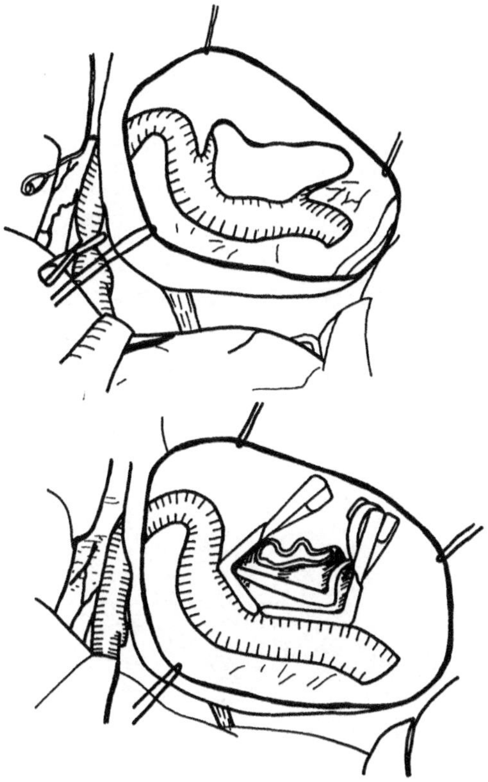

Fig. 7. Operative diagram. Upper: The cavernous sinus and aneurysm was cut open after trapping of internal carotid artery. The aneurysm was examined inside. Lower: Reconstruction of the internal carotid artery was done with Sugita clips

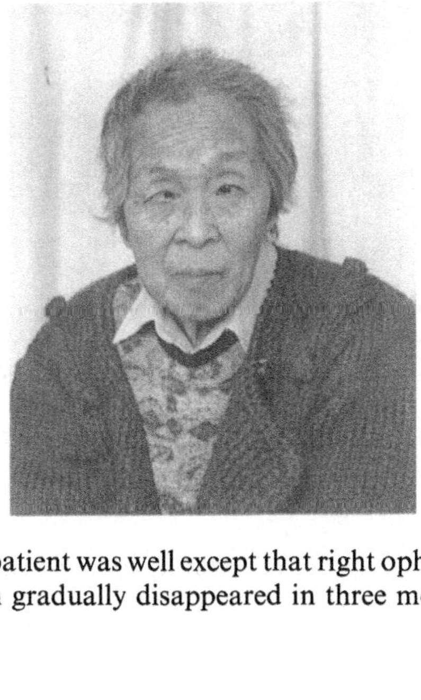

Fig. 8. Postoperatively patient was well except that right ophthalmoplegia appeared which gradually disappeared in three months

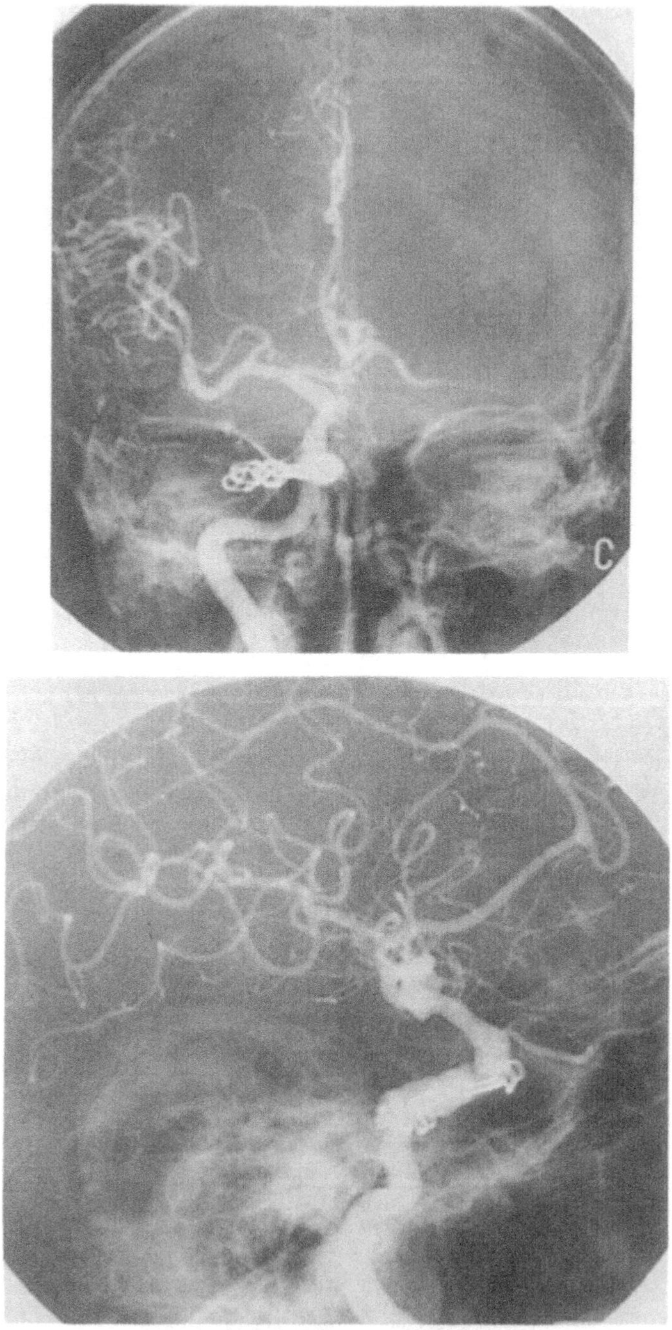

Fig. 9. Postoperative angiogram of right internal carotid artery showed the aneurysm had disappeared. The internal carotid artery remained

Discussion

The cavernous sinus is the most difficult area to be explored by neursurgeons [1–11]. Carotid ligation with or without EC-IC bypass surgery has been a common procedure for intracavernous carotid aneurysms [3, 9].

Problems of intracavernous surgery are:

1. how to control the bleeding from the cavernous sinus;
2. how to preserve nerves;
3. how to maintain the cerebral blood flow if one uses a temporary clip.

We shall discuss these three problems. Regarding the control of bleeding, a giant aneurysm blocks the cavernous sinus by itself. If we operate in the aneurysmal cavity after trapping, there is no bleeding. Therefore we only have to control bleeding at the site of preparation of the aneurysm from the cavernous sinus. Thus, the bleeding is not a problem at all.

As regards preservation of the nerves, we can find the nerve's entrance into the cavernous sinus. If we approach intra-aneurysmally, we can prepare just around the entrance of the internal carotid artery and still preserve nerves between the aneurysm wall and the sinus dural wall. Actually in our case though ophthalmoplegia appeared after the operation it disappeared 3 months afterwards.

Since the aneurysm has to be opened to work inside the cavity, the trapping of the internal carotid artery is essential during the procedure. How to maintain CBF during this period is the most important problem. Using the balloon Matas test EEG, SEP and clinical symptoms were monitored for about 15–20 minutes. Although left carotid occlusion produced δ-activity one minute after occlusion no neurological deficit appeared. Right carotid occlusion, however, revealed no adverse effect. This indicates that EEG monitoring is more sensitive than clinical symptoms. Angiogram showed that the right side had better collateral circulation and the aneurysm was bigger on the right side. So the right aneurysm was selected to be operated on first. We thought that the case could tolerate ischemia without previous EC-IC bypass surgery. However, this may not always be the case and in that case simultaneous EC-IC bypass surgery will be necessary.

Another interesting point of intracavernous giant aneurysm is the aneurysm wall. While usually the wall of an intracranial giant aneurysm is very thick, an intracavernous giant aneurysm wall is very thin. It may be torn during the preparation. As the wall of the intracavernous giant aneurysm is reinforced by the cavernous sinus wall, it is not necessary to strengthen the aneurysm wall.

References

1. Barr HWK, Blackwood W, Meadows SP (1971) Intravenous carotid aneurysms. A clinical pathological report. Brain 94: 607–622
2. Dolenc VV (1983) Direct microsurgical repair of intracavernous vascular lesions. J Neurosurg 58: 824–831
3. Gelber BR, Sundt TM Jr (1980) Treatment of intracavernous and giant carotid aneurysms by combined internal carotid ligation and extra-intracranial bypass. J Neurosurg 52: 1–10
4. Harris FS, Rhoton AL Jr (1976) Anatomy of the cavernous sinus. A microsurgical study. J Neurosurg 45: 169–180
5. Jefferson G (1938) On the saccular aneurysms of the internal carotid artery in the cavernous sinus. Br J Surg 26: 267–302
6. Johnston I (1976) Direct surgical treatment of bilateral intracavernous internal carotid artery aneurysms. Case report. J Neurosurg 51: 98–102
7. Lombardi G, Passerini A, Migliavacca F (1963) Intracavernous aneurysms of the internal carotid artery. AJR 89: 361–371
8. Mason TH, Swain GM, Osheroff HR (1954) Bilateral carotid cavernous fistula. J Neurosurg 11: 323–326
9. Matsuda M, Matsuda I, Hanada H et al (1979) Intracavernous giant aneurysm associated with Marfan's syndrome. Surg Neurol 12: 119–121
10. Seltzer J, Hurteau EF (1957) Bilateral symmetrical aneurysms on internal carotid artery within the cavernous sinus. Case report. J Neurosurg 14: 448–451
11. Wilson CB, Myers FK (1963) Bilateral saccular aneurysms of the internal carotid artery in the cavernous sinus. J Neurol Neurosurg Psychiatry 26: 174–177

Treatment of intracavernous aneurysms of the ICA and CCFs by direct approach

V. V. Dolenc, M. Čerk, J. Šušteršič, R. Pregelj, and M. Škrap

University Department of Neurosurgery, University Medical Centre, Ljubljana, Yugoslavia

Twenty-five patients with intracavernous vascular lesions were treated by a direct operative approach and microsurgical repair. Fifteen patients of this series had an intracavernous carotid aneurysm, which in five cases was due to trauma. Ten patients had carotid-cavernous fistulas (CCFs).

The same approach to the lesion of the internal carotid artery (ICA) in the cavernous sinus (CS) was used in all patients [8].

Aneurysms and/or CCFs were excluded from the circulation by clipping in 18 cases, and by reconstruction of the arterial wall by means of interrupted sutures in seven cases.

Vascular lesions were excluded in all cases. Carotid patency was preserved in 16 of the total of 25 patients.

One patient only was treated by ligation of the carotid artery in the neck.

In our series, four patients died: one patient with a CCF, who had been comatose prior to surgery, and one patient with a traumatic intracavernous aneurysm of the ICA, who had been comatose and artifically ventilated since the accident. Another two deceased harboured a giant aneurysm of nontraumatic origin; one died 2 weeks after the operation from a large brain infarction resulting from carotid occlusion, and another 3 months postoperatively from generalised infection. Of the 21 patients surviving the operation, one is unable to care for himself and depends on the assistance of others, while 12 patients have resumed their previous work, or a job similar to the original one.

Introduction

The cavernous sinus (CS) and its structures: the third through the sixth cranial nerves, the internal carotid artery (ICA) and the venous canals show most interesting topographic anatomy.

The structure of the CS, especially its architecture, has been described in detail in several neurosurgical reports [14, 23, 24, 29, 33]. As shown by recently published studies, the topographic anatomy of the CS and the relationships between the intracavernous structures are still controversial [2].

Saccular aneurysms may arise from the ICA in the CS, through less frequently than from other intracranial vessels. The literature abounds in reports on such lesions, yet they differ widely as to the therapeutic technique used [1, 4, 11, 15, 16, 18, 20, 26, 28, 30, 35].

Besides other injuries, a skull base fracture may involve also a lesion to the ICA in the CS. Such an injury may produce either rupture of the ICA wall, or may completely interrupt the vessel. A traumatic aneurysm of the ICA or a CCF occurs as a result of an injury to the intracavernous segment of the ICA. Whether an aneurysm or a CCF will result depends on the condition of the structures surrounding the ICA, and on the extent of the injury to the bone sinuses.

A traumatic aneurysm of the ICA usually manifests itself by a massive epistaxis. Frequently, only emergency tamponade can prevent death from massive bleeding [3, 5, 13, 19, 21, 22, 27]. Most traumatic aneurysms remain asymptomatic for several days, or even months, after the accident [17, 34]. Patients with a traumatic intracavernous ICA aneurysm frequently show impaired vision on the side of the lesion.

Another type of lesion due to an injured ICA wall is a CCF.

Arterial blood failing to find its way out from the ICA leaves the CS via the venous system. A CCF is not a life-threatening lesion, yet it becomes a serious problem because of the annoying, unrelenting bruit due to permanent shunt it creates. The condition is further complicated by the orbital veins congestion with resulting pulsating exophthalmos, ophthalmoplegia and visual deterioration or even complete loss of vision. The CCF usually occurs immediately or soon after the accident, and only exceptionally at a later date. Exclusion of an intracavernous vascular lesion through a direct attack on the CS and microsurgical reconstruction of the arterial wall along with preservation of carotid patency [8], is the ideal therapeutic technique. These vascular lesions can also be excluded by the technique of the detachable balloon catheter [7, 6, 31]. These two techniques, which have many advantages as well as drawbacks, have been increasingly used as complementary procedures, rather than techniques excluding each other.

Thrombogenic techniques and, especially, extra- and intracranial ligation of the ICA in combination with an extra-intracranial bypass procedure, should also be mentioned in this context.

Occlusion of the CCF with a muscle embolus and intraluminal occlusion of the ICA should be definitively excluded from the modern neurosurgical repertoire, but unfortunately the technique of ligating and clipping the ICA central and peripheral to the aneurysm is frequently the only feasible life-saving procedure in the treatment of traumatic aneurysms of the intracavernous ICA [17, 34]. Yet, in patients submitted to this operative procedure who show poor cross circulation, as a rule, an additional extra-intracranial bypass procedure should be done.

Today, any direct operative approach to the CS can be accomplished with a patient under normal neuroanaesthesia, and no special measures such as hypothermia, hypotension, extracorporeal circulation and/or cardiac arrest have to be taken. And finally, neuroradiologic interventions using the detachable balloon catheter are feasible without anaesthesia.

Patients, methods, and results

Table 1 shows our patients with intracavernous vascular lesions. In the majority of patients, the diagnostic evaluation included a CT scan of the brain. Angiographic cross-flow studies were done in all our patients. All patients with a vascular lesion situated in the CS, were treated by a direct microsurgical approach, as described in our previous reports [8, 9,].

No special measures, such as hypotension, hypothermia or extracorporeal circulation and cardiac arrest were taken during surgery. Of the 25 patients treated for an intracavernous ICA lesion, only one underwent ligation of the carotid artery in the neck.

Traumatic intracavernous ICA aneurysms

In all five patients, lesion of the ICA wall was due to fracture of the skull base. In four of them, the ruptured traumatic aneurysm in the CS produced bleeding in the bone sinuses and skull base with a resulting massive epistaxis. Severe nosebleed occurred from 10 days to 2 months after trauma. Two patients had had a single episode, one two, and one three episodes of epistaxis by the time the cause of bleeding was discovered. In all four patients epistaxis was heralded by a sensation of pressure or even pain in the cheek and nasal area, which warned the patients that a life-threatening bleeding was imminent. In all our patients the epistaxis was successfully controlled by emergency packing. Blood transfusion was required in all patients. Immediately after injury, all four patients developed loss of vision ipsilateral to the traumatic aneurysm. In one of the four patients, the

Table 1. Summary of patients operated

Lesion	Sex	Lesion excluded by		Clipping of the ICA	Patency of the ICA following surgery
		clip-ping	resection and recon-struction of the ICA		
Traumatic Aneurysms	2 F	2	0	2	0
	3 M	3	0	3	0
CCFs	2 F	2	0	0	1
	8 M	4	4	0	6
Saccular Aneurysms	5 F	2	3	0	2
	5 M	5	0	0	4
	25	18	7	5	13

traumatic intracavernous aneurysm of the ICA did not cause epistaxis but SAH. In this profoundly comatose woman this unusual complication was discovered by a routine CT scan of the brain, instead of a suspected epidural or subdural hematoma (Fig. 1).

Angiographic studies were indicated despite the poor condition of the patient. The carotid angiogram revealed a traumatic intracavernous aneurysm of the ICA (Fig. 2). Cross-circulation studies showed adequate contralateral blood flow via the anterior communicating artery. During the operation, a large rupture of the ICA wall and dura of the CS was found. Adequate reconstruction of the ICA was not feasible and therefore the aneurysm was excluded from the circulation by clipping the ICA proximally and distally to the lesion. Eighteen days after the accident the patient succumbed to sequelae of primary brain trauma involving a severe brain stem injury.

As regards the remaining four patients, preoperative angiographic studies showed complete severance of the ICA in two patients, and rupture on for intracavernous vascular lesion

Blind in the eye ipsilateral to the lesion: preop.	postop.	Other neurol. deficits postop.	Lesion excluded	Lesion persisting	Died	Survived	Living Normally
2	2	0	2	0	1	1	1
3	3	0	3	0	0	3	3
1	1	0	2	0	0	2	2
1	1	one patient: hemiplegic one patient: paresis of the sixth nerve	7	1	1	7	6
0	0	0	5	0	2	3	3
0	1	0	5	0	0	5	5
7	8	2	24	1	4	21	20

of the ICA wall with preserved patency of the vessel in the other two. Operative repair of the damaged ICA was not possible in any of them. In all four cases the lesion was excluded by clipping the intracavernous segment of the ICA centrally and peripherally to the aneurysm, yet always proximally to the point of origin of the ophthalmic artery. Exclusion of the ICA in the CS by clipping was indicated by adequate preoperative cross-circulation in all patients. Four patients with a traumatic intracavernous aneurysm treated by the above mentioned technique, who developed blindness in the ipsilateral eye immediately after trauma, remained blind after the operation.

Movements of the blind eye, however, were within normal limits. In all of them, the aneurysm was completely excluded from circulation and epistaxis did not recur. Their neurological status was normal, apart from loss of vision in the eye on the side of the lesion. All the four patients perform the same work as before the accident.

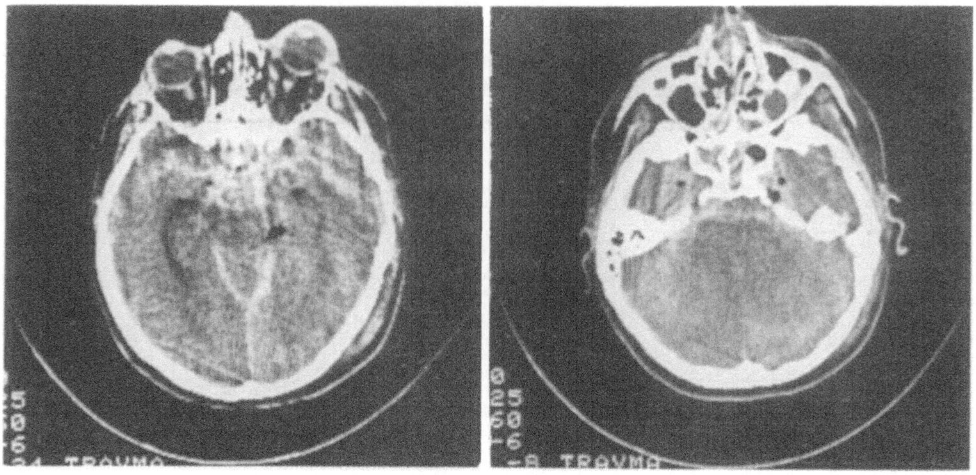

Fig. 1. CT scan of brain shows right-sided exophthalmos, SAH and air bubbles on the right side of the skull base as well as on the right aspect of the brain-stem

Carotid-cavernous fistulas

With the exception of a patient with a CCF resulting from stab wounding of the CS and its ICA with a metal umbrella rib, nine patients developed a CCF as a result of an ICA injury due to a skull base fracture.

In all patients a characteristic bruit and a more or less pronounced exophthalmos occurred immediately after trauma. Two patients became blind in the eye ipsilateral to the CCF. One showed bilateral loss of vision in the presence of a unilateral CCF. One patient only had bilateral CCF, which, however, did not produce deterioration of vision of either eye.

All our patients with CCFs had angiographic cross-flow studies, which were of great value in planning surgery. In all cases but one (a patient with a bilateral CCF), we managed to completely exclude the lesion, either by clipping the ICA or reconstructing its wall. In six patients, the CCF was excluded from circulation by clipping (Fig. 3), and in four by a direct repair of the ruptured ICA wall using interrupted sutures. Patency of the ICA was

---

Fig. 2. Right carotid angiograms: anteroposterior view (**a**) showing a traumatic ICA aneurysm (lower two arrows) and poor filling of the ICA (upper arrow); lateral view (**b**) showing the same lesion in a very different dimension. Notice: the arrow points to the fracture line through the floor of the sella

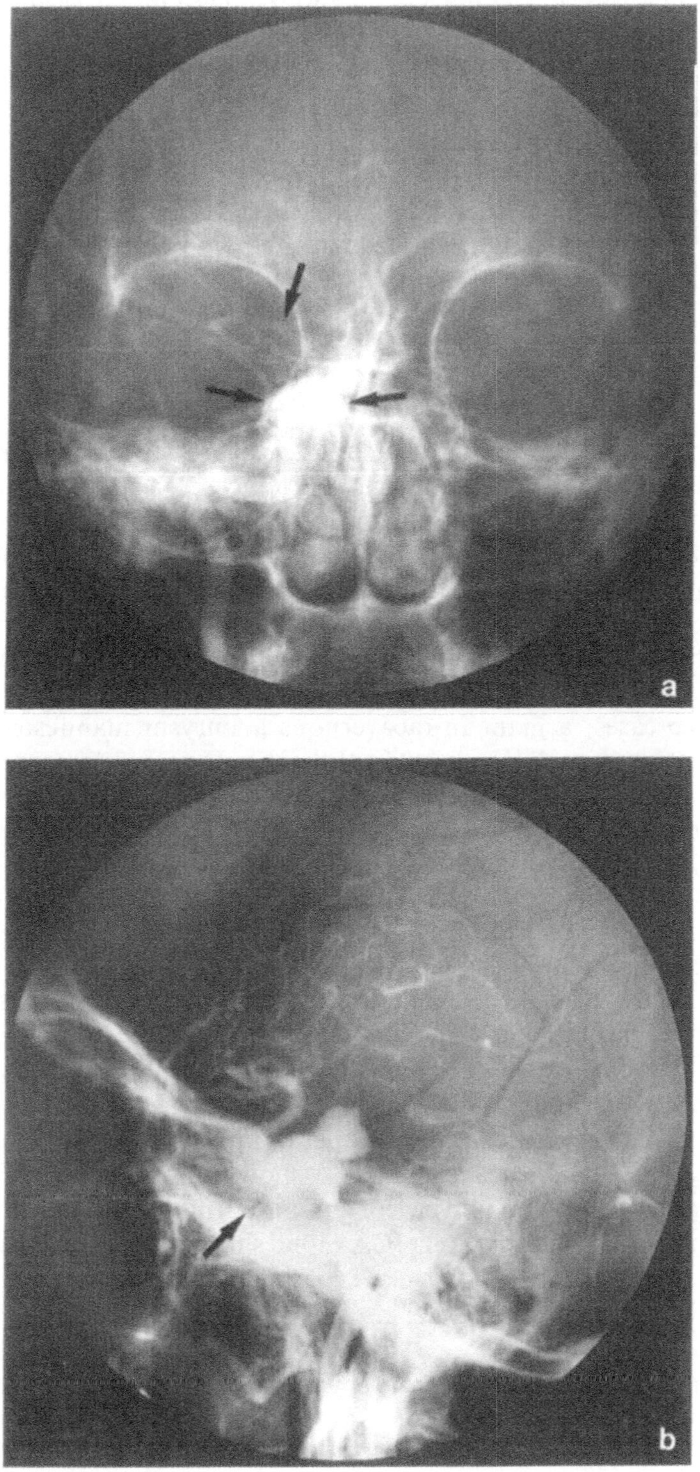
a
b

preserved in seven cases. One patient with bilateral loss of vision, who had the CCF excluded by reconstruction of the vessel with no preservation of patency, died 3 weeks after surgery. Of the nine survivors, one with a bilateral CCF is bedridden because of hemiplegia and occlusion of the ICA on the operated side. In addition, he has a persistent contralateral CCF. The eight patients surviving the operation are free of motor deficits. All these patients, except one with persistent paresis of the sixth nerve, have normal eye movements and show no deficits in function of the third through the sixth cranial nerves. Two of the eight patients are blind in the eye ipsilateral to the CCF, yet they have resumed their previous work, like the other six patients.

Nontraumatic intracavernous ICA aneurysms

Of the ten patients treated for saccular intracavernous ICA aneurysms, five harbored small and five giant lesions. In four cases, a small intracavernous aneurysm was discovered accidentally by angiography of intracranial vessels, which was done to identify SAH due to rupture of another intracranial aneurysm. In three cases, bleeding occurred as a result of rupture of a saccular aneurysm located in the CS, with its smaller part protruding into the intradural space. Two of these three lesions were giant, while one was small in size.

In three cases, a giant intracavernous aneurysm manifested itself by retro-orbital pain and progressive ophthalmoplegia due to compression of the third through the sixth cranial nerves by a tumor-like aneurysm. We decided on occlusion of the ICA, according to the cross circulation situation shown by preoperative angiographic studies. In seven patients the lesion was excluded by clipping, and in three by resection and reconstruction of the ICA by interrupted sutures.

Two patients with a giant aneurysm treated by resection and reconstruction of the ICA died, one 2 weeks, and another 3 months after the operation. Eight patients made an uneventful recovery and resumed their previous job. One of them is blind in the eye ipsilateral to the operated aneurysm. In this, and another patient with a giant aneurysm, occlusion of the ICA in the CS occurred after the operation. Six patients operated on for an aneurysm of the intracavernous ICA show normal patency of the ICA. Of the eight patients who underwent an uneventful operation for a saccular aneurysm of the intracavernous ICA, none show any deficit in function of the third through sixth cranial nerves. Preoperative or transient postoperative paresis of the cranial nerves in these patients regressed within 3 months.

Pain in the area supplied by the V/1 and V/2 branches of the fifth nerve experienced by patients with a giant aneurysm, settled down soon after the operation and has never recurred.

Discussion

The first reports on successful treatment of intracavernous vascular lesions by direct operative approach appeared in the literature fairly early. In the ensuing years, a number of modifications have been proposed in order to solve the problems connected with this technique [8, 11, 16, 23, 25, 28, 34]. Safer conditions for operative management of this area were ultimately afforded by a risk-free exploration of the ICA before its entrance to the CS [12]. A combination of three approaches, the pterional [36], the subtemporal [10] and exposure of the intrapetrous segment of the carotid artery [12], with certain modifications [8, 9], has made it possible for the surgeon to attack the CS from all sides. Thanks to thorough anatomical studies of this structure, the CS could finally be entered in a really safe way [2, 14, 24, 29, 32, 33]. Introduction of the neuroradiological technique of the detachable balloon catheter in the management of intracavernous vascular lesions has made the direct operative approach less popular [6, 7, 31]. The new technique of the detachable balloon catheter has definitively replaced the treatment of CCFs by occlusion of the ICA with a Fogarty catheter. In the future, thrombogenic techniques will most likely be supplanted by the detachable balloon catheter technique, too [23].

The new operative approach, which includes exposure of most of the CS structures without even opening the CS [8], safe elective occlusion of the CS, and exposure of the ICA within it, has made unnecessary the use of hypotension, hypothermia, extracorporeal circulation and cardiac arrest. Treatment of traumatic aneurysms of the ICA located in the CS, which produce massive epistaxis [3, 13, 17, 19, 22, 34] commonly requires occlusion of the ICA centrally and peripherally to the traumatic lesion [17, 34, and authors experience]. In principle, the technique of the detachable balloon catheter is employed unless the ICA has been completely ruptured. Patients with a completely ruptured ICA are at risk of retrograde bleeding from the peripheral stump due to cross circulation. For this reason, occlusion of the ICA peripherally but, as a rule, proximally to the ophthalmic artery origin, is imperative. Insertion of the detachable balloon catheter in the orifice of the fistula is preferable in CCFs. Yet, the aim of this procedure, which is to occlude the fistula and preserve patency of the ICA, is often not attainable. Even in the hands of the most experienced and skilled surgeons, this technique fails to preserve patency of the ICA in more than 50% of cases [7]. The use of the detachable balloon catheter is elderly, however, the method of choice in elder and poor-risk patients.

The ideal method of treating saccular aneurysms of the ICA in the CS is still controversial. It is hard to believe that in cases of giant aneurysms the use of the detachable balloon catheter could adequately reduce compression of the adjacent structures and thus relieve pain or ophthalmoplegia. On the

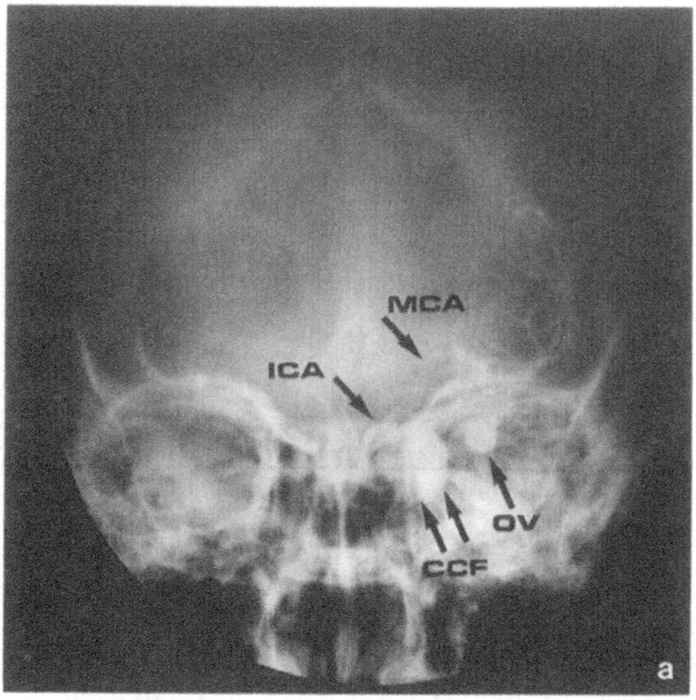

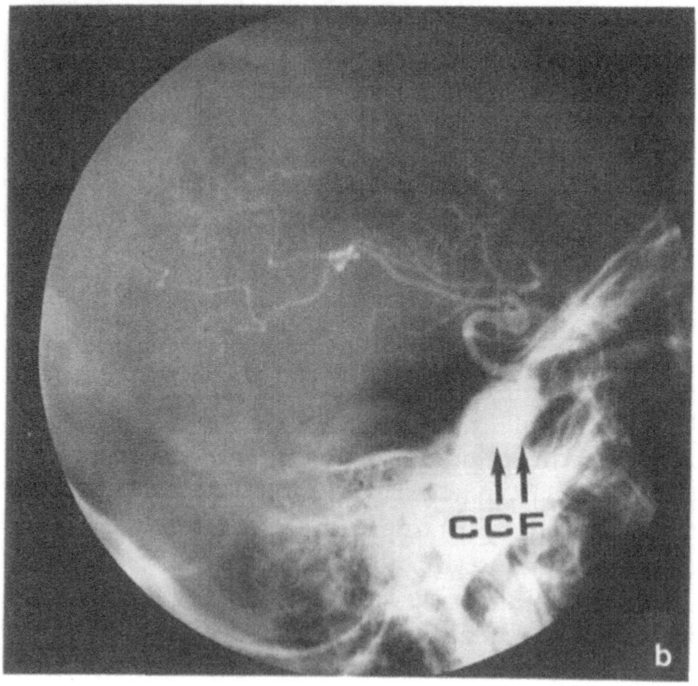

Fig. 3. Left carotid angiograms anteroposterior views (**a, c**) and lateral views (**b, d**). **a, b** Preoperative angiograms showing a typical carotid-cavernous fistula. Note the

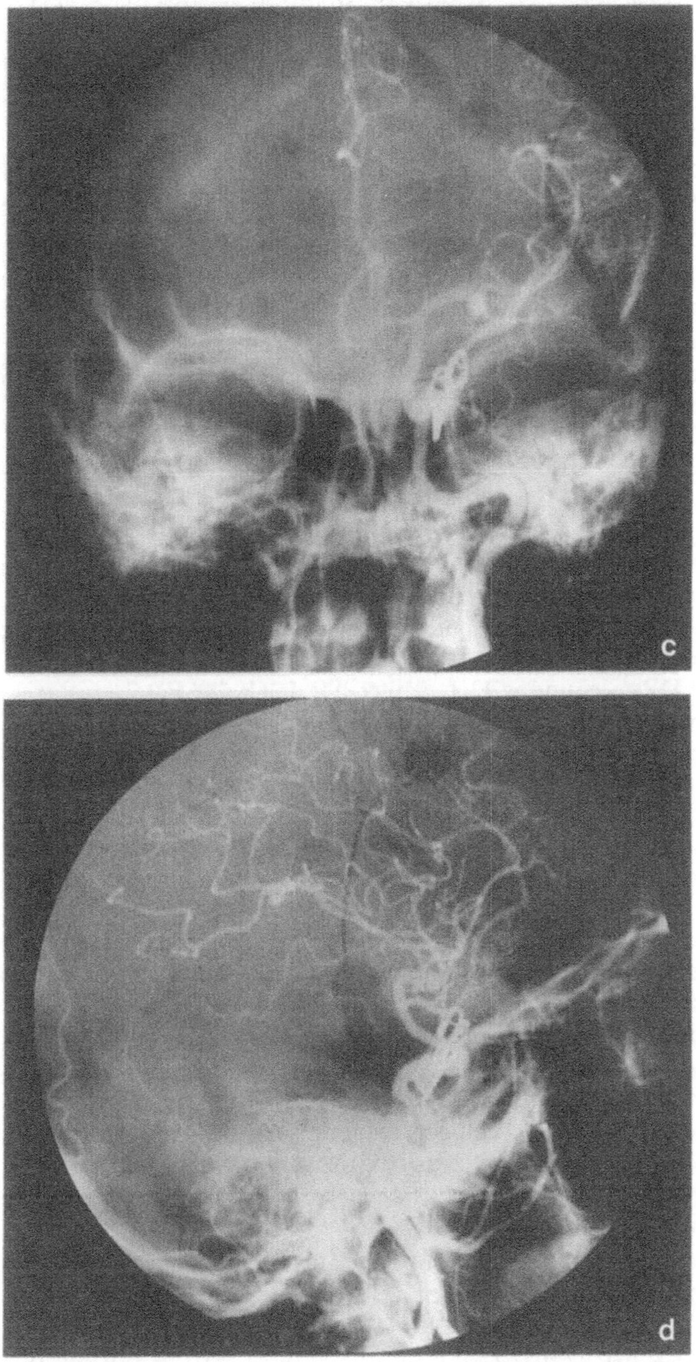

engorgement of the orbital vein (*OV*). **c, d** Postoperative angiograms showing two clips on ICA, no CCF and normal ICA and much better filling of its branches in comparison to the preoperative angiograms other hand, proper insertion of the balloon represents a very demanding task in patients with small aneurysms. Management using the detachable balloon catheter should therefore be reserved for those patients who, because of their advanced age or for other reasons, would poorly tolerate the direct approach and prolonged operative treatment.

The technique of the detachable balloon catheter has certain advantages which cannot be denied. The same holds true of the direct microsurgical approach. Nevertheless, in certain cases the surgeon will still be obliged to have recourse to the technique of extra- and intracranial anastomosis and to the thrombogenic technique. In the future, the most rational policy would to be further refine the existing operative techniques and to use them discriminately, weighting all the pros and cons for each particular case.

References

1. Barr HWK, Blackwood W, Meadows SP (1971) Intracavernous carotid aneurysms. A clinical pathological report. Brain 94: 607–622
2. Brassier G (1984) Anatomie microchirurgicale du sinus caverneux. Thèse, Université de Rennes
3. Busby DR, Slemmons DH, Miller TE Jr (1968) Fatal epistaxis via carotid aneurysm and eustachian tube. Arch Otolaryngol 87: 295–298
4. Cabezudo JM, Carrillo R, Vaquero J et al (1981) Intracavernous aneurysm of the carotid artery following transsphenoidal surgery. Case report. J Neurosurg 54: 118–121
5. Chambers EF, Rosenbaum AE, Norman D et al (1981) Traumatic aneurysms of cavernous internal carotid artery with secondary epistaxis. AJNR 2: 405–409
6. Debrun G (1978) Detachable balloon and calibrated leak balloon technique in the treatment of cerebral vascular lesions. J Neurosurg 49: 635–649
7. Debrun G, Lacour P, Viñuela F et al (1981) Treatment of 54 traumatic carotid-cavernous fistulas. J Neurosurg 55: 678–692
8. Dolenc VV (1983) Direct microsurgical repair of intracavernous vascular lesions. J Neurosurg 58: 824–831
9. Dolenc VV (1985) A combined epi- and subdural direct approach to carotid-ophthalmic artery aneurysms. J Neurosurg 62: 667–672
10. Drake CG (1978) Treatment of aneurysms of the posterior cranial fossa. Prog Neurol Surg 9: 122–194
11. Gelber BR, Sundt TM Jr (1980) Treatment of intracavernous and giant carotid aneurysms by combined internal carotid ligation and extra- to intracranial bypass. J Neurosurg 52: 1–10
12. Glasscock ME (1969) Exposure of the intra-petrous portion of the carotid artery. In: Hamberger CA, Wersäall J (eds) Disorders of the skull base region. Proceedings of the 10th Nobel symposium. Almqvist and Wiksell, Stockholm, pp 135–143

13. Handa J, Handa H (1976) Severe epistaxis caused by traumatic aneurysm of cavernous carotid artery. Surg Neurol 5: 241–243
14. Harris FS, Rhoton AL Jr (1976) Anatomy of the cavernous sinus. A microsurgical study. J Neurosurg 45: 169–180
15. Jefferson G (1938) On the saccular aneurysms of the internal carotid artery in the cavernous sinus. Br J Surg 26: 267–302
16. Johnston I (1979) Direct surgical treatment of bilateral intracavernous internal carotid artery aneurysms. Case report. J Neurosurg 51: 98–102
17. Liw MY, Shils CJ, Wang YC et al (1985) Traumatic intracavernous carotid aneurysm with massive epistaxis. Neurosurgery 17: 569–573
18. Lombardi G, Passerini A, Migliavacca F (1963) Intracavernous aneurysms of the internal carotid artery. AJR 89: 361–371
19. Mahmoud NA (1979) Traumatic aneurysm of the internal carotid artery and epistaxis. Review of literature and report of a case. J Laryngol Otol 93: 629–656
20. Matsuda M, Matsuda I, Handa H et al (1979) Intracavernous giant aneurysm associated with Marfan's syndrome. Surg Neurol 12: 119–121
21. Mc Cormick WF, Beals JD (1964) Severe epistaxis caused by ruptured aneurysm of the internal carotid artery. J Neurosurg 21: 678–686
22. Moore D, Budde RB, Hunter CR et al (1979) Massive epistaxis from aneurysm of the carotid artery. Surg Neurol 11: 115–117
23. Mullan S (1979) Treatment of carotid-cavernous fistulas by cavernous sinus occlusion. J Neurosurg 50: 131–144
24. Ono M, Ono M, Rhoton AL Jr et al (1984) Microsurgical anatomy of the region of the tentorial incisura. J Neurosurg 60: 365–399
25. Parkinson D (1973) Carotid cavernous fistula: direct repair with preservation of the carotid artery. Technical note. J Neurosurg 38: 99–106
26. Parkinson D, West M (1980) Traumatic intracranial aneurysms. J Neurosurg 52: 11–20
27. Petty JM (1969) Epistaxis from aneurysm of the internal carotid artery due to a gun shot wound. Case report. J Neurosurg 30: 741–743
28. Reddy SVR, Sundt TM Jr (1981) Giant traumatic false aneurysm of the internal carotid artery associated with a carotid—cavernous fistula. Case report. J Neurosurg 55: 813–818
29. Rhoton AL Jr, Hardy DG, Chambers SM (1979) Microsurgical anatomy and dissection of the sphenoïd bone, cavernous sinus and sellar region. Surg Neurol 12: 63–104
30. Seltzer J, Hurteau EF (1957) Bilateral symmetrical aneurysms of internal carotid artery within the cavernous sinus. Case report. J Neurosurg 14: 448–451
31. Serbinenko F (1974) Wound catheterization and occlusion of major cerebral vessels. J Neurosurg 41: 125–145
32. Taptas JM (1982) The so-called cavernous sinus: a review of the contraversy and its implications for neurosurgeons. Neurosurgery 11: 712–717
33. Umansky F, Nathan H (1982) The lateral wall of the cavernous sinus, with special reference to the nerves related to it. J Neurosurg 56: 228–234
34. van Dellen JR (1980) Intracavernous traumatic aneurysms. Surg Neurol 13: 203–207

35. Wilson CB, Myers FK (1963) Bilateral saccular aneurysms of the internal carotid artery in the cavernous sinus. J Neurol Neurosurg Psychiatry 26: 174–177
36. Yaşargil MG, Fox JL, Ray MW (1975) The operative approach to aneurysms of the anterior communicating artery. In: Krayenbühl H et al (eds) Advances and technical standards in neurosurgery, vol 2. Springer, Wien New York, pp 113–170

The antero-external approach to the internal carotid artery at the base of the skull and intrapetrously

F. Lesoin[1], A. Autricque[1], L. Villette[1], K. Franz[1], M. Jomin[1], and P. Pellerin[2]

[1] Department B of Neurosurgery, and [2] Department of Plastic and Reconstructive Surgery, C.H.R.U., Lille, France

The authors report the use of the antero-external approach for the intrapetrous and skull base portion of the carotid artery. They underline its advantages and limits and report its indications.

Introduction

Depending on the type of lesion to be treated, it may be necessary to approach the internal carotid artery at the base of the skull or overt its entire intrapetrous part. The lateral approaches enable exposure of the artery at the base of the skull and if necessary over its entire intrapetrous portion up to the point of entry in the cavernous sinus involving the sacrifice of the hearing function [3, 5, 6, 7, 10, 16]. The superior approach only enables the exposure of the horizontal segment of the intrapetrous carotid artery [8, 17]. The antero-external approach, which we propose, is an extension of this approach and enables the exposure of the carotid from the base of the skull to the cavernous sinus without the drawback of sacrificing the hearing function as in Fisch's infratemporal approach [5]. There is no doubt that it involves certain technical difficulties. The indications for this technique are discussed.

Technique

The approach to the intrabasal internal carotid artery using the antero-external pathway can either be restricted to the horizontal portion or cover the entire intrabasal section freeing the carotid backwards from the cavernous sinus to its point of entry in the base of the skull. Its purpose is to permit as extensive as possible an approach while cutting down the postoperative sequelae to a minimum (Figs. 1, 2, 3, and 4).

The approach to the horizontal segment comprises 4 stages designed to free the carotid artery separated from the dura mater of the middle cerebral fossa by a thin osseous wall which is sometimes absent and belongs to the anterosuperior face of the petrosal bone. Surgery is performed with the patient under general anaesthetic. The patient is ventilated with negative pressure and placed on a mannitol drip which facilitates the pushing back of the temporal lobe. The supine position is used with the head rotated through 90°. The frontotemporal skin incision is taken down to the malar arch. The scalp is detached from the epicranium and from the temporal aponeurosis as far as the external upper orbital edge and the malar arch along which the periosteum is incised and retracted. Subperiosteal dissection enables the branches of the facial nerve to be left intact.

The anterior half of the temporal muscle and the masseter is retracted and the orbit dissected. The temporal flap bone is then cut and removed. Then with three osteotomy strokes of the vibrating saw, the detached periorbit being protected with a malleable strip, the body of the malar, the orbital apophysis of the frontal and the malar arch, are sectioned, enabling mobilization of the orbitozygomaticomalar flap. The temporal muscle can then be pushed outwards right out of the way and we get an excellent view to the pterygomaxillary fossa and the solum of the temporal fossa. The dura mater is only incised to drain the cisterns and to obtain a reduction of the CSF and a brain collapse.

The second stage of the operation involves the exposure of the anterosuperior face of the petrosal bone using an extradural approach. This is achieved by gradually detaching the dura mater under the microscope. Hemostases are obtained with bipolar coagulation. Detachment is performed from the back and by working forwards and may be hampered by the existence of fibrous strips around the petrosquamous suture which are cut with microscissors as are those around the arcuate eminence. Further forwards detachment is easier but also more dangerous. It uncovers the 2 petrosal nerves coming out of the Fallopian hiatus and the accessory hiatus. They appear like two whitish strips stretched between the dura mater and the bone. They are sectioned in order to prevent traction on the nerve VII and secondary facial paralysis. Further forward the foramen spinosum is uncovered and the middle meningeal artery is coagulated. The detachment of the dura mater is continued as far as Meckel's cavity and the infraorbital nerve which enters the oval hole and constitutes the anterior limit of the detachment process. The anterolateral face of the petrosal bone is exposed between the arcuate eminence at the rear and the infraorbital nerve at the front, inside the superior edge of the petrosal bone which contains the

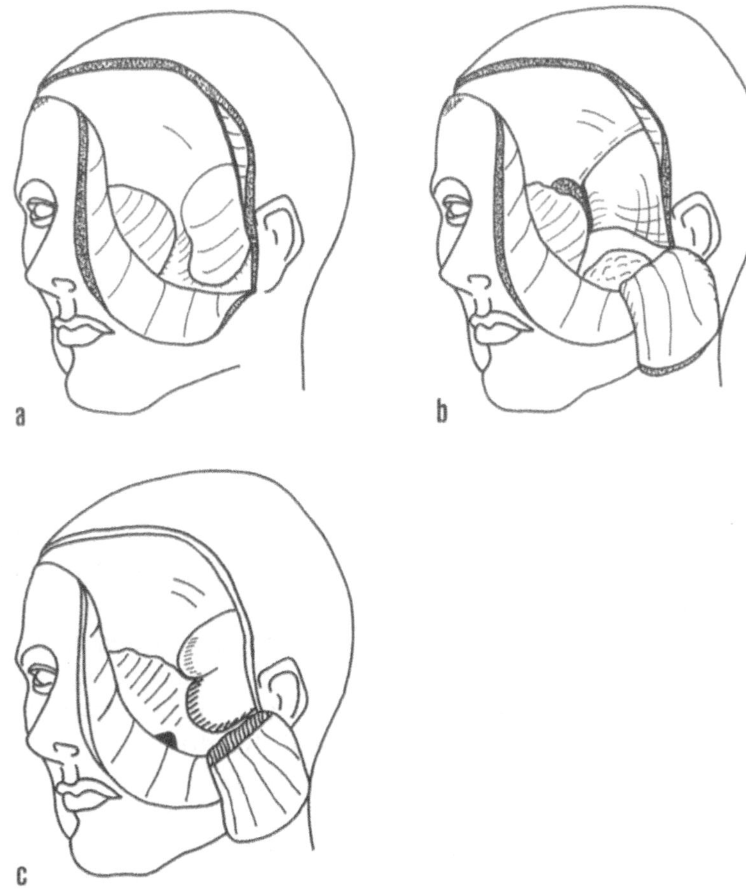

Fig. 1. Diagrams showing the different stages for orbitozygomaticomalar bone flap

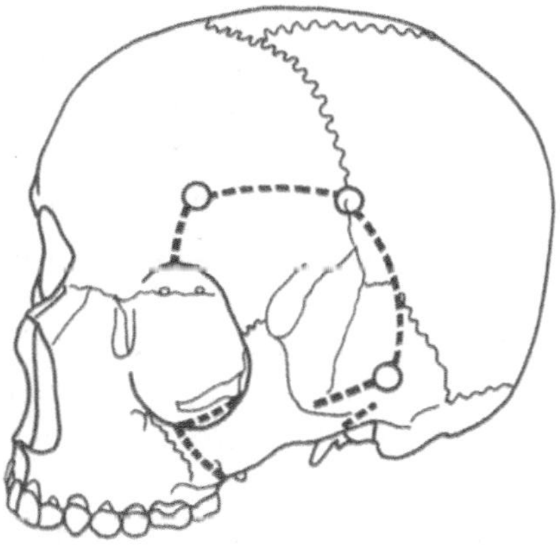

Fig. 2. Limits of the bone flap

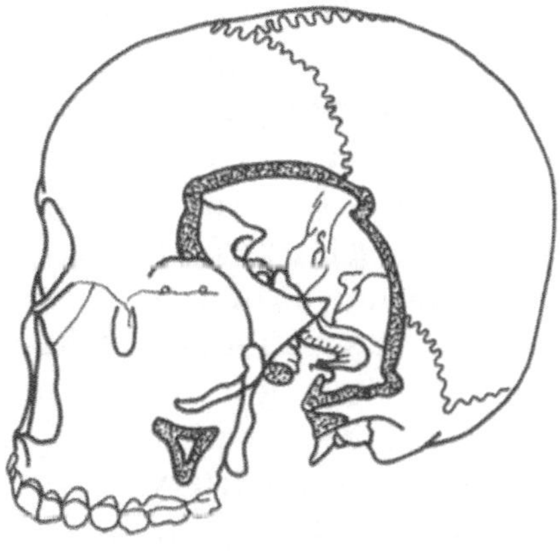

Fig. 3. Exposure of the intrapetrous artery in its horizontal segment

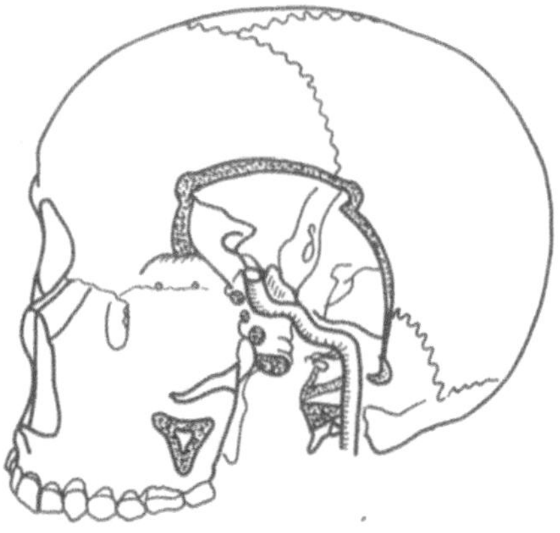

Fig. 4. Exposure of the intrapetrous artery in its vertical segment

superior petrous sinus wrapped in the dura mater. An antistatic retractor is installed to push back the dura mater and the temporal lobe. The third stage of the procedure involves locating the horizontal portion of the carotid canal. Three elements are used to locate the carotid: the greater superficial petrosal nerve, the middle meningeal artery, the infraorbital nerve. The internal carotid artery is cast into this triangle with a certain degree of variability as shown by Paullus, Pait, and Rhoton [11]. The greater superficial petrosal nerve is parallel to the horizontal segment of the internal carotid artery.

The point of origin of the infraorbital nerve is located in 98% of cases behind and in 2% of cases in front of the carotid canal. The middle meningeal artery covers a distance of 4.7 mm outside the carotid canal.

Gradual drilling under the microscope of the petrosal bone opposite to the origin of the infraorbital nerve enables the fourth stage of the operation to be undertaken, which consists in exposing the proximal part of the superior face of the horizontal segment of the intrapetrous internal carotid artery. The bone is not very thick at this point. In some cases, there is no bone at all and this makes it easier to locate the carotid canal. The exposure of the superior face can be continued laterally for 1 cm to the infraorbital nerve enabling the carotid to be exposed as far as the bend which separates the horizontal portion from the vertical portion. At this stage of the operation the superior face of the carotid artery is exposed. Its mobilization requires the freeing of its external face and therefore the opening of the Eustachian tube which follows a path parallel to the intrapetrous segment of the internal carotid artery.

The exposure of the entire basal carotid artery involves the exposure of the horizontal portion together with bone resection of the posterior root of the great wing carried out progressively with bone forceps or a diamond drill, the limits of it being at the front and inside the infraorbital nerve, and at the rear and inside the internal carotid artery at its point of entry in the base of the skull. This bone resection is, however, hampered at the rear by the temporomaxillary articulation. It is possible to luxate the lower jaw forwards or to section its condylus by resecting the glenoid fossa [1, 2, 9]. The dissection of the carotid artery can then be continued by opening the anterior wall of the vertical portion of the intrapetrous segment in a retrograde fashion from the bend which should have been located and freed prior to this.

At his level, the bend is directly linked with the cochlea and the geniculate ganglion at the rear; the vertical portion with the entire middle ear is at the rear. It is therefore imperative to free the carotid artery in these segments, opening only the anterior wall of the carotid canal so as to preserve the hearing function. The artery thus exposed can be progressively separated from the periosteum of the carotid canal and translated forwards after bipolar coagulation of the periarterial venous plexi and the intrapetrous branches of the carotid artery [15].

Depending on the lesion to be treated, it is then possible to mobilize the carotid artery to perform a vascular suture if necessary. The exposure of the horizontal segment only permits a terminolateral suture, whereas the dissection of the entire intrapetrous portion of the carotid artery makes a terminoterminal suture possible.

The closing procedure involves obliteration of the Eustachian tube with temporal fascia or its reconstruction with a bone graft, the replacement and osteosynthesis of the temporal flap bone and orbitozygomaticomalar bone.

Discussion

The regular practice of craniofacial surgery with collaboration between neurosurgeons and plastic surgeons prompted us to treat benign or malignant tumorous lesions of the base of the skull which extended to the lateral sector in contact with the internal carotid artery [12, 13, 14]. Progressively we were prompted to dissect the horizontal segment followed by the vertical segment as far as the foramen lacerum.

The antero-external approach to the internal carotid artery which we propose enables:

considerable enlargment of the field of vision by reducing the retraction of the temporal lobe, thereby enabling an extracerebral approach. This is explained by the removal in first intention of the orbitozygomaticomalar flap bone [12] which represents the main bone impediment to access to the temporal solum. The forward luxation of the lower jaw or the condylus section by resecting the glenoid fossa using the technique employed by Batzdorf and Gregorius [1] gets the temporomaxillary articulation out of the way which otherwise hampers the freeing of the vertical portion;

control of the carotid artery in the cavernous sinus at the base of the skull contrary to Glasscock who only frees the horizontal portion [8] and without the drawbacks of Fisch's infratemporal approach [5]: the deroutation of the facial nerve in the 2nd and 3rd portions inevitably leads to a paralysis which according to Fisch regresses after a few months, but above all this approach calls for the sacrifice of the middle ear.

Its disadvantages are:

the necessary opening of the Eustachian tube which may cause the secondary appearance of a serious otitis, which can be avoided by repairing the solum of the tube with a bone graft or by the secondary installation of a transtympanic aerator. This sacrifice is also necessary with Glasscock's anterosuperior and with Fisch's infratemporal approach;

the need to section the two petrosal nerves in order to avoid facial paralysis secondary to traction on the nerve VII.

Its indications are:

resection to benign or malignant tumors which have spread to the lateral sector of the base of the skull and are compressing the carotid artery. If in fact for tumors affecting the ear and the petrosal bone a transpetrous approach to the carotid artery is the most logical, tumors starting anteriorly and at the middle of the base of the skull are best treated by this anterolateral approach. We were prompted to use this approach for 8 patients: 5 of them presented with a meningioma and the other three with a craniofacial epithelioma with infiltration of the base (Figs. 5, 6);

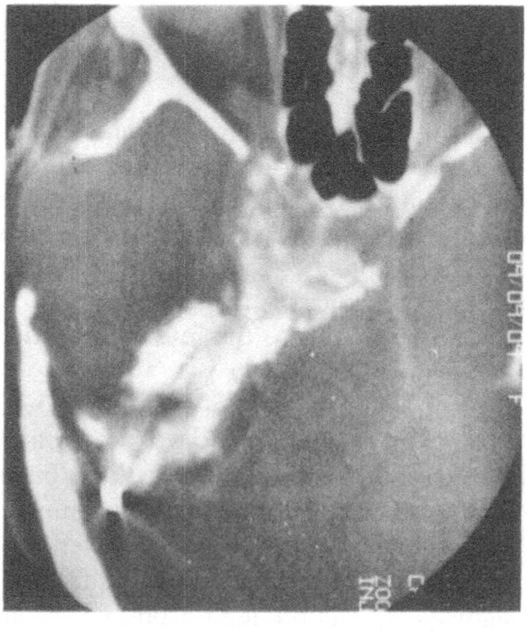

Fig. 5. CT scan: meningioma with extension of the skull base ot the petrous bone

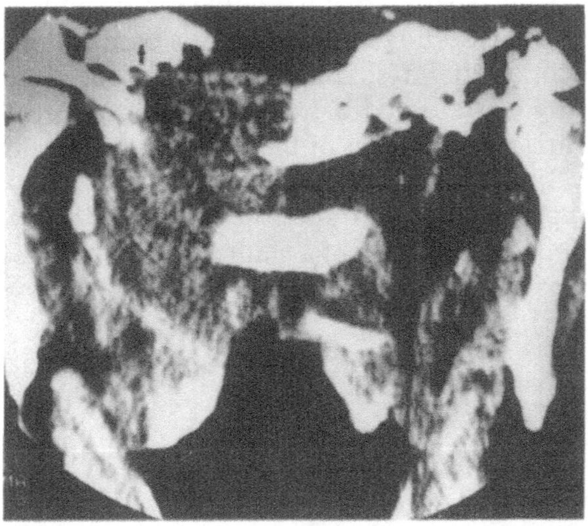

Fig. 6. CT scan (frontal view): epithelioma with extension to the petrous bone (*t*)

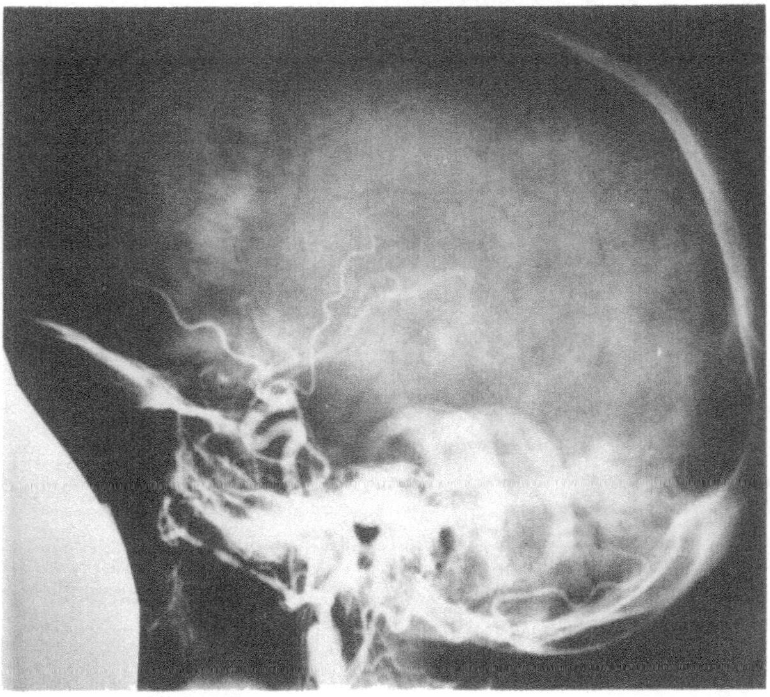

Fig. 7. Arteriography (lateral view): aneurysm of the skull base

treatment of intrapetrous vascular malformations. A true aneurysm is rare and we have no experience of it. On the other hand, we have used this approach to treat a dissecting aneurysm of the base of the skull in a patient who presented an arterial dysplasia extending to the vertical intrapetrous portion. Bridging was effected between the internal carotid artery at the neck and the horizontal segment of the intrapetrous portion of the carotid artery (Figs. 7, 8);

lastly, the approach to the intrapetrous portion of the carotid artery was necessary to control it upstream of a giant aneurysm of the cavernous sinus in two patients, as performed by Dolenc [4] and in intracavernous tumorous pathology (Fig. 9).

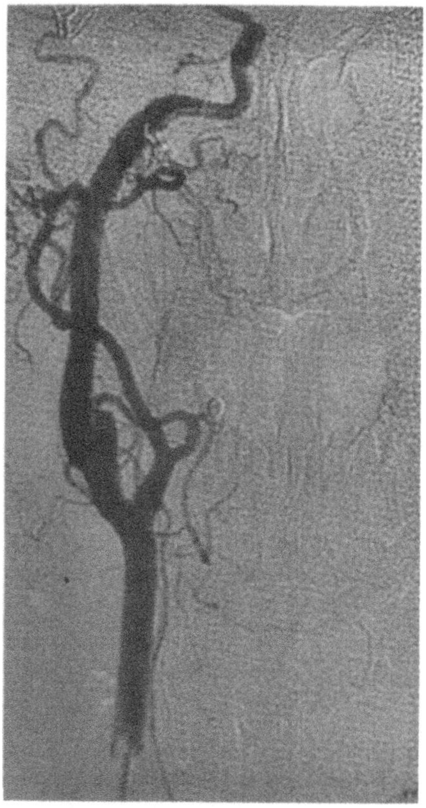

Fig. 8. Control arteriography showing the saphene venous graft going to the intrapetrous portion of the carotid artery

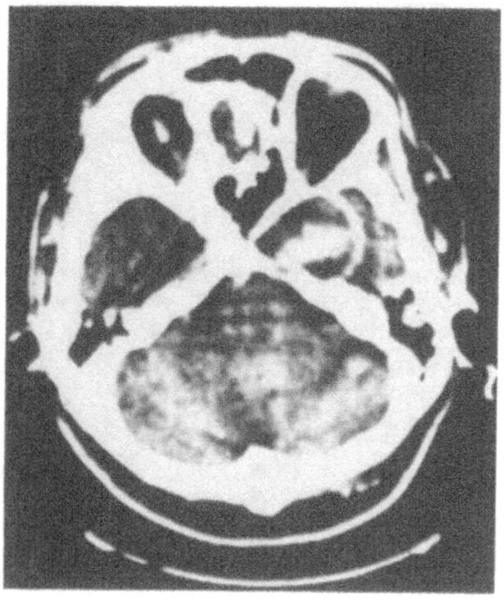

Fig. 9. CT scan: intracavernous giant aneurysm

References

1. Batzdorf U, Gregorius FK (1983) Surgical exposure of the high cervical carotid artery: experimental study and review. Neurosurgery 13: 657–661
2. Batzdorf U, Bentson JR, Mechleder HI (1979) Blunt trauma to the high cervical carotid artery. Neurosurgery 5: 195–201
3. Denecke HJ (1978) Die Chirurgie ausgedehnter Tumoren des Felsenbeins und der Otobasis. Laryngol Rhinol 57: 287–290
4. Dolenc V (1983) Direct neurosurgical repair of intracavernous vascular lesions. J Neurosurg 58: 824–831
5. Fisch U (1978) Infratemporal fossa approach to tumors of the temporal bone and base of the skull. J Laryngol Otol 92: 949–967
6. Fisch U, Oldring DJ, Senning A (1980) Surgical therapy of internal carotid artery lesion of the skull base and temporal bone. Otolaryngol Head Neck Surg 88: 548–554
7. Fisch U (1977) Die Mikrochirurgie des Felsenbeines. HNO 25: 193–197
8. Glasscock ME, Jackson CG (1979) Temporal fossa approach: surgical anatomy, difficulties and complications. Laryngol Otol Rhinol 100: 21–25
9. Hershey FB (1974) Operation for aneurysm of the internal carotid artery high in the neck. A new and an old technique. Angiology 25: 24–30
10. House WF (1977) Transcochlear approach to the petrous apex and clivus. Trans Am Acad Ophthalmol Otolaryngol 84: 927–931
11. Paullus WS, Pait RG, Rhoton AL (1977) Microsurgical exposure of the petrous portion of the carotid artery. J Neurosurg 47: 713–726
12. Pellerin P, Lesoin F, Dhellemmes P, Donazzan M, Jomin M (1984) Usefulness of the orbito fronto malar approach associated with bone reconstruction for frontotemporosphenoid meningiomas. Neurosurgery 15: 715–718
13. Pellerin P, Lesoin F, Auffret P, Dhellemmes P, Jomin M (1985) Tumeurs malignes étendues à la base du crâne. Principes d'exérèse et de reconstruction. Soc Neurochir Française. Communication orale
14. Queval P (1982) L'abord chirurgical de la carotide interne à la base du crâne et dans le rocher. Thèse, Université Lille
15. Quisling RG, Rhoton AL (1979) Intrapetrous carotid artery branches. Radioanatomic analysis. Radiology 131: 133–136
16. Simon C, Gazel P, Wayoff M (1980) Extension to the base of the skull of the benign tumors of the petrous pyramid. On 9 cases. Rev Otoneuroophthalmol 52: 220–230
17. Vaneecloo FM, Jomin M, Camuzet JP, Janssen B (1984) Abord de la face antéro-superieure du rocher par voie sus-pétreuse. Son intérêt pour le traitement des lesions rares interessant la sphénoïde, le nerf trijumeau, l'artère carotid interne. Ann Otolaryng Chir Cervicofac 101: 95–101

Tumor surgery

The direct microsurgical approach to intracavernous tumors

F. Lesoin[1], P. Pellerin[2], A. Autricque[1], J. Clarisse[3], and M. Jomin[1]

[1] Department B of Neurosurgery, [2] Department of Plastic and Reconstructive Surgery, and [3] Department of Neuroradiology, C.H.R.U., Lille, France

Strictly intracavernous tumors remain rare and their management is still a subject of controversy. The authors expose the direct surgical approach to these lesions. They consider this to be necessary in order to determine the exact nature of the intracavernous process. The subsequent treatment, in particular radiotherapy, will depend to it.

Progress in surgical technique for intracavernous lesions has mainly concerned vascular pathology since the work done by Parkinson [2]. The approach to the cavernous sinus has considerably benefited from the microsurgical anatomical studies carried out, which have enabled the relationship between the cavernous sinus, carotid artery and nerves III, IV, V, and VI to be clearly defined [15, 21]. Paradoxically, the direct approach for tumorous lesions is envisaged with much more circumspection [10, 22], although they doubtless pose fewer problems from the technical standpoint.

Since 1983, we have developed a direct surgical approach technique for this sinus which has been used in 21 patients presenting with a strictly intracavernous tumorous lesion. We discuss here its implementation, indications and results.

Patients and methods

Between January 1, 1983, and September 1, 1985, 21 cases were dealt with (Table 1). The average age of the 12 male and 9 female patients was 43 and the age range was 25 to 70.

The clinical findings enabled the patients to be classed into three groups:

15 of the patients presented with a progressive syndrome of the cavernous sinus with unilateral damage to the nerves III, IV, V or VI, with

Table 1. Results of the direct surgical approach technique

Case	Sex	Development time	Clinical symptomatology	Treatment	Histology
1	M	6 months	III incomplete exophthalmos	Resection of tumor	Meningioma
2	F	12 months	III complete exophthalmos	Resection of tumor	Meningioma
3	M	12 months	Exophthalmos	Ditto	Meningioma
4	M	1 month	III incomplete headaches	Ditto	Metastasis
5	F	10 months	III incomplete exophthalmos	Ditto	Meningioma
6	M	1 month	Complete cavernous syndrome	Exclusion	Metastasis
7	F	8 months	III complete exophthalmos	Resection of tumor	Meningioma
8	F	3 months	III complete exophthalmos	Ditto	Meningioma
9	M	Transient	III incomplete	Ditto	Meningioma
10	M	6 months	III incomplete exophthalmos	Ditto	Meningioma
11	M	Transient	III incomplete	Ditto	Meningioma
12	M	Transient	III incomplete	Ditto	Meningioma
13	F	14 months	III incomplete	Ditto	Meningioma
14	F	10 months	Cavernous syndrome with damage to III, IV	Denudation of carotid artery	Meningioma
15	F	16 months	Exophthalmos	Resection of tumor	Neurinoma
16	M	Transient	III incomplete	Ditto	Meningioma
17	M	2 months	Complete cavernous syndrome	Exclusion	Metastasis
18	F	Transient	III incomplete headaches	Resection of tumor	Meningioma
19	M	18 months	III incomplete	Ditto	Chondroma
20	F	9 months	III incomplete	Ditto	Meningioma
21	F	Acute	III incomplete headaches	Ditto	Meningioma

or without retro-orbital pain. The exophthalmos found in 8 cases remained moderate. The visual acuity and the field of vision were normal;

1 patient presented with an acute syndrome of the cavernous sinus with a rapidly appearing oculomotor deficit accompanied by headaches, this being linked to a rapid increase in the size of the lesion due to the highly vascularized nature of the tumor, a part of which was necrosed;

5 patients had a transient syndrome with the oculomotor damage appearing suddenly then regressing within a few days.

16 meningiomas were responsible for a partial cavernous syndrome as were the condroma and the neurinoma. On the other hand, 2 of the 3 metastases were accompanied by a complete cavernous syndrome.

An angiographic assessment was done for all the patients and this showed a tumorous blush in 15 meningiomas. The frontal and sagittal section of the CT scan showed a full, hyperdense cavernous sinus in the case of a meningioma, metastasis or neurinoma together with intracavernous calcifications in the case of the chondroma (Figs. 1 and 2).

Surgical technique

Initially we used the pterional approach together with a temporal flap bone, but we now use essentially on orbitozygomaticomalar flap. The skin incision is that recommended by Cairns-Unterberger. The scalp is detached from the epicranium and the temporal aponeurosis as far as the external superior orbital edge and from the malar arch, along which the periosteum is incised and retracted. Subperiosteal dissection allows the branches of the facial nerve to be left intact. The anterior half of the temporal muscle and the masseter is retracted, the orbit being dissected. The frontotemporal flap bone is then cut and removed. Then with three osteotomy strokes of the vibrating saw, while protecting the detached periosteum with a malleable strip, the body of the malar, the orbital apophysis of the frontal bone and the malar arch are cut, thus enabling the mobilization of the frontozygomaticomalar flap bone. The temporal muscle can then be pushed outwards right out of the way so as to obtain an excellent view of the pterygomaxillary fossa, the sphenomaxillary fissure and the floor of the temporal fossa.

Behind the cavernous sinus the lesser wing of the sphenoid is removed all the way to the anterior clinoid, which is resected. This enables the optic canal and the sphenoid fissure to be opened. The surgeon then controls the anterior part of the cavernous sinus, the anterior carotid artery behind it, the ophthalmic artery, nerves III and IV and the ophthalmic branch of nerve V.

In front of the cavernous sinus the intrapetrous carotid artery (ICA) is exposed extradurally around Glasscock's triangle [5]. The dura mater is only incised to drain the cisterns and deplete the CSF so as to obtain a brain collapse. The exposure of the anterosuperior face of the petrous bone extradurally is achieved by progressive detachment of the dura mater under the operating microscope. Hemostasis is produced by bipolar coagulation. Detachment started backwards is then continued by working forwards and may be hindered by the existence of fibrous bands around the petrosquamous suture and the arcuate eminence which will be cut with microscissors. Further on detachment becomes much easier, but also much more hazardous. It uncovers the 2 petrosal nerves coming out of Fallop's hiatus and the innominate foramen. They appear like two whitish cords stretched between the dura mater and the bone. They are cut without traction so as to avoid any facial paralysis. Further forward the foramen spinosum is uncovered and the meningeal artery coagulated. The detachment of the dura is continued as far as Meckel's cavity and the infraorbital nerve which enters the oval foramen and constitutes the upper limit of the detachment procedure. The anterosuperior face of the petrous bone is exposed with the arcuate eminence behind, the infraorbital nerve in front, and on the inside the superior edge of the petrous bone which contains the superior petrous sinus, wrapped in the dura mater. A selfretaining retractor is installed to push back the dura and the temporal lobe. The next step is to locate the horizontal portion of the carotid canal and three landmarks are used to do this: the greater superficial petrosal nerve, the middle meningeal artery and the infraorbital nerve. The internal carotid enters this triangle with a certain variability [14].

The greater superficial petrosal nerve is parallel to the horizontal section of the inner carotid. In 90% of cases the infraorbital nerve has its origin under, in 2% of cases in front of the carotid canal, while the middle meningeal artery is located 4.7 mm outside the carotid canal. Progressive drilling under the microscope of the petrous bone opposite the point of origin of the infraorbital nerve enables the proximal part of the superior face of the intrapetrous inner carotid artery to be exposed along its horizontal section. The bone is not very thick at this point. In some cases, it does not exist at all, which makes it easier to locate the carotid canal. The exposure of the superior face can be continued laterally for a further 1 cm to the infraorbital nerve and this enables the carotid to be exposed as far as the band separating the horizontal section from the vertical section. At this point in the procedure, the superior face of the carotid artery is unroofed. Its mobilization requires the freeing of its external face and therefore the opening of the Eustachian tube, whose path is parallel to the section of the intrapetrous internal carotid artery.

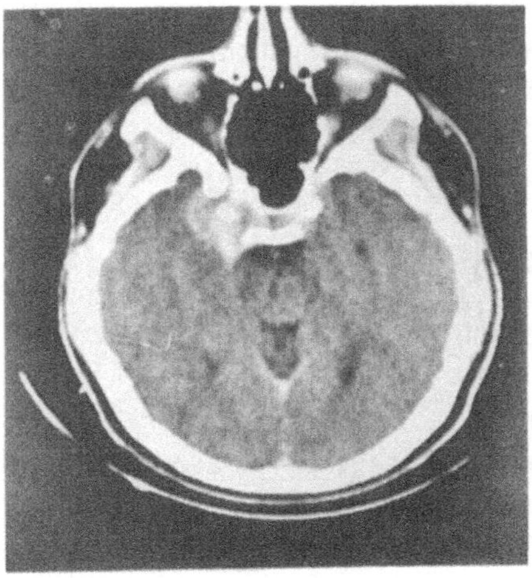

Fig. 1. CT scan: intracavernous meningioma

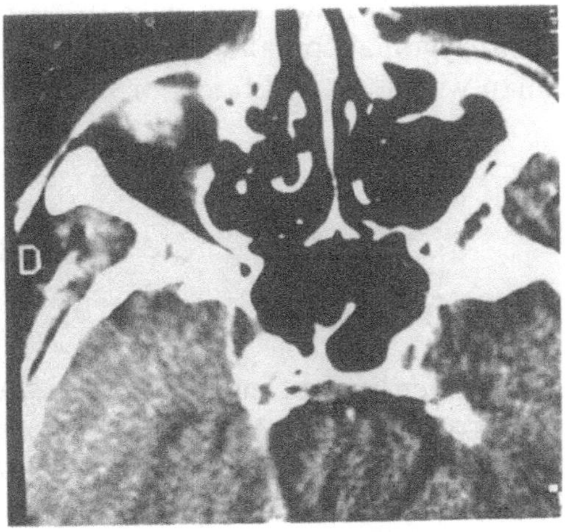

Fig. 2. CT scan: intracavernous chondroma

The cavernous sinus is then opened at the superior part of Parkinson's triangle [12] parallel to nerves III and IV whose paths have already been localized by the opening of the sphenoid fissure. Very often, nerves III and IV are pushed back towards the inner part of the cavernous sinus and the ophthalmic nerve towards the outer part through the bulging of the tumorous growth. Venous bleeding is virtually non-existent because the afferent and efferent sinuses are filled with tumorous tissue. The linear incision is kept open with threads taken each side of the external wall of the cavernous sinus. At this stage, the surgeon can either:

perform a progressive resection of the intracavernous tumor making allowance for the special situation of nerve VI along the intracavernous carotid.

Resection is made more or less difficult by the consistency of the expansive process and its bleeding. Very often, if the resection is large, the freeing of the afferent and efferent sinuses leads to venous bleeding which can be controlled by packing with Surgicel, muscle or bone dust.

In all cases sealing the external wall will provide definitive hemostasis;

or lay bare the intracavernous carotid including the sacrifice of all the nervous elements and the resection of the walls of the sinus;

or exclude the cavernous sinus after installing a clip on the carotid, upstream in the intrapetrous portion and downstream before the point of origin of the ophthalmic artery. In this case we carry out the classic preoperative tests with compression of the carotid at the neck: EEG, Doppler test and recording of the residual pressure after a clamping test.

Sealing includes steel wire osteosynthesis of the frontotemporal and orbitozygomaticomalar flap bones following the obliteration of the Eustachian with temporal fascia or its reconstruction with a bone graft.

Results

All the patients were treated by a direct surgical approach. Surgery comprised:

18 extensive but incomplete resections;

2 exclusions for 2 patients who presented with a metastasis with total ophthalmoplegia and a satisfactory alternative network;

1 denudation of the intracavernous carotid was performed in one patient presenting with a meningioma with major oculomotor damage with no valid alternative network.

The treatment was completed by radiotherapy at a dose of 3400 rads for the metastases and the 5 grade III or IV meningiomas. Two patients with a grade I or II meningioma came in for regular clinical and CT scan checks every six months and the same applied to the chondroma.

Five patients experienced a transient worsening of their oculomotor condition. Eleven patients are currently stabilized and 10 patients have in the main improved.

Comments

The direct surgical approach to the cavernous sinus in tumorous pathology has, in our experience, considerably benefited from the cooperation between maxillofacial surgeons and neurosurgeons, as has the treatment of meningiomas of the sphenoid ridge with invasion of the cavernous sinus [15] and the treatment of malignant craniofacial tumors with secondary extension to this same sinus. We will comment on the technical problems before going on to discuss the usefulness of this direct approach.

The technical control for residual intracranial pressure regularly used in vascular surgery is a very important means of finding out whether definitive clamping of the carotid artery is possible should the surgeon wish to perform an exclusion. The use of the operating microscope enables the nervous elements to be located and this even before the sinus is opened after bone resection of the superior edge of the sphenoid fissure.

The general technical approach which we have gradually developed enables control of both the anterior and the posterior parts of the sinus. It seems important to carry out a histopathological study of any intracavernous tumorous process. It is in fact in vain to think that the use of computed tomography will provide a histopathological diagnosis [23]. A meningioma is certainly the most likely etiology but it is essential to determine its grade [2, 6, 9] as this will govern its subsequent development and management. The limits of resection through the direct approach depend first of all on the nature of the tumor. In the case of meningiomas it is rather in vain to think that it is possible to completely cut away the intracavernous tumor without aggravating the oculomotor symptoms. This can be understood in as far as the anatomical studies [1, 13, 18] have shown that the arachnoid tissue lines the whole of the inner face of the sinus and surrounds the carotid artery and that there are many arachnoid islands disseminated between the nervous elements. Resection can be more or less extensive depending on the hemorrhagic nature of the tumor, its consistency and above all its adhesion to the vascular elements. In our experience total resection of a meningioma or an intracavernous metastasis remains therefore very difficult. On the other hand, in the case of a neurinoma resection was facilitated by the splittable and nonhemorrhagic nature of the lesional process. In the case of the chondroma, it was easy to remove the fleshy tumorous portion, but the calcified portion had to be left because of its adhesion to the nervous elements. The limits of resection through the direct approach are linked to the criteria expounded by Laine et al. [10]. True exclusion can only be offered when there is complete ophthalmoplegia, damage to nerve V, thrombosis of the carotid artery or an alternative and effective contralateral system, currently checked out by taking the residual pressure following upstream clamping of the carotid. Should this not be the case and if the oculomotor symptomatology is extensive, denudation of the intracavernous carotid artery may be performed. This takes away the walls of the sinus, the intracavernous nervous elements and the tumorous process while leaving the intracavernous carotid intact.

Whether we are dealing with a metastasis or a meningioma of grade III or IV or of the hemangiopericytic type, this surgical approach is followed up with radiotherapy. The efficacity of radiotherapy has in fact now been proved [4, 7, 8, 21, 22] without lifting the doubt surrounding possible parietal fragilization of the inner carotid artery and long-term repercussions on the hypothalmo-hypophyseal axis.

A grade I or II meningioma rules out radiotherapy at the outset but calls for regular clinical, ophthalmological and CT scan monitoring [11, 18, 20].

Conclusions

Surgery of the cavernous sinus remains difficult but its usefulness in tumorous pathology should not be underestimated. From the technical standpoint the classical notion of considerable venous bleeding occurring should be made light of in tumorous pathology. It only occurs in fact at the end of the procedure once the sinus has been freed. The resection remains limited, especially if the oculomotor symptomatology is incomplete. The usefulness of a histological study and of grading the tumors, especially the meningiomas, is considerable given the possibility of secondary radiotherapy which will certainly gain in refinement with the advent of the multibeam technique.

References

1. Bedford MA (1986) The "cavernous sinus". Br J Ophthal 50: 1–46
2. Christensen D, Laursen H, Klinken L (1983) Prediction of recurrence in meningiomas after surgical treatment. Acta Neuropathol 61: 130–134
3. Dolenc V (1983) Direct microsurgical repair of intracavernous vascular lesions. J Neurosurg 58: 824–831
4. Fukui M, Kitamura H, Nakagari Y, Yamakawa Y, Kinoshita N, Hayabuchi K, Jingu Y, Nnuaguchi K, Matsuura K, Watanabe K (1980) Irradiated meningiomas: a clinical evaluation. Acta Neurochir 54: 33–43
5. Glasscock ME (1969) Exposure of the intrapetrous portion of the carotid artery. In: Hamberger CA, Wersäall J (eds) Disorders of the skull base region. Proceedings of the 10th Nobel symposium. Almqvist and Wiksell, Stockholm, pp 135–143
6. Jaaskelainen J, Halta M, Laasonen R, Wahlstrom T, Valtonen S (1985) The growth rate of intracranial meningiomas and its relation to history. An analysis of 43 patients. Surg Neurol 24: 165–172
7. Kepes JJ (1982) Meningiomas. Biology, pathology and differential diagnosis. Masson monographs in diagnostic pathology. Masson, New York, pp 112–113
8. Kind KL, Chang CH, Pool JL (1966) Radiotherapy in management of meningiomas. Acta Radiol 5: 87–90
9. Kline LB, Acker JD, Post JD (1982) Computed topographic. Evaluation of the cavernous sinus. Ophthal Rochester 89: 374–385
10. Laine E, Galibert P, Pruvo J, Christiaens JL (1965) Possibilités d'éxèrese des méningiomes envahissant le sinus caverneux. Soc Neurochir Française, Paris 19: 564–566
11. Melamed S, Sahar A, Bellar AJ (1979) The recurrence of intracranial meningiomas. Neurochirurgia (Stuttg) 22: 47–51
12. Parkinson D (1973) Carotid cavernous fistula: direct repair with preservation of the carotid artery. Technical note. J Neurosurg 38: 99–106
13. Patouillard P, Vaneuville G (1972) Les parois du sinus caverneux. Neurochirurgie 18: 551–560
14. Paullus WS, Pait RG, Rhoton AL Jr (1977) Microsurgical exposure of the petrous portion of the carotid artery. J Neurosurg 47: 713–726
15. Pellerin P, Lesoin F, Dhellemmes P, Donazzan M, Jomin M (1984) Usefulness of the orbito-frontomalar approach associated with bone reconstruction for fronto-temporosphenoid meningiomas. Neurosurgery 15: 715–718

16. Rhoton A, Hardy S, Chambers M (1979) Microsurgical anatomy and dissection of the sphenoid bone, cavernous sinus and sellar region. Surg Neurol 12: 63–104
17. Spallone A, Gagliardi M, Vagozzi R (1979) Intracranial meningiomas related to external irradiation. Surg Neurol 12: 153–159
18. Taptas JN (1949) La loge du sinus caverneux. Rev Otoneuro Ophthalmol 21: 197–199
19. Tytus JS, Laserohn T, Reifel E (1967) The problem of malignancy in meningioma. J Neurosurg 27: 551–557
20. Umansky F, Nathan H (1982) The lateral wall of the cavernous sinus with special reference to the nerves related do it. J Neurosurg 56: 228–234
21. van Effentere JP, Bataini E, Cabanis M, Iba-Zizen J (1979) High energy radiotherapy in the treatment of meningiomas of the cavernous sinus. Acta Neurochir (Wien) 28: 464–467
22. Wara W, Shelline H, Newman J, Townsend E, Boldrey B (1975) Radiation therapy of meningiomas. Am J Roentgen Radium Ther Nucl Med 123: 453–458
23. Zozulla Y, Romodanov A, Partski Y (1979) Diagnosis and surgical treatment of benign cranio-basal tumours involving the cavernous sinus. Acta Neurochir (Wien) 28: 387–390

Usefulness of the orbitofrontomalar approach associated with bone reconstruction for frontotemporosphenoid meningiomas

F. LESOIN[1], P. PELLERIN[2], P. DHELLEMMES[1], and M. JOMIN[1]

[1] Department B of Neurosurgery, and [2] Department of Plastic and Reconstructive Surgery, C.H.R.U., Lille, France

Twenty-five cases of frontotemporosphenoid meningioma are reported. The principles of the orbitofrontomalar approach and of reconstruction of the orbital cone and of the frontomalar region with an orbitotemporal flap are discussed.

Introduction

Sphenotemporoorbital meningiomas pose diagnostic and therapeutic problems. The extent of invasion towards the anterior fossa, the middle fossa, the orbit, the sellar region, the cavum, the zygomatic fossa, and the pterygomaxillary fossa can now be determined by computed tomography. Several investigators have shown that the excision of these tumors requires a radical surgical approach.

Since 1980, with cooperation between maxillofacial surgeons and neurosurgeons, we have operated on frontotemporosphenoid meningiomas using the orbitofrontomalar approach. This approach requires first the cutting of a frontoorbitomalar flap and then the resection of the osteoma and the meningioma with bone reconstruction. This procedure is based on three-dimensional visualization of the region and comprises reconstruction of the orbital cone and the frontomalar region with an orbitotemporal prop. The principles of this approach and the method of bone reconstruction are detailed in this report.

Clinical material and method

Between 1980 and 1985, twenty-five patients presented with a sphenoid meningioma and underwent this surgical procedure. Eighteen were female and seven were male. The average age was 51. In seven of the patients, the operation was performed for a recurrent tumor after the first operation had been limited to resection of the meningioma without total resection of the osteoma. Three of the patients had meningiomas en plaques and this procedure was used in first intention for fifteen patients.

The clinical symptoms developed gradually over a period of 4 years (on average). They included ophthalmological symptoms (exophthalmos in twenty-five patients, oculomotor damage in twenty patients, and decrease in visual acuity in eight patients, two of whom suffered from blindness), convulsive seizures in two patients, contralateral hemiparesis in one patient, and neuralgia of nerve V in one patient.

Standard X-ray films revealed osteosclerosis in en plaques meningiomas and osteolysis in other meningiomas. Computed tomography including axial and frontal sections showed orbital intracranial extension to the pterygomaxillary fossa, to the sphenoid bone, and sometimes to the temporal muscle. Carotid angiography showed the effect of the tumor on vascular structures, especially the cavernous sinus (in five cases, considerable stenosis was observed in the cavernous sinus). It also revealed which vessels, such as branches of the internal maxillary artery and the ophthalmic artery, can be embolized before operation, thus reducing blood loss during surgery. It is sometimes difficult to control intraoperative bleeding through intraosseous vessels. We consider it essential to examine the contralateral carotid system to check for compression due to invasion of the sphenoid sinus.

An ophthalmological assessment includes determination of visual acuity, evoked response testing, campimetry, and Lancaster's test.

Surgical procedure

A bitemporal scalp incision is made anterior to the tragus on the side of the lesion. Dissection at the level of the temporalis aponeurosis is extended to the zygomatic protrusion and the superior orbital edge. The bifrontal bone flap is either free or attached to the contralateral temporalis muscle. The roof of the orbit is dissected on both sides: on the intracranial side through the subdural pathway and on the orbital side through the subperiosteal pathway. The temporalis is detached from the malar bone, the pterion, and the temporal bone, and the periosteum is removed from the malar arch. With the use of a vibrating saw, a frontoorbitomalar free flap including the superior orbital edge is removed (Fig. 1). The malar bone and the malar arch provide access to the orbit and the pterygomaxillary fossa (Fig. 2). With a

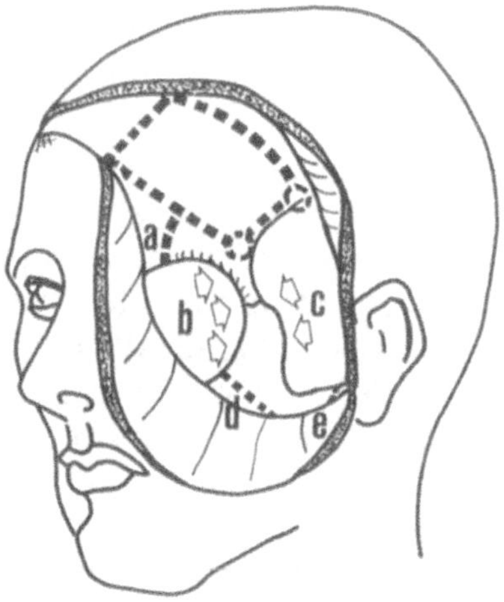

Fig. 1. With a vibrating saw, a frontoorbitomalar free flap including the superior orbital edge is removed. **a** Vertical orbital section; **b** horizontal orbital section; **c** external orbital section; **d** malar section; **e** zygomatic section

rongeur, working from the outside to the inside, the great and the lesser wings of the sphenoid bone are excised, taking with them the diseased bone and opening up the lateral segments of the frontal and temporal fossae and the extradural part of the middle cerebral fossa.

When the tumor is circumscribed, the dura mater is opened and the tumor is separated from the cerebral parenchyma and then removed. Musculoaponeuroplasty is then performed. We use the epicranium for defects of average size. For areas greater than 4 × 4 cm, we use the sural aponeurosis centered on the tensor muscle of the fascia or the abdominal aponeurosis (oblique muscles) lined with a 5 to 8 mm thick layer of fatty, cellular tissue sutured by direct overcasting. The orbital tumor is resected after the carotid artery and the cranial nerves are located. The rest of the diseased bone is removed systemically, including the whole of the lesser wing with in two roots, which exposes the optic canal and the top edge of the sphenoid fissure, and the great wing and its roots, which exposes the large, round, and oval holes to free the maxillary and infraorbital nerves and the bottom edge of the sphenoid fissure. The remainder of the excision is dependent on the extension of the tumor (lateral mass of the ethmoid bone, sphenoid sinus, pterygoid apophysis, and maxilla) and is continued until macroscopically sound bone is found. When the excision is completed, at least the following will have been removed: the roof and the internal wall of the orbit, the orbital apex, the roof of the temporal fossa and a segment of the frontotemporal vault, and the adjacent regions.

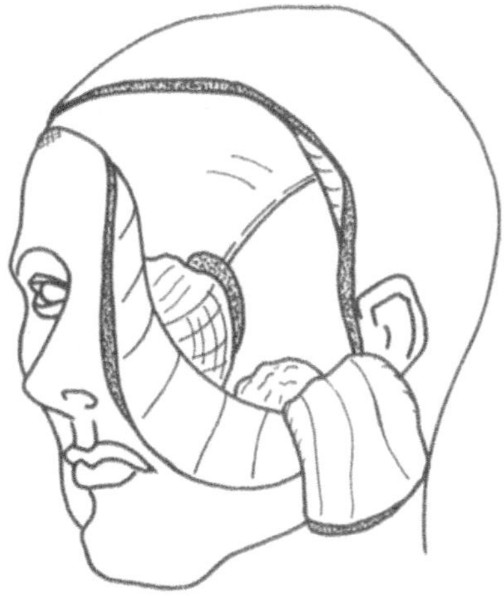

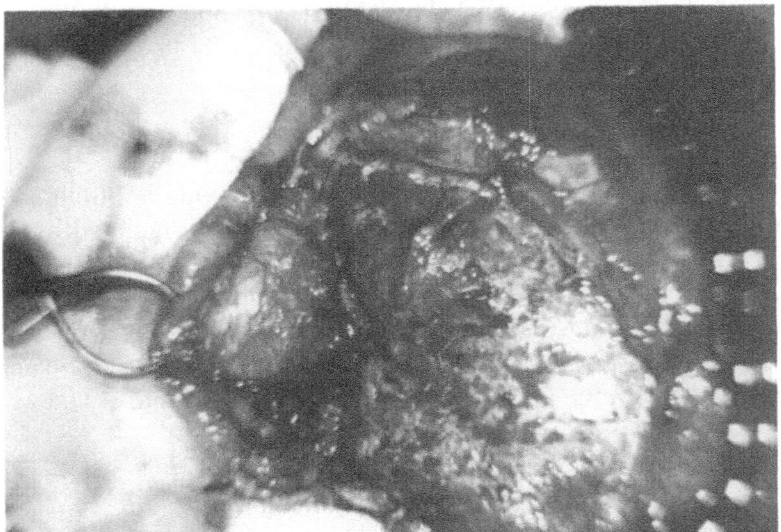

Fig. 2. After the frontoorbitomalar free flap and the frontotemporal flap are removed, access to the orbit and the pterygomaxillary fossa is possible

The second step requires reconstruction using iliac bone for grafting. An iliac graft is advantageous because the material for the graft is cortico-spongious. The spongious bone is responsive to the cutaneoperiosteal zones, which vascularize rapidly. The graft is taken from the internal cortical part, leaving the external half of the iliac crest untouched. Dissection of the internal table is done subperiosteally, pushing the iliac muscle inward.

This procedure provides a large graft, 10 to 13 × 6 to 8 cm. The necessary segments are cut from the large graft in solid blocks as required. The "scrap" material is arranged as required to fill in the remaining gaps in the nonvisible zones (under the temporal muscle and the hairy area of the vault).

Reconstruction of the roof of the temporal fossa

A wedge-shaped graft (Fig. 3) is inlaid between, anteriorly, the maxillary tuberosity and, posteriorly, the inside part of the root of the zygoma; under this graft, the maxillary and infraorbital nerves will pass. Because the graft is held between the temporal lobe and the pterygoid muscles, it does not need to be fixed in place.

Reconstruction of the orbital walls

A piece of bone shaped as a half-frustrum of a cone is obtained from a curved iliac fragment. It is then placed in position (Fig. 3) with the inside edge resting on the roof of the ethmoid bone and the outside edge resting on the pyramidal apophysis of the maxilla, to which it is attached with a steel wire ligature. The outer radius corresponds to the orbital periphery and the inner radius corresponds to the orbital apex and allows the optic nerve and the components of the sphenoid fissure to pass through.

Reconstruction of the pterion

A graft cut from a fragment of internal table (Fig. 4) is placed in the form of a prop between the squama temporalis and the junction of the cone, with crosswise stabilization.

Frontomalar reconstruction

If undamaged, the frontomalar frame is laid in place and attached with three steel wire sutures (Fig. 4). In the event of segmental invasion, the fragment is

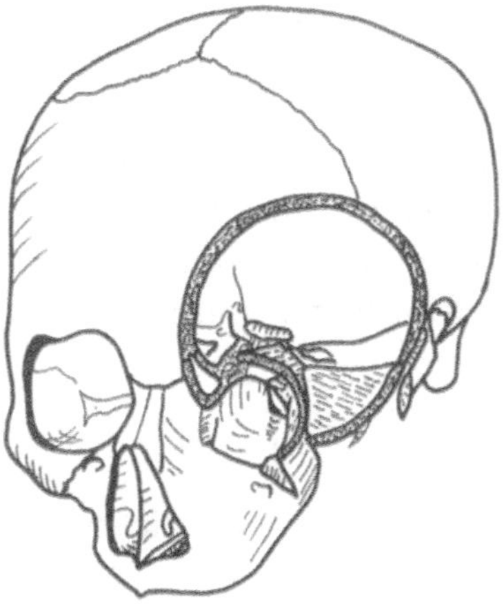

Fig. 3. Reconstruction of the roof of the temporal fossa and the orbital walls

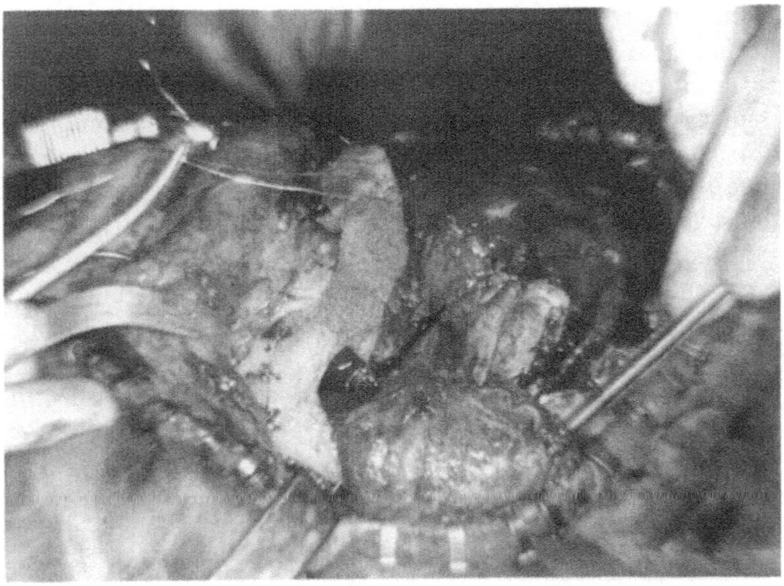

Fig. 4. Reconstruction of the pterion and the frontomalar frame

excised and replaced with an iliac graft. In four of our cases, we replaced the top and the external orbital edges while preserving the body of the malar bone and the malar arch. In two cases, we replaced the whole of the frontomalar flap with a large single graft that we curved and cut as required and then attached to the frontal bone, maxilla, and orbital cone (graft) along with a fragment of the malar bone. The remaining graft material was arranged to reconstruct the temporal vault.

Finally, the retrofrontal or pterygomaxillary empty spaces (in a broad-based excision) are filled with free grafts of fatty, cellular tissue.

Results

We assessed the results based on functional (ophthalmological and neurological) and esthetic criteria. We obtained three groups. Eleven patients had very good results: no neurological sequelae, excellent esthetic results, and disappearance of the exophthalmos (Fig. 5). Thirteen patients had good results: no neurological sequelae, good esthetic results and lessening of the exophthalmos. One of the patients died of postoperative cerebral ischemia, which was confirmed by a computed tomographic (CT) scan. Autopsy revealed that this patient had suffered thrombosis of the internal carotid artery in the cavernous sinus on the side of operation and that the lumen of the artery was greatly reduced, probably because of extrinsic tumorous compression. Furthermore, the contralateral carotid artery had severe acquired dysplasia; angiographic evaluation of the artery had not been done before the operation. A local infection occurred 15 days after operation in one patient and was treated by irrigation of the operative zone and systemic antibiotic therapy. We do not use prophylactic systemic antibiotic therapy despite the length of the operation.

The patients experienced an immediate postoperative functional oculomotor paralysis. This completely regressed after 3 months, but orthoptic rehabilitation was required.

All patients underwent CT scanning before and after excision. In all cases, one CT scan was judged sufficient.

Discussion

The excision of tumors of the base of the skull centered on the sphenoid bone poses many technical problems, as was described by Derome [3] in 1972. The orbitofrontomalar approach broadens the operative field and makes it easier to evaluate the vascular and neural structures and the tumor extension in the periorbit, the maxilla, the pterygomaxillary fossa, the pterygoid apophyses, and the parapharyngeal regions. Furthermore, the

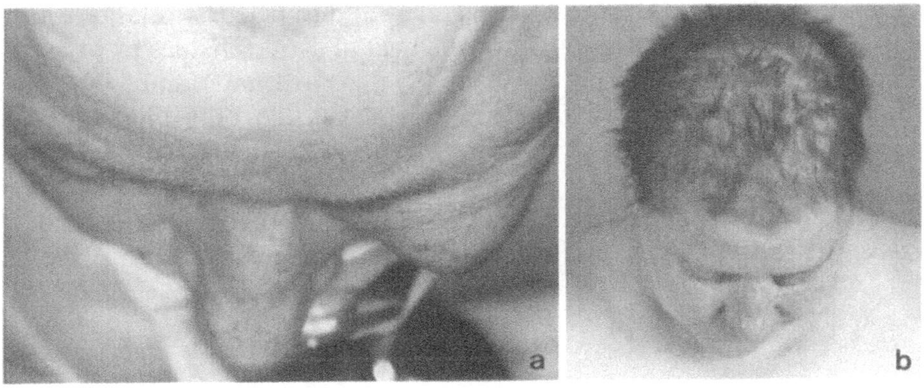

Fig. 5. The patient before (**a**) and 6 months after (**b**) the complete excision of a frontotemporosphenoid meningioma

conventional frontal or frontotemporal approach requires brain retraction or even frontal or temporal brain resection [1]. Like Yaşargil [7], we think that a tangential approach enables an extracerebral approach. Carrizo proposed a dual approach: transmalar or frontotemporal [2]. The choice of just one frontoorbitomalar approach seems preferable because the risk of sepsis is reduced.

Bone reconstruction is performed with the iliac bone, which seems better than costal graft material or acrylic prostheses. The natural shape of the internal cortical part of the iliac wing is a curve similar to that of the structures to be reconstructed. The plasticity of the iliac bone enables us to reproduce exactly the structures under reconstruction by arching it with Tessier's forceps. Rib grafts require the juxtaposition of several fragments, which never fuse together perfectly, whereas iliac graft material enables us to reconstruct continuous, single piece structures. The disadvantages of using iliac graft material (pain, hematoma, area of anaesthesia in the femorocutaneous zone, crural paralysis) are avoided if certain precautions are taken: the insertions for the gluteal muscles on the external cortical part must be left untouched, the external part of the iliac crest must be left untouched, the insertions of the oblique muscles of the abdomen must be fixed to the remaining half-crest, the femorocutaneous nerve must be left untouched, and an external drain must be installed to prevent the formation of a hematoma, which might cause crural paralysis.

The indications for this type of operation have been limited. However, Bonnal showed in 1961 that, after the subtotal resection of an en plaque or mass meningioma, recurrences occurred within a short time (14 months to 5 years) [1]. Progress in the field of anaesthetics and broadening of surgical approach methods have enabled teams representing several branches of surgery to tackle these tumors satisfactorily and to perform total resection with reconstruction. Dismantling of the orbital frame enables us to check intraorbital extension. The problem of the cavernous sinus remains, however, extension into the cavernous sinus is the only limit to total resection of the tumor. In 1956, Laine proposed the deliberate sacrifice of the cavernous pit and its components after ligation of the carotid artery at the clinoid process [6]. This technique can be used if one is certain of revascularization of the hemisphere from another area.

References

1. Bonnal J, Sedan R, Paillas JE (1961) Problèmes cliniques, évolutifs et thérapeutiques soulevés par les méningiomes envahissants de la base du crane. Neurochirurgie 7: 108–117
2. Carrizo A, Basso A, Dickman G, Chersi J, Kreutel A (1981) Combined approach to sphenoorbital tumors. Presented at the int cong neurosurg in Munich, Germany
3. Derome P (1972) Les tumeurs sphéno-ethmoïdales: possibilité d'exérèse et de réparation chirurgicale. Neurochirurgie 18 [Suppl] 1: 1–161
4. Guiot G, Derome P (1966) A propos des méningiomes en plaques du pteryon de traitement chirurgical des méningiomes osseux hyperostosants. Ann Chir 20: 19–20
5. Guyot JF, Vouyouklakis D, Pertuiset B (1967) Méningiomes l'arête sphénoïdale: à propos de 50 cas. Neurochirurgie 13: 571–584
6. Laine E, Galibert P, Pruvot J, Christiaens JL (1965) Possibilités d'exérèse des méningiomes envahissant le sinus caverneux. Presented at the Soc Neurochir de Langue Française, in Paris, France
7. Yaşargil MG, Fox JL (1975) The microsurgical approach to intracranial aneurysms. Surg Neurol 3: 7–14

An orbitozygomaticomalar bone flap approach: a technical note

F. LESOIN[1], K. FRANZ[1], P. PELLERIN[2], L. VILLETTE[1], A. AUTRICQUE[1], and M. JOMIN[1]

[1] Department B of Neurosurgery, and [2] Department of Plastic and Reconstructive Surgery, C.H.R.U., Lille, France

The authors describe an orbitozygomaticomalar bone flap approach which gives lateral extra-cerebral access to the internal base of the skull. The technique is described, and some of the situations in which it has been used are discussed.

Introduction

Depending on the size of the extracerebral intracranial lesion to be operated upon, there are two very different approaches available to the neurological surgeon: if the lesion in question is very small, he can use microsurgical techniques, which reduce the size of the operating field [2, 7, 8], or he can instead open a large extended area if wide access is necessary for thorough treatment [3, 5]. Regardless of the size of the field of operation, treatment of an extracerebral intracranial lesion necessitates access to the affected area without causing damage to the surrounding healthy brain tissue. For example, tumors of the temporal fossa which lie on the greater wing of the sphenoid and which are largely vascularized by arteries arising from the external carotid artery are quite difficult to isolate with the traditional temporal bone flap approach [2, 7, 8]. Fujitsu and Kuwabara [3] devised a zygomatic arch bone flap which opens the way to anterior tumors; our approach lends itself to temporal tumors of the internal base of the skull.

Surgical procedure

Using an enlarged Cairns-Unterberger incision (Fig. 1), the operating field is exposed by extending the incision and reflecting the skin along the zygomatic arch flap to the superior edge of the orbit (Fig. 2). Careful

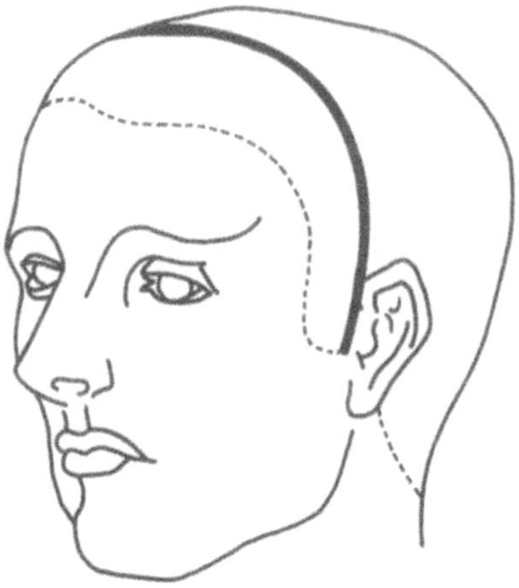

Fig. 1. The Cairns-Unterberger skin incision

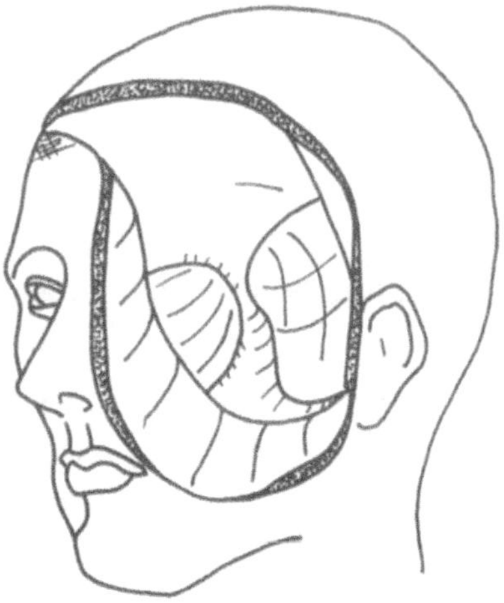

Fig. 2. The scalp incision is extended to the zygomatic protuberance and the superior orbital ridge

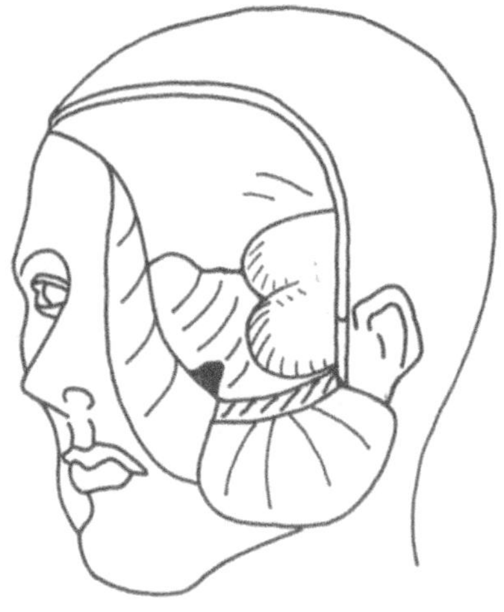

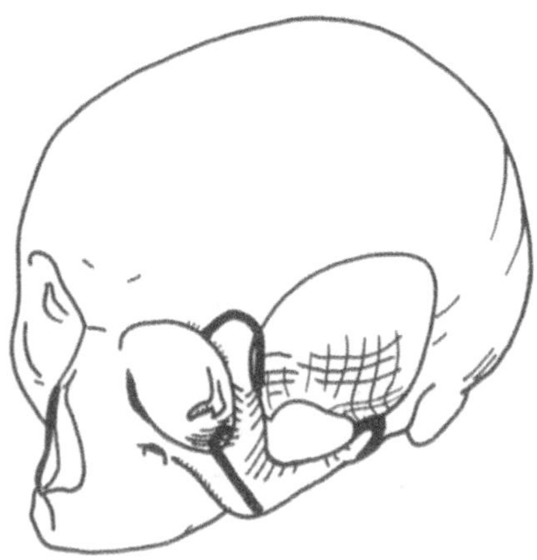

Figs. 3 and **4.** Dissection of the superior orbital ridge, the malar bone, and the zygomatic arch with a vibrating saw

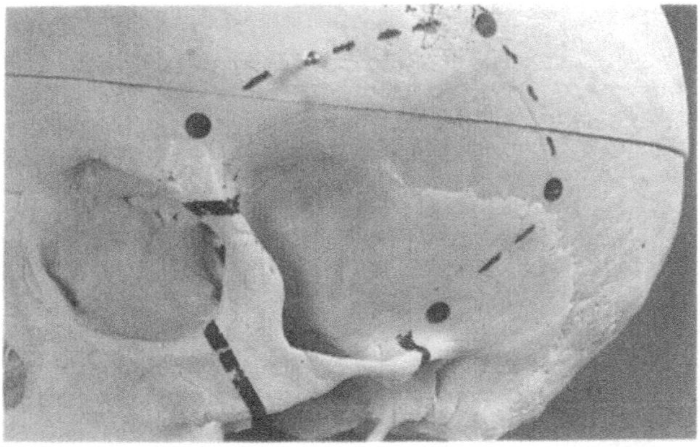

Fig. 5. The operating field of the orbitozygomaticomalar bone flap

dissection of the subperiosteum exposes the branches of the facial nerves which can then be protected from surgical injury. The masseter, the orbital, and the anterior half of the temporal muscles are then dissected free, and a vibrating saw is used to section the malar bone, the superior orbital ridge, and the zygomatic arch (Figs. 3, 4). With the temporal muscle retracted, the following structures are visible: the zygomatic fossa, the floor of the temporal fossa, and the sphenomaxillary fissure. A temporal bone flap is then made, giving access to the internal base of the skull and a clear view of the area to be operated upon, with a minimum of damage to the brain itself. If necessary, a ronguer can be used to clear the floor of the middle cranial fossa if greater access is required. After removal of the orbitozygomatico-malar bone flap, the maxillary nerve is freed and protected, and the middle meningeal artery can then be coagulated (Fig 5).

Removal of a bone flap is useful in treatment of lesions situated on the middle cranial fossa floor, but is not necessary for disorders of the interpeduncular cistern, such as aneurysms of the vertebrobasilar system, craniopharyngiomas, or chondromas.

The dura mater is closed in the usual manner, and the bone flap is replaced and secured with two or three wire sutures, i.e., a frontal, a zygomatic, and if necessary a malomalar. Sometimes an iliac graft is required to reconstruct the floor of the middle cranial fossa. The pericranium is then closed, and after suction drainage, final skin closure is done.

Discussion

In addition to being less traumatic than other approaches to the internal skull base, the orbitozygomaticomalar bone flap technique gives a better view of, and wider access to, the middle cranial fossa floor and the temporal lobe. We have used this in the treatment of two cases of vertebrobasilar

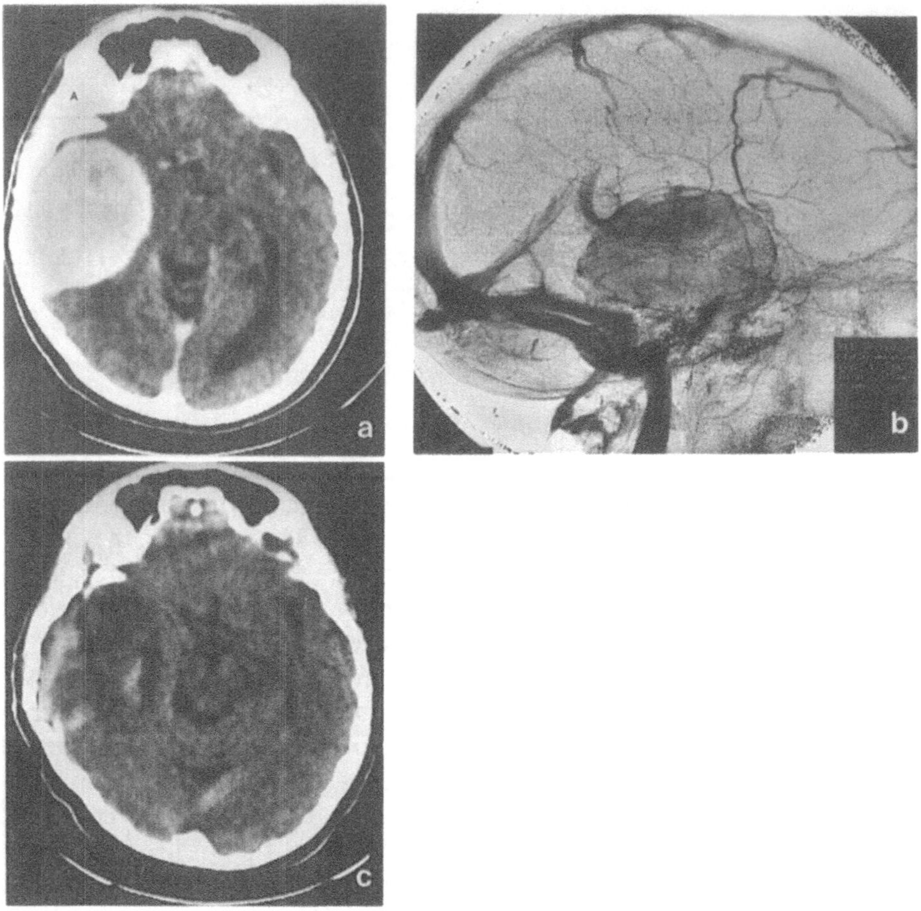

Fig. 6. A widely spread meningioma of the floor of the temporal fossa invading the dura mater: an ideal indication for this approach. Preoperative CT scan (**a**), preoperative angiography (**b**), immediate post operative CT scan (**c**)

aneurysms and we feel that it is superior to the removal of the chondromas and the craniopharyngiomas of the interpeduncular region as proposed Fujitsu and Kuwabara [3].

Branches of the external carotid artery (especially the internal maxillary and the middle meningeal) which supply tumors of the middle cranial fossa are easily isolated, and tumoral infiltrations of surrounding bone tissue and/or dura mater can be removed and the affected structures grafted and reconstructed if necessary. We have removed large tumors of the greater wing of the sphenoid (Fig. 6) with this technique, as well as tumors situated at the apex of the petrous bone, or in the cavernous sinus.

References

1. Dhellemmes P, Pellerin P, Jomin M, Laine E, Donazzan M (1980) Les fractures fronto-sphéno-temporales entités anatomocliniques. Rev Stomatol Chir Maxillofac 81: 246–252
2. Drake CG (1979) The treatment of aneurysms of the posterior circulation. Clin Neurosurg 26: 96–144
3. Fujitsu K, Kuwabara T (1985) Zygomatic approach for lesions in the interpeduncular cistern. J Neurosurg 62: 340–343
4. Pellerin P, Queval Ph, Donazzan M (1984) Voie d'abord supéro-externe vers la fosse ptérygo-maxillaire et ses extensions. Rev Stomatol Chir Maxillofac 1: 46–50
5. Pellerin P, Lesoin F, Dhellemmes P, Donazzan M, Jomin M (1984) Usefulness of the orbitofrontomalar approach associated with bone reconstruction for frontotemporosphenoid meningiomas. Neurosurg 15: 715–718
6. Vaneecloo FM, Jomin M, Camuzet JP, Janssen B (1984) Abord de la face antéro-supérieure du rocher par voie sous-pétreuse. Son intérêt pour les lésions rares intéressant le sphénoide, le nerf trijumeau, l'artère carotide interne. Ann Otolaryngol 101: 95–101
7. Sugita K, Kobayashi S, Shintani A et al (1979) Microneurosurgery for aneurysms of the basilar artery. J Neurosurg 51: 615–620
8. Yamaura A, Ise H, Makino H (1983) Surgical approach of the transsylvian approach to the aneurysm arising from the terminal portion of the basilar artery. In: Ichii S (ed) Proc second annu meeting jpn congr neurosurg. Japanese Congress of Neurosurgeons, Tokyo, pp 142–158

Skull base approaches for meningiomas invading the cavernous sinus

T. Kawase[1], S. Toya[1], R. Shiobara[1], C. Kimura[2], and H. Nakajima[3]

Departments of [1] Neurosurgery, of [2] Ophthalmology, and of [3] Plastic Surgery, Keio University School of Medicine, Tokyo, Japan

Two kinds of surgical approach via the skull base were introduced for meningiomas arising around the cavernous sinus. The aim of those approaches are to minimize brain retraction, having a wide exposure for radical surgery. The transzygomatic approach was applicable for orbit-cranial boundary meningiomas extending to the cavernous sinus. The zygomatic arch, orbital wall and middle cranial base were removed in the procedure. The transpetrosal approach was beneficial for meningiomas arising from clivus or anterior pyramidal bone, and extending to the posterior cavernous sinus. The anterior pyramidal bone was resected extradurally through the temporal craniotomy. Nineteen surgical examples and results are mentioned in this study.

Introduction

Meningiomas arising from the major sphenoid wing or from the medial wall of the middle fossa often extend into the orbit and into the anterior part of the cavernous sinus (CS). The tumors from the upper clivus or from the tentorium sometimes involve the posterior part of the CS. As many cranial nerves from II to VI and the carotid artery run through the area, it is a surgical challenge to remove the tumor radically with preservation of those structures. When those tumors are accessed by the standard frontotemporal, subtemporal or suboccipital craniotomy, the surgical field does not extend wide enough to expose the whole tumor, and further brain retraction with cutting of the bridging veins is hazardous to the patient. In this report, two surgical approaches via the skull base, the transzygomatic approach and transpetrosal approach are mentioned. The principle of those surgical procedures are to access the tumor extradurally low enough to expose the skull base, from where the tumor is growing. Those approaches have been performed in 19 patients out of 45 skull base meningiomas in the last five years. In this report our experience with nine patients with meningioma extending to CS is mentioned. We believe those approaches have some advantages in the removal of these tumors.

Transzygomatic approach

This approach is acceptable for orbit-cranial boundary tumors, such as sphenoid wing meningiomas or parasellar tumors. Collaboration between neurosurgeons, ophthalmologists and plastic surgeons is ideal for this surgery.

Surgical procedure

The main surgical procedures are the removal of the zygomatic arch, upperlateral orbital roof and the temporal skull base extradurally (Fig. 1 a). The scalp is incised coronally, being extended along the radix of auricule on the side of the tumor, to spare damage on the frontal branches of the facial nerve. The frontal periosteum is incised along the orbital rim and the whole zygomatic arch is exposed. The supraorbital nerve is freed from the orbital notch. Frontal periosteum and fascia of the temporal muscle are dissected from the skull in one layer, for substantial use of the dural defect on closure. Next the fronto-temporal craniotomy is made, the dura mater being dissected from the anterior and middle fossa, and one block of the orbital rim with zygomatic arch is cut off from the craniotomy site with a oscillating saw. Protection of the orbital contents is necessary during sawing. After this, temporal muscle can be completely turned down at its radix of muscle process of the mandibula. Next the basal dura mater is further dissected from the skull base, and the whole sphenoid ridge and the lateral orbital wall are removed with a small rongeur and an air drill extradurally until the orbital fissure is completely opened. When the tumor is widely invading the basal cranium, it is resected until the foramen rotundum and foramen ovale are opened (Fig. 1 b). If the tumor is invading the orbit, the periorbita is removed with the tumor. When it invades beyond the periorbita, orbital contents, especially the muscle cone, must be carefully preserved.

After the orbital tumor is cleared, the dura is incised along the margin of the tumor. When the tumor attaches to the wall of the CS, the outer wall of the CS is removed. When the CS is swollen, being packed with the tumor, it is opened along the first branch of the trigeminal nerve. Venous hemorrhage is controllable by elevating the head and packing with a piece of oxycel cotton. Every effort must be made to confirm the location of cranial nerves

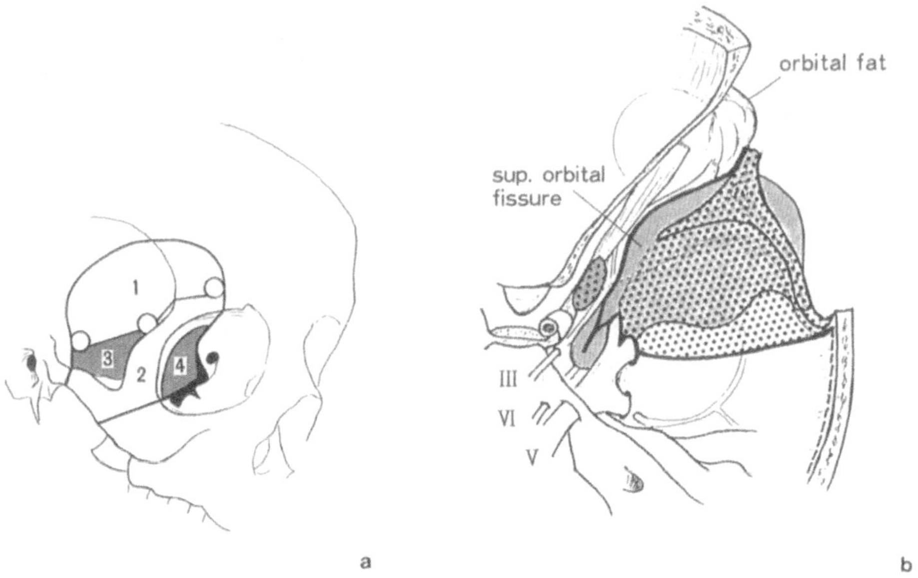

Fig. 1. **a** Surgical process of the transzygomatic approach. Frontotemporal craniotomy (*1*), cutting the zygomatic arch with orbital rim (*2*), resection of the temporal base (*3*), and resection of superolateral orbital wall (*4*). **b** Illustration of surgical exposure according to the above procedure. Intraorbital and intracranial tumors (shaded) are exposed in one surgical field. The cranial invasion site is further removed (dotted). A broad line indicates the dissected periorbita and the site of dural incision

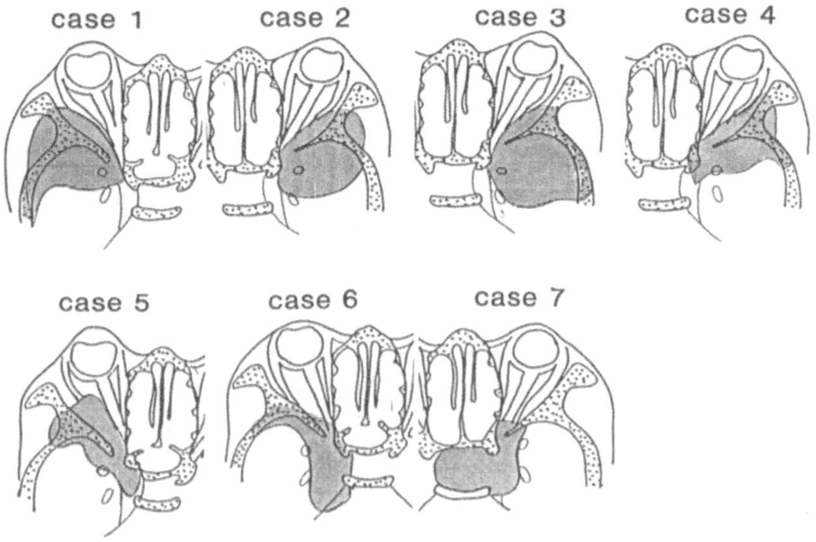

Fig. 2. Tumor extension on the CS (shaded)

and the carotid artery. An intracavernous tumor is usually very hard to remove, being mixed with trabeculas in the sinus, and an ultrasonic surgical aspirator is useful. When the carotid artery is shifted backwards, the location is carefully confirmed by a finger or by intracranial Doppler sonography. The abducens nerve, running freely in the CS, is the most vulnerable during manipulation.

A living membrane of the preserved temporal fascia graft is more acceptable than a dural substitute for repair of the dural defect on the skull base. The orbital wall is reconstructed with free pieces of the iliac bone. When the skull defect is very wide, pieces of costal bone or the outer layer of the cranium are implanted.

Cases and surgical results

Seven patients were operated upon by this approach. All patients were female, between 32 and 58 years of age. Five of them had unilateral exophthalmos as their chief complaint. Three had disturbance of unilateral visual acuity. Extraocular movment was disturbed in two patients, whereas they did not complain of double vision because of their visual loss on the affected side. Only one patient complained of facial hypesthesia (Table 1). On CT scan, the tumor extended both into the retrobulbar space and into the subdural space. All had a tumor attachment on the wall of the CS, and three had a tumor invasion into the CS. The intracavernous carotid siphon was displaced on angiograms in two of them. The basal cranium was widely infiltrated by the tumor in most cases, and optic canal was involved in one case (Fig. 2).

In five patients the tumor was totally removed, whereas in two patients, whose CS had been completely packed by the tumor, it was not possible to remove the tumor completely, even when the CS was opened. The postoperative recovery was prompt in all the patients. Exophthalmos disappeared after surgery, and a common postoperative symptom was facial hypesthesia caused by the manipulation of the trigeminal nerve around the CS. Permanent oculomotor palsy was present in one patient, whose CS was completely filled by the tumor. Visual deterioration was seen in one patient.

Transpetrosal approach

This approach is considered to be useful for meningiomas arising from the upper clivus, tentorium or from the anterior part of the petrosal bone and extending into the CS.

Surgical procedure

The patient is positioned laterally and the head is elevated higher than the heart. The scalp incision and position of the bone window are almost the same as in the standard subtemporal approach (Fig. 3 a). The dura of the middle fossa base is peeled from the skull until the petrosal ridge is identified. The anterior pyramidal bone is drilled to create a 2 × 1 cm groove (Fig. 3 b). The area of drilling is surrounded by the trigeminal ganglion anteriorly, the cochlear organ posteriorly, the sphenopetrosal groove laterally, and the carotid canal and internal auditory canal inferiorly. The dura mater in the internal auditory canal must be preserved to avoid damage to the nerves VII and VIII. The resection of the petrosal rim reduces the retraction damage in the temporal lobe, and the extradural subtemporal access minimizes the possibility of damage on temporal bridging veins, such as the vein of Labbé. After resection of the petrosal rim, small dural incisions are made above and below the superior petrosal sinus, and double Weck clips are applied to the sinus. The tentorium is incised between cranial nerves V and VII until the tentorial notch is opened. Bilateral leaflets of the tentorium are folded, and the tumor is visualized just below. The anterior surface of the brain stem can be directly seen by this approach. The dural incision is then extended on the nerve V, along the lateral wall of the CS. The location of cranial nerves in the CS should be carefully identified. The trigeminal nerve runs on the wall of the CS, and the oculomotor nerve usually runs just below the roof of the CS. The abducens nerve is easily involved in the tumor, being vulnerable in the course of the tumor resection. Ultrasonic suction is beneficial for resection of the tumor in the CS. When the tumor is removed completely from the CS, venous bleeding results and is controlled with oxycell cotton mixed with Biobond glue. The dural opening on the petrosal rim is packed with a graft of the temporal muscle.

Case report

This approach was performed in twelve patients with clivus or cerebellopontine angle meningiomas. Two clival meningiomas invaded the CS, and they were removed totally. One case is presented below.

This 49 year old woman noticed double vision and numbness in her right cheek for five months. Neurological examination on admission revealed right abducens palsy and hypesthesia in the right 1st and 2nd branch of the trigeminal area with decrease of her corneal reflex. Computerized tomography demonstrated an upper clival meningioma invading the CS (Fig. 4 a). The cavernous portion of the internal carotid artery was displaced forward and downward with mild luminal narrowing. Radical surgery was

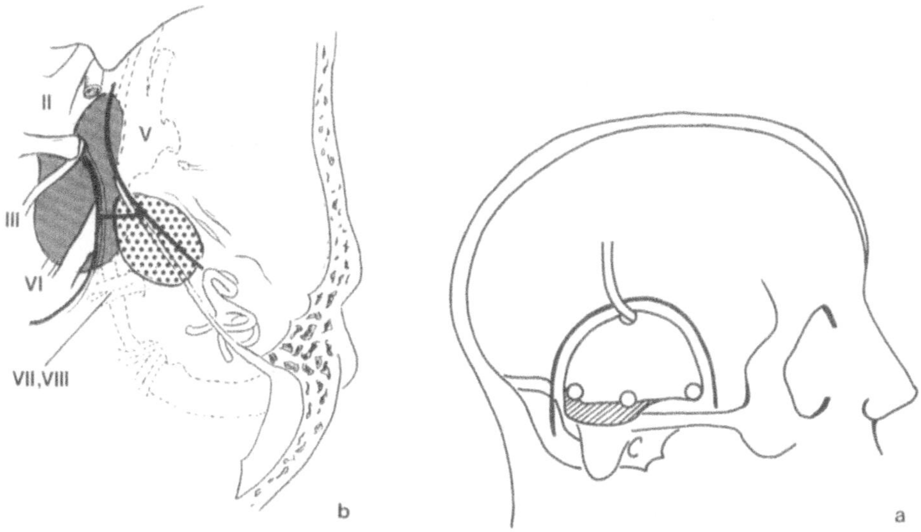

Fig. 3. Illustrations of the transpetrosal approach. **a** Skin incision and craniotomy site; **b** Anterior pyramidal bone is resected (dotted) extradurally. Broad lines indicate the dural incision and tentorial notch

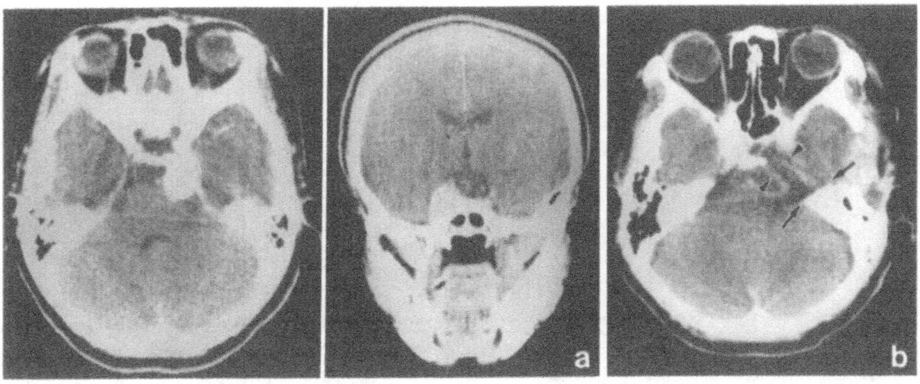

Fig. 4. a Clival meningioma invading the CS. **b** Contrast CT after surgery. Resected pyramidal bone (arrows) and opened cavernous wall (arrowheads) are demonstrated

Table 1. Clinical data in 7 patients undergoing the transzygomatic approach

Case	Age	Sex	Symtoms	Plain X-P Angiography	Surgical Findings cranio-dural invasion	orbital mass	sub-dural mass	CS in-vasion	Surgical Results
1	O. R. 48	F	L exophthalmos	hyperostosis	+ + +	+ +	+ +	CS wall	total removal L facial hypesthesia (V/2, V/3)
2	F. M. 53	F	R exophthalmos	hyperostosis	+ + +	+ +	+ + +	CS wall	total removal R facial hypesthesia (V/1, V/2)
3	K. E. 44	F	R exophthalmos	hyperostosis	+ + +	+ +	+ + +	CS wall	total removal R facial hypesthesia (V/1)
4	S. H. 32	F	R exophthalmos	hyperostosis narrowing of optic canal	+ + +	+ +	+ +	CS wall	total removal R visual loss
5	T. K. 45	F	L exophthalmos L visual disturbance	hyperostosis	+ + +	+ +	+ + +	anterior 1/3 CS	total removal L vision unchanged L facial hypesthesia (V/1)
6	F. J. 57	F	L facial hypesthesia L visual disturbance	skull erosion IC displacement	+ + +	—+	—+	whole CS	80% removal L facial hypesthesia (V/2, V/3) L vision unchanged
7	T. N. 58	F	R visual disturbance (severely impaired)	IC displacement and encasement	+	+	+ + +	whole CS	60% removal no recovery of vision with palsy of nerve VI R facial hypesthesia (V/2, V/3)

CS Cavernous sinus; *R* right; *L* left

performed by the transpetrosal approach. After the subtemporal craniotomy, the anterior part of the pyramidal bone was drilled extradurally. The internal auditory canal was not opened. The superior petrosal sinus was clipped and the tentorium was incised until the tentorial notch was opened. The tumor was located between nerves III and V, and nerve VI was involved in the tumor. The anterior part of the tumor extended into the CS, along nerve V. The basilar artery was adjacent to the tumor. After the margin of the tumor was dissected, an ultrasonic surgical aspirator was used to remove the tumor. When the posterior fossa was cleared venous hemorrhage occurred from the inferior petrosal sinus, and it was controlled with pieces of oxycell cotton. Then the dural incision was extended anteriorly along nerve V, and the CS was opened. It was filled with the tumor, and the lateral side of the posterior clinoid process was eroded. The internal carotid artery, encased by the tumor, was dissected carefully. Nerve VI could not be confirmed in the sinus. When the tumor was completely cleared, venous hemorrhage came from the anterior CS, and was controlled in the same maneuver.

Postoperative recovery was prompt without any temporal symptoms. She had incomplete palsy of nerve III and complete palsy of nerve VI with right facial hypesthesia. She discharged 19 days after surgery. Her oculomotor palsy and abducents palsy were recovered one year later, whereas slight hypesthesia in her mouth were not recovered. The tumor disappeared on CT after surgery (Fig. 4 b), and she has been working during the 3 years follow-up.

Discussion

Tumors arising from the sphenoid ridge, or from the anterior middle fossa, have commonly been reached subdurally through the standard fronto-temporal or temporal craniotomy. However, in a case when the orbit and related structures, such as orbital fissure and the CS are widely involved in the tumor, surgical excision through the craniotomy has been difficult. A wider exposure including the orbital rim were described recently for those tumors [1, 2, 3, 4, 5]. Further opening with removal of the zygomatic arch was beneficial to minimize the retraction of the brain, because of lower access than the standard craniotomy. This exposure also offers a combined surgical field between the orbit and the CS with an easy anatomical understanding. The surgical reconstruction of the orbital wall is not difficult with the technical knowledge of plastic surgery.

When the tumor arises more posteriorly, from the upper clivus or from the anterior pyramidal bone, it has been commonly reached via the suboccipital or subtemporal-transtentorial route, whereas the suboccipital approach does not offer a sufficient surgical field because of the many cranial nerves in the way. The subtemporal-transtentorial route may be more acceptable, while retraction of the temporal lobe has the possibility of sacrificing significant temporal bridging veins such as the vein of Labbé, when the tumor extends down into the posterior fossa.

Surgical removal of the pyramidal bone has been used for excision of acoustic neuromas since 1970 [6, 7, 8, 9, 10, 11]. This approach gives the surgeon the possibility of reaching the clival region with minimum brain retraction. However, in this approach, auditory function was sacrificed because of the resection of the posterior part of the pyramidal bone. When the resection is confined to the anterior part of the pyramidal bone, it is possible to preserve the auditory function, as shown in this report. The authors introduced the transpetrosal approach for lower basilar aneurysms in 1985 [12]. By cutting the tentorium, it offered sufficient exposure even in clival meningiomas. It also offered sufficient exposure when the tumor in the CS was removed.

References

1. Bickham US, Phar M (1974) Operative surgery. Saunders, Philadelphia, pp 692–693
2. Brihaye J (1976) Neurosurgical approaches to orbital tumors. In: Krayenbühl M et al (eds) Advances and technical standards in neurosurgery, vol 3. Springer, Wien New York, pp 103–121
3. Jane JA, Park TS, Poberskin LH, Winn HR, Butler AB (1982) The supraorbital approach: technical note. Neurosurgery 11: 537–542
4. Maroon JC, Kennerdel JS (1984) Surgical approaches to the orbit. Indications and techniques. J Neurosurg 60: 1226–1235
5. Al-Mefty OA, Fox JL (1985) Superolateral orbital exposure and reconstruction. Surg Neurol 23: 609–613
6. King TT (1970) Combined translabyrinthine-transtentorial approach to acoustic nerve tumors. Proc R Soc Med 63: 780–782
7. Morrison AW, King TT (1973) Experiences with a translabyrinthine-transtentorial approach to the cerebellopontine angle. Technical note. J Neurosurg 38: 382–390
8. House WF, Graham MD (1973) Surgery of acoustic tumors. Otolaryngol Clin North Am 6: 245–266
9. Bochenek Z, Kukwa A (1975) An extended approach through the middle cranial fossa of the internal auditory meatus and the cerebellopontine angle. Acta Otolaryngol 80: 410–414
10. Hakuba A (1978) Total removal of cerebellopontine angle tumors with combined transpetrosal-transtentorial approach. No Shinkei Geka 6: 347–354
11. Shiobara R (1980) A modified extended middle cranial fossa approach for acoustic tumors. Neurol Med Chir 20: 173–182
12. Kawase T, Toya S, Shiobara R, Mine S (1985) Transpetrosal approach for aneurysms of the lower basilar artery. J Neurosurg 63: 857–861

Trigeminal neurinomas. A special type of cavernous sinus tumors

M. Sindou and I. Pelissou

Neurological Hospital, Lyon, France

The first case of primary tumor of nerve V was reported by R. W. Smith in 1838 (cited in [43]). Trigeminal neurinomas are not frequent, as they only represent 0.2% of all intracranial tumors [43]. They constitute a special type of cavernous sinus (CS) tumors explained by the anatomical situation of the nerve V, both in Meckel's cave and the adjacent cerebellopontine angle (CPA) (Fig. 1).

This report is a summary of a review of 131 cases published or quoted in the literature since 1970 and will be illustrated with a recent personal case that led us to discuss their surgical peculiarities.

Anatomical features

From a histological point of view, the majority of trigeminal neurinomas are benign schwannomas (Fig. 2). However, on some rare occasions, 7 published cases [10, 12, 18, 21, 30], they may present a high cellular density and caryocinetic activity suggesting a certain degree of malignancy. In one case the neurilemmoma presents mesenchymal differentitation [22].

These tumors always arise from the Schwann sheath of the sensory root. They essentially grow from the immediate retrogasserian part of the root, *i.e.* centrally to the ganglion, like most neurinomas; although occasionally they may develop from the Gasserian ganglion itself or even its peripheral branches [5]. Following Jefferson's classification [5, 20] 3 groups may be distinguished in relation to their anatomical extension.

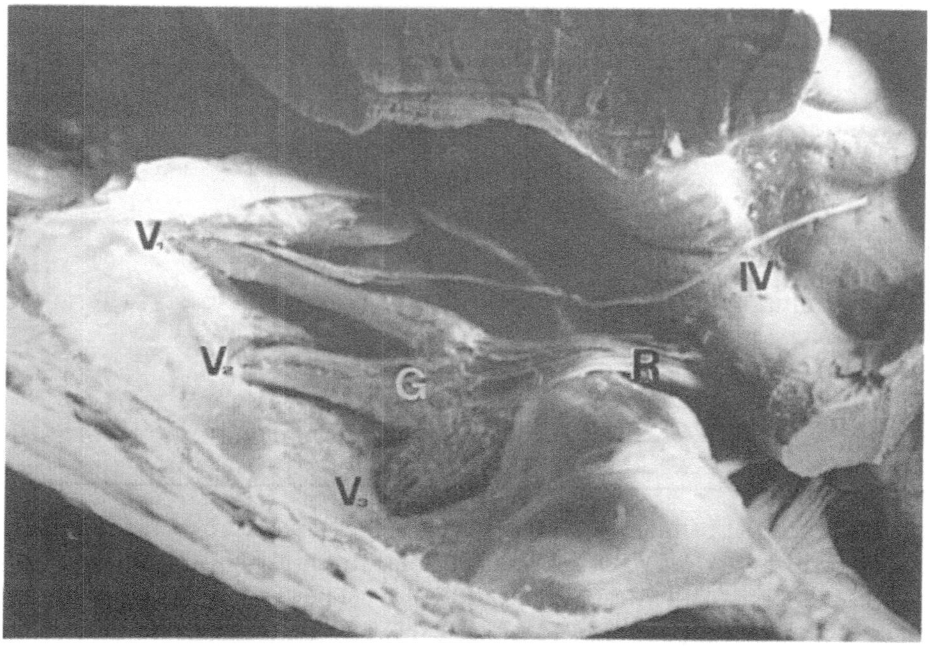

Fig. 1. Lateral anatomical view of the trigeminal nerve (from BALE Museum). First (*V*/1), second (*V*/2) and third (*V*/3) divisions; Gasserian ganglion (*G*); triangular plexus (*TP*); sensory root (*R*), trochlear nerve (*IV*); common oculomotor nerve (*III*)

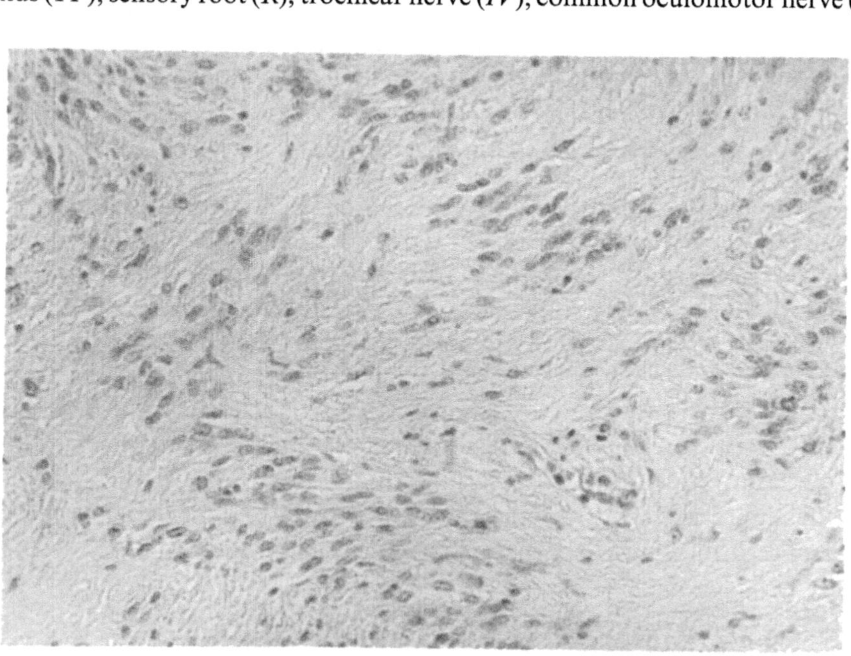

Fig. 2. Trigeminal neurinoma; schwannoma of Antoni A type characterized by interlacing bundles of Schwann cells with nuclear palisading

Type A

It corresponds to neurinomas arising from the Gasserian ganglion inside Meckel's cave. They develop upwards and laterally into the middle fossa, the dura of which may be perforated, as well as internally into the cavernous sinus, thus compressing and/or invading its vascular and cranial nerve contents. In the most advanced cases, extensions can penetrate into the orbit through the sphenoïdal fissure, into the infratemporal space [2] and/or erode the foramina rotundum and ovale. Because the apex of the petrous bone is generally worn away, the tumor is almost always adjacent to the carotid artery at the foramen lacerum as well as the anterior part of the carotid canal, its superior wall being eroded.

Type B

Neurinoma of this type arise from the trigeminal root itself and predominantly extend into the CPA.

Type C

This corresponds to the association of type A and B and undergoes a hourglass anatomical extension on both sides of the petrous apex. Although type A is considered as the most frequent anatomical variety (63.41%), surgical explorations have shown that a majority of trigeminal neurinomas extend not only into the middle fossa but also, at least to a certain degree, into the CPA, as described in type C. Because this anatomical classification has surgical implications, type C frequency should not be underestimated.

Surprisingly enough, only 3 cases of Recklinghausen's disease with trigeminal neurinoma have been reported in the literature [5, 38].

Clinical data

Material

This study is a review of 131 cases published in the literature, whose sex, age and tumor location are detailed in Table 1.

The sex ratio was biased forwards females rather than males (59.7% versus 40.3%).

Peak frequency was more evident between 30 and 40 years of age. The small incidence during childhood [9, 36, 42, 48] is probably due to the slow growth of these benign tumors. Another related consequence is the fact that they often reach a large volume before causing sufficient symptoms to lead the patient to a neurosurgical clinic.

Table 1.

Material

(131 cases reported in the literature, bibliographic citation, list generated by Medlars II 1971–1985)

Sex distribution (data on 67 cases)	Females	Males
	40 (59.7%)	27 (40.3%)

Age (data on 70 cases)

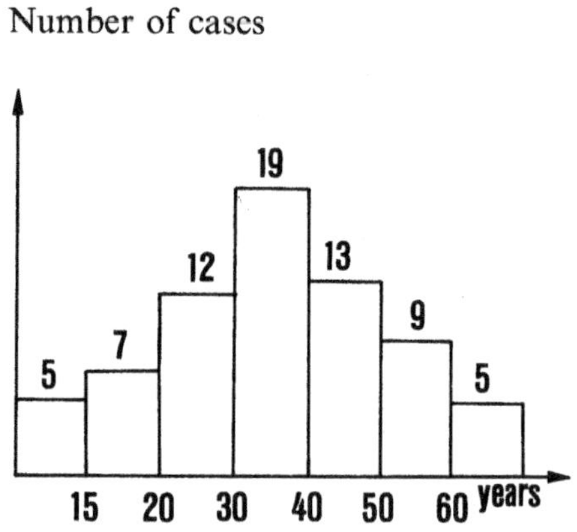

Locations		Gasserian	Root	"Dumb-bell"
Schisano-Olivecrona	1958	11	4	—
Paillas	1974	2	4	2
Arseni	1975	3	1	2
De Benedittis	1977	5	1	1
Vidovsky	1979	5	—	—
		26 (63.4%)	10 (24.4%)	5 (12.2%)

	Benign	Malignant
Histology (data on 118 cases)	110	8

Clinical description

Due to the fact that these tumors generally extend to several anatomical regions, clinical symptomatology is rich and initial symptoms may be of various types, as shown in Table 2.

According to most authors [1, 3, 5, 11, 14, 24, 27, 29, 31, 34, 43] trigeminal sensory disturbances are the most frequent revealing symptoms (58.7%). When it corresponds to a trigeminal neuralgia (which occurred in 34.9% of the 63 cases in whom the clinical description was detailed), a hypesthesia and/or a decrease corneal reflex was most often present, suggesting the diagnosis of symptomatic trigeminal neuralgia [50]. In our series of 650 patients referred in the 10 past years for "tic douloureux" only one out of the 14 trigeminal neuralgias due to a tumor or a vascular malformation was found in relation with a trigeminal neurinoma [45]. Numbness was a revealing symptom in 23.8%. For some authors [11, 44] the initial symptom would be most frequently numbness in type B and pain in type A neurinomas, whilst for others, like Jannetta [54] there would be no significant difference according to the origin of the tumor.

Diplopia was the second revealing symptom in frequency (20.63%). A VIth nerve palsy alone was responsible in 17.46% whilst its association with both a IIIrd and IVth nerve palsies was noticed in the other 3.17%. Predominance of the VIth nerve palsy can be explained by the fact that the nerve is directly compressed down to the petrous bone.

Surprisingly enough, VIIth and VIIIth disturbances were revealing symptoms in a rather large percentage of cases (14.27%). This was noticed either when the tumor predominantly developed in the CPA or when it was accompanied with a huge extension to the petrous bone leading to a compression of the Eustachian tube and/or an erosion of the Fallopian canal.

Although present at clinical examination, palsy of the masticatory muscles was not a frequent revealing symptom (3.17%), probably because it was often unknown to the patient.

When others symptoms [6, 10, 26, 42, 52] like intracranial hypertension (4.76%) revealed the tumor, it should be pointed out that the anamnestic inquiry actually showed a relatively long process of trigeminal disturbances. Indeed, the detailed analysis of the series' clinical data confirmed that trigeminal disturbances were always present, with the exception of 7 cases [3, 9, 15, 38, 53].

Radiological findings

1. On plain radiographies sharply circumscribed erosion of the petrous apex

Table 2. Clinical description

Neurological signs		Initial and revealing symptoms 63	Signs at admission 114
V	Trigeminal neuralgia	22 (34.9%)	27 (23.7%)
	Sensory loss	15 (23.8%)	41 (36%)
	Palsy of masticatory muscles	2 (3.17%)	17 (15%)
VI nerve palsy		13 (20.63%)	25 (22%)
III nerve palsy		2 (3.17%)	18 (15.8%)
IV nerve palsy		2 (3.17%)	10 (8.8%)
Sight impairment		7 (11.1%)	10 (8.8%)
Exophthalmos		2 (3.17%)	13 (11.4%)
Otalgia		3 (4.76%)	3 (2.6%)
Serous otitis (by occlusion of the Eustachian tube)		1 (1.58%)	2 (1.75%)
VIII disturbances		6 (9.52%)	27 (23.7%)
VII	Facial nerve palsy	2 (3.17%)	18 (15.8%)
	Facial hemispasm	1 (1.58%)	3 (2.6%)
IX, X, XI disturbances		—	1 (0.9%)
Cerebellar signs		—	6 (5.3%)
Headaches		6 (9.52%)	10 (8.8%)
Intracranial hypertenstion		3 (4.76%)	4 (3.5%)
Other signs	Alternating hemiplegic episodes	1 (1.58%)	1 (0.9%)
	Hemiplegia	—	1 (0.9%)
	Pathological laughs	1 (1.58%)	1 (0.9%)
	Nasal stuffiness	1 (1.58%)	1 (0.9%)

was the most frequent abnormality (77.19%). Erosion of the clivus lateral aspect, considered as pathognomonic of tumor extension in the posterior fossa, was only apparent in 1.75%. A clearly delimited sharp-edged bone defect (Figs. 3, 4) in the floor of the middle fossa was present in 35.1% and enlargement of the foramen rotundum and ovale in 27.19%. A significant radiological abnormality, even in a tomogram, couldn't be found in more than 6.1% [11, 37, 39].

2. CT scan abnormalities were significant in 87.5% showing an evident

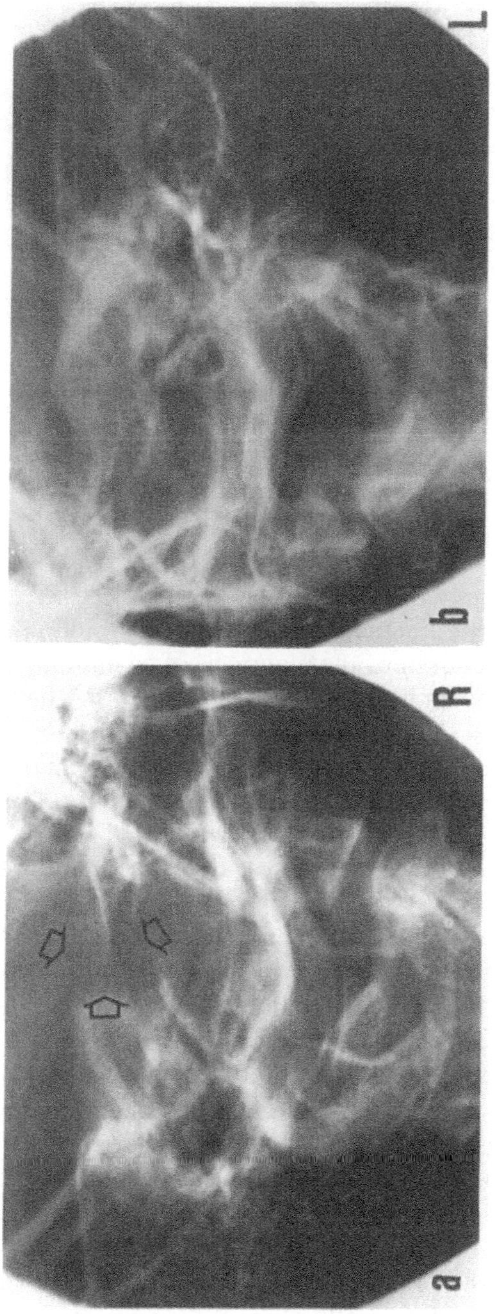

Fig. 3. Stenvers' projection: in **a** notice the sharp destruction of the right petrous bone by the tumor (arrows) in comparison with the contralateral side (**b**)

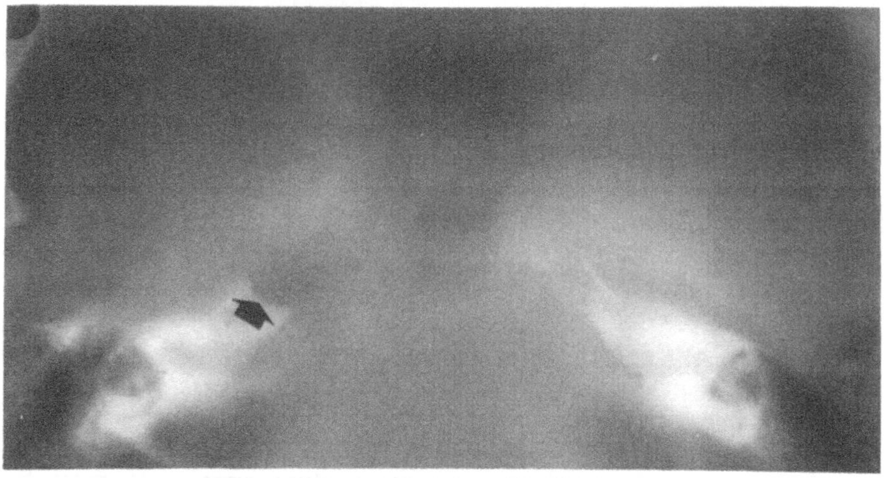

Fig. 4. Tomogram in submentovertical projection showing erosion of the right petrous bone apex (arrow)

mass with contrast enhancement in the trigeminal area. When the tumor straddled the petrous apex the diagnosis of trigeminal neurinoma was more suggestive than when it predominated in the CPA or the middle fossa [29] (Fig. 5).

In the smallest tumors, high resolution CT may show distortion or obliteration of Meckel's cave which normally has a fairly constant elipsoid shape [8].

3. Angiographic studies demonstrated vascular abnormalities in 93% of cases.

As trigeminal neurinomas most often invade Meckel's cave, the parasellar and/or the juxtasellar portion of the internal carotid artery is usually stretched and displaced medially, anteriorly and/or inferiorly, as shown in Table 3 (Figs. 6, 7) [35, 37, 39].

Abnormal pedicles to the tumor, usually not visible in normal arteriographies, as well as neovessels can be clearly seen on the angiograms with subtractions (Fig. 6) (25% of cases in this study). These pedicles most often arose from branches of Bernasconi's artery or the inferior cavernous sinus artery which normally supplies Gasserian ganglion.

When neurinoma extends into the posterior fossa, this leads to a significant displacement of the superior cerebellar artery (SCA) which is shifted upwards and medially (Fig. 7). This is the same for the posterior cerebral artery (PCA), especially when the tumor straddles the tentorial incisure [35]. When the tumor develops downwards in the CPA, the antero-inferior cerebellar artery may be stretched down [51].

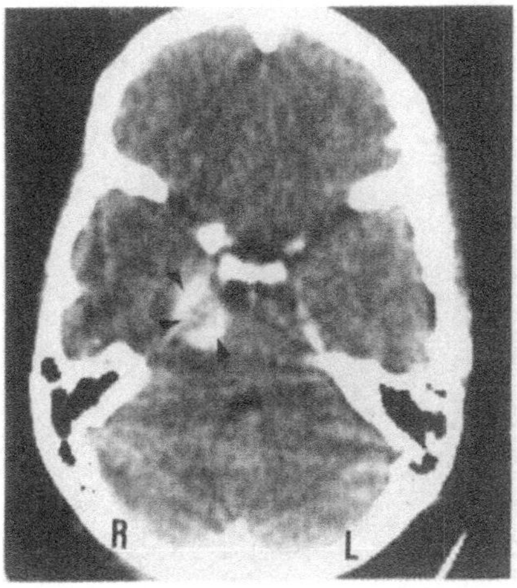

Fig. 5. Preoperative CT scan showing a typical trigeminal neurinoma with contrast enhancement developing into hour-glass both in the right CPA and cavernous sinus (triangles)

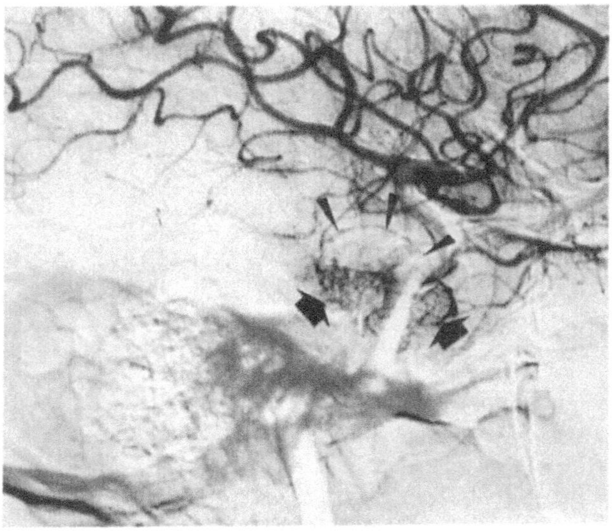

Fig. 6. Lateral view of the right carotid angiogram after substraction showing tumorous network (arrows) and abnormal pedicles (triangles) arising from the cavernous carotid portion

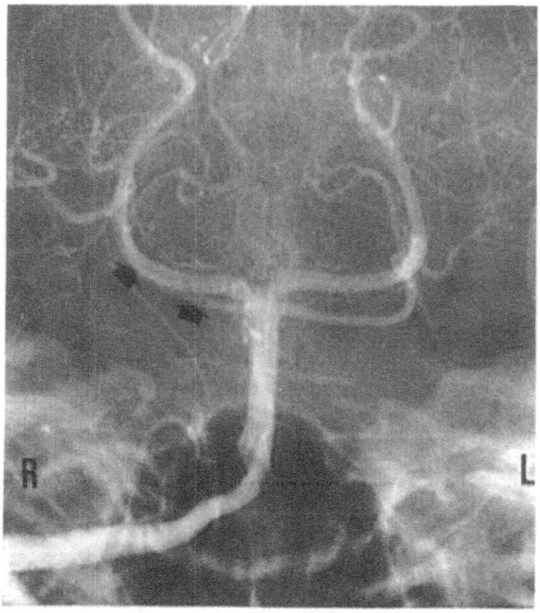

Fig. 7. AP view of the right vertebral angiogram demonstrating the medial and upward displacement of the superior cerebellar artery (arrows)

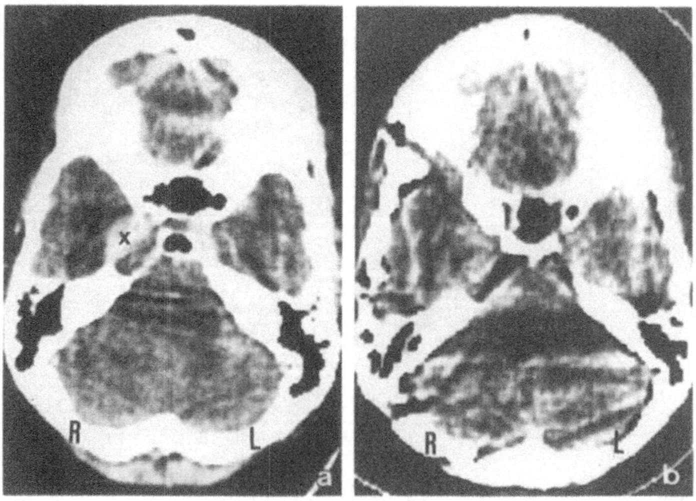

Fig. 8. **a** Control CT scan after the first stage suboccipital approach showing the remaining Meckel's cave cavernous part of the tumor (*X*); **b** Control CT scan after the second stage subtemporal approach demonstrating total removal

Tumorous extension into the middle fossa may give significant displacements of the temporal branches of the middle cerebral artery, especially when the tumor has ruptured the dural cavernous sinus walls (Table 3).

Surgical techniques

The choice of the most adequate approach according to the topography of the tumor is of primary importance to allow a safe dissection of the tumor adhesions to the surrounding blood vessels and adjacent cranial nerves. As a matter of fact, the study of the surgical results reported in the literature shows that incomplete removals as well as surgical complications were related to insufficient exposure of the lesion. It must be recalled that trigeminal neurinomas almost always straddle the petrous apex even when they predominantly extend into the middle fossa or the CPA.

As shown in Table 4, the extradural or intradural subtemporal approaches allowed complete removal in 14 out of the 23 parasellar neurinomas, whilst none of the six hour-glass neurinomas could be totally removed through this approach.

As regard to the suboccipital approach the study of the results found that this approach allowed complete removal of the tumor in 8 of the 12 cases mainly developed in the CPA, while it always resulted in incomplete removal in the 3 cases in which the tumor extended into the middle fossa.

Surprisingly enough, through the pterionotemporal transtentorial approach, the surgeons could achieve a total removal in only 5 of the 13 cases.

When a combined suboccipital and temporal approach was used total removal was obtained in 2 out of the 3 cases.

The relatively high percentage of incomplete removal is probably explained by the fact that a significant number of cases of this study were operated upon before the microsurgical era.

Although microsurgical techniques provide more efficient and safer means to deal with these difficult lesions, a rigorous analysis of topographical extensions and the anatomical relationships of the tumor is needed before adopting the most adequate approach.

The suboccipital retromastoidian route is the most logical approach for the tumors which mainly develop into the posterior fossa. A good visual control allows a sharp dissection of the lesion from the brain stem, the antero-inferior and superior cerebellar arteries, as well as the acoustic and facial nerves. But it is not always sufficient for achieving a safe removal of the supratentorial part of the tumor and a rigorous hemostasis of its pedicles arising from the intracavernous carotid artery. Moreover, as in 84% of cases only a single sheath of the dura mater separates Meckel's floor from the nearby intrapetrous carotid [17], this approach involves serious risks of injuring the carotid artery itself, especially in case of invasive tumors.

Table 3. Radiological findings

	No. of cases		No. of cases		No.of cases
Plain radios	114	CT scan	16	Angiography	72
Normal	7	Normal	2	Normal	5
Erosion of the apex	88	Tumor of the middle fossa or parasellar tumor	5	Abnormal vessels	18
Erosion of petrous bone (other than apex)	11	CPA tumor	3	— Accessory meningeal pedicle	1
Bone defect in the floor of the middle fossa	40	Tumor of the cavernous sinus	1	— Bernasconi pedicle	1
Enlargement of the foramen ovale	18	Tumor into the sphenoidal sinus	1	— Inferior cavernous sinus pedicle	2
Enlargement of the foramen rotundum	5	Hour-glass tumor both in the middle and posterior fossa	4	Displacement of the intra-cavernous carotid	
Enlargement of the superior orbital fissure	4			— forwards	12
				— backwards	8
				— medially	23
				— upwards	3
				— downwards	1

Enlargement of the foramen spinosum	13	Displacement of the ganglion part of the siphon anteriorly, medially, and inferiorly	1
Enlargement of the foramen lacerum	1	Displacement of the basilar artery	
Erosion of dorsum and base sellae	5	— contralaterally	3
Distortion of the sphenoidal sinus	7	— backwards	4
Erosion of the clivus	2	— forwards	3
Calcifications	1	Displacement of SCA	
		— upwards	6
		— medially	3
		— downwards	3
		Displacement of AICA	3
		Displacement of the veins of the posterior fossa	4

Table 4. Results (removal) in relation to surgical approaches

Approaches \ Locations	Parasellar (Gasserian)	CPA (root)	Hour-glass neurinoma
Extradural subtemporal approach (5 cases)	Subtotal 1; Total 4		
Intradural subtemporal approach (20 cases)	Incomplete 3; Subtotal 2; Total 8	Total 1	Incomplete 2; Subtotal 4
Intradural pterional approach (5 cases)	Incomplete 2; Subtotal 1; Total 2		
Intradural pterionotemporal and transtentorial approach (13 cases)	Incomplete 4; Subtotal 3; Total 3	Subtotal 1; Total 1	Total 1
Suboccipital approach (15 cases)	Subtotal 1	Incomplete 3; Subtotal 1; Total 8	Incomplete 2
Two stage temporal and suboccipital approach (1 case)			Subtotal 1
Two stage suboccipital and temporal approach (1 case)		Total 1	
One stage combined temporooccipital approach (1 case)			Total 1

Incomplete Subtotal Total

As regard to the temporal approach, the procedure can be performed using different modalities.

1. The extradural subtemporal variety theoretically allows a good exposure of the entire Meckel's cave. As a matter of fact, Meckel's cave, which consists of an evagination of the posterior fossa dura mater, surrounding the Gasserian ganglion and lying under the middle fossa dura mater, can be anatomically cleaved [41]. However, as the tumor size is most often large, its extradural approach does not provide sufficient access to the neighbouring structures. Therefore an intradural approach seems preferable.

2. In addition to an easy exposure of Meckel's cave through the tumor dome, the intradural subtemporal approach offers the possibility of opening the cavernous sinus at Parkinson's triangle in case of intracavernous invasion [40]. Its main risks is an excessive retraction of the temporal lobe as well as of its venous pedicles to the superior petrosal sinus.

3. Another alternative is the pterionotemporal approach. The opening of the sylvian fissure does facilitate retraction of the temporal lobe with lesser stretching of the posterior temporal veins. This pterionotemporal transsylvian approach offers in addition a good control of the supraclinoidian carotid artery.

4. Intradural temporal approaches can be associated with an opening of the tentorium, which provides an access to the retrogasserian part of the fifth root. Such a transtentorial approach is sufficient for tumors with only small posterior extensions that may be lifted up from the posterior fossa. But it cannot offer a sufficiently safe control for tumors occupying the entire CPA.

The limitations of either the suboccipital or the temporal approach for the tumors which develop on both sides of the petrous ridge and of course especially for the real hour-glass neurinomas, justify the combined approach [16]. Combined suboccipital and temporal approaches may be performed in the same stage, using a supra and infratentorial route through the same bone flap centered on the lateral sinus. They may be also performed in two different stages. In this eventuality, we find it safer to begin with suboccipital dissection and removal of the posterior pole of the tumor. This allows us in addition to detect whether some healthy rootlets of nerve V can be preserved [42, 54].

Although less frequently than when dealing with CS meningiomas, total removal of trigeminal neurinomas may benefit from an interruption of the internal carotid circulation. This can be easily achieved, as classically, by a cervical supraclinoidian temporary trapping or as introduced by Dolenc [13] by exposing the intrapetrous carotid artery in its canal at Glasscock's triangle. In addition to allow there a direct proximal clamping of the carotid artery, Dolenc's procedure makes it easier to identify its intracavernous course after leaving the carotid canal.

Surgical results

As previously detailed in the chapter dealing with the surgical approaches (Table 4) a total removal of the tumor was achieved in only 50% cases (30 out of the 61 cases in whom surgical results were mentioned). Long term evolution of the 31 cases with incomplete removal was not described in most publications, with the exception of 2 cases in whom reoperation, 3 and 8 years later, obtained a successful result.

As the evolution of initial symptoms after surgery was generally not mentioned by most authors, it is impossible to know precisely how much the removal of the tumor resulted in their favorable outcome. However, 9 publications [10, 15, 23, 42, 43, 44, 49, 52, 53] which mentioned their data could provide some slight idea about the problem. According to them initial deficits were only scarcely improved after surgery: from 1.8% for nerves III, IV and VII, 3.6% for the VIIIth disturbances and 9.1% for the nerve VI and the trigeminus.

Frequency of surgical complications (Table 5) has been difficult to estimate, as not all the papers reported them precisely. Out of the 55 cases with available data 6 died after operation in 3 cases from temporal or CPA hematoma; in the 3 others cause of death was not mentioned. The high percentage of mortality (10.9%) as well as majority of the complications were probably due, at least in the oldest series, to surgical problems related to the lack of microsurgical equipment.

Some complications were in direct relation to surgery:

Rhinorrhea (5.4%) through the mastoid cells or the Eustachian tube spontaneously dried up with a lumbar drainage twice and required a surgical closure in the other case.

Temporal complications, related to an excessive retraction were reported in 9 cases (16.36%). They consisted of psychological disturbances (2 cases) [11], aphasia (3 cases) [19, 43], hemiparesis (2 cases) [19, 43], attacks of dreamy state (1 case) [43], and epileptic seizures (4 cases) [29, 38, 43].

Frequency of oculomotor palsies directly related to surgery has been difficult to evaluate, as in a significant number of patients diplopia was already present on admission. However, a careful analysis of the 55 cases in whom pre- and postoperative data were detailed has led us to estimate postoperative oculomotor complications at 7.27%, 9.1%, and 1.8% for nerves IV, VI, and III respectively.

Postoperative VIIth and VIIIth deficits or aggravations were noticed in 7.27% and 9.1% respectively.

Table 5. Surgical complications (data of 55 cases)

		Complications related to surgery
	Trigeminal pain	5 (9.1%)
	Sensory loss	20 (36.36%)
V	Corneal complications	5 (9.1%)
	Palsy of the masticatory muscles	4 (7.27%)
	Herpetic lesions	1 (1.8%)
Palsy of nerve VI		5 (9.1%)
Palsy of nerve IV		4 (7.27%)
Ophthalmoplegia		1 (1.8%)
II		2 (3.6%)
Facial nerve palsy		4 (7.27%)
VII disturbances		5 (9.1%)
"Temporal" complications		9 (16.36%)
Rhinorrhea		3 (5.4%)
Recurrence		3 (5.4%)
Death		6 (10.9%)

Surgery of trigeminal neurinomas, almost always resulted in aggravation of trigeminal deficits [50]. Only three well-documented publications, reporting a total of 4 cases, presented convincing data on significant preservation or improvement of the Vth nerve function [15, 42, 54]. Findler [15] has stressed the interest of repeated studies of trigeminal evoked potentials to predict recovery of the facial sensation.

Although mentioned by most authors disability due to long term persisting trigeminal disturbances after the operation seems to have been underestimated. Atypical facial pain was evaluated at 9.1% and occurred mostly in patients with incomplete removal of the lesion. Authentic trigeminal neuralgias were exceptionally noticed. Three cases of these have been reported after partial removal of the tumor [18, 19, 43] with only one after its total removal. But in the later case there was some conservation of trigeminal rootlets [11]. Three of them underwent a secondary rhizotomy [11, 18, 43] which succeeded in relieving neuralgia in 2. Surprisingly, anaesthesia dolorosa following complete resection of the trigeminal nerve was mentioned by only one author [43]. The same was true for numbness in the face! Corneal trophic complications were estimated at 9.1% and masticatory disturbances at 7.27%.

The review shows that surgery of trigeminal neurinomas still entails a high rate of complications and severe trigeminal disturbances. The systematic use of microtechniques as well as adequate combined approaches when necessary must minimize nervous structure retraction and injury of the surrounding vessels and cranial nerves. Nevertheless, only a much earlier diagnosis will be able to reduce the functional disability related to trigeminal disturbances in allowing a complete removal with conservation of some intact rootlets.

Conclusions and summary

Fifth nerve neurinomas, which are more often benign schwannomas arising from the Gasserian ganglion or the root, constitute a special type of cavernous sinus tumors. Trigeminal anatomy explains their frequent extension both to the posterior and middle fossa. Initial clinical symptoms may be of various types, but trigeminal sensory disturbances are predominant. Neuroradiological abnormalities are very often suggestive. Among them, clear-sharped petrous bone apex and/or middle fossa floor erosions, corresponding to well-delineated homogenous contrast-enhanced mass in CT scan are evocative, if not specific. Angiographic studies with substraction can be helpful in showing abnormal pedicles and neovessels originating from intracavernous branches of the internal carotid artery; displacements of surrounding vessels in the cerebellopontine angle and/or temporal fossa, testifying to their voluminous extension, can be seen. A precise evaluation of the neuroradiological data is of prime importance as it conditions the surgical approach. Unless the tumor predominantly develops either into the cerebellopontine angle or the middle fossa, justifying a suboccipital or a temporal approach a combined route must be preferred. As a matter of fact, hour-glass trigeminal neurinomas (far from the most numerous) which straddle the petrous bone apex can be better removed in performing a combined approach. The suboccipital stage provides good control of its posterior pole, while the intradural subtemporal approach gives a possible access to the cavernous sinus, through Parkinson's triangle, in case of intracavernous extension of the tumor; in addition it allows exposure of the intrapetrosal carotid at Glasscock's triangle.

Sequels due to oculomotor palsies and to a greater extend trigeminal disturbances, which remain frequent and provide a severe disability, will only be reduced through an earlier diagnosis allowing us to preserve some intact rootlets of the trigeminal nerve.

Case report

This 33 year old woman was referred a right trigeminal neuralgia with atypical paresthesias and diplopia episodes. Neurological examination showed a right facial hypoesthesia, superficial keratitis, masticatory deficit and abducens nerve palsy. As neuroradiological findings were typical of a trigeminal neurinoma of the nerve V (Figs. 3, 4, 5, 6, 7), of the hour-glass type, a two-stage combined approach was decided. The cerebellopontine angle portion of the tumor was removed first through a suboccipital approach (Fig. 8a). As no intact trigeminal rootlet could be found, a complete section of the nerve was performed at its root entry zone into the pons. The total removal of the remaining Meckel's cave and cavernous extension was achieved three weeks later through an intradural pterionotemporal approach (Fig. 8b). A CSF rhinorrhea which occurred soon after the second operation, was dried up with a 10 day lumbar drainage. The right VIth nerve palsy progressively recovered within 3 months. The total sensory trigeminal loss fortunately did not result in anaesthesia dolorosa, but only in an unconfortable sensation of numbness.

References

1. Amirkhanina SE, Lebedev AN (1979) Clinical diagnosis of neurinomas of Gasserian ganglion. Zh Nevropatol Psikhiatr 79: 559–562
2. Arena S, Hilal Ey (1976) Neurilemmomas of the infratemporal space: report of a case and review of the literature. Arch Otolaryngol 102: 180–184
3. Arseni C, Dumitrescu L, Constantinescu A (1975) Neurinomas of the trigeminal nerve. Surg Neurol 4: 495–503
4. Bloch S, Danziger J (1973) Neurinoma of the Gasserian ganglion. Report of a case and review of the literature. S Afr Med J 47: 1467–1470
5. Bonnal J (1978) Trigeminal tumors. In: EMC Neurologie Fasc 17376, A-10. Editions Techniques SA, Paris
6. Bouvier A, Chevalier JF, Brion S (1981) Pathological laughing and posterior fossa tumours. Encephale 7: 83–94
7. Chkili T, Medejel A, El Ouarzazi A, Bellakhdar F (1979) Neurinomas of the trigeminal nerve. Report of a case of "hour-glass" neurinoma occupying the posterior and middle fossa. Maroc Med 1: 223–228
8. Chui M, Tucker W, Hudson A, Bayer N (1985) High resolution CT of Meckel's cave. Neuroradiology 27: 403–409
9. Comninos S (1981) Neurinomas of the Gasserian ganglion and the trigeminal nerve. Arch Psychiatr Nervenkr 230: 171–177

Acknowledgements to Doctors J. Pialat (Neuropathology Laboratory) and J. Duquesnel (Neuroradiological Department) for their contributions to this study and to Mrs. Lozat for her technical assistance.

10. Dany A, Pefferkorn JP, Vallat JN, Loubet R, Maudoux M (1970) Neurinoma of the Gasserian ganglion with temporal development. Neurochirurgie 16: 349–356
11. De Benedittis M, Bernasconi V, Ettore G (1977) Tumours of the fifth cranial nerve. Acta Neurochir (Wien) 38: 37–64
12. Dinakar I, Rao SB, Rao KS (1971) Malignant schwannoma of the trigeminal nerve. Neurol India 19: 43–44
13. Dolenc V (1983) Direct microsurgical repair of the intracavernous vascular lesions. J Neurosurg 58: 824–831
14. Fee WE Jr, Epsy CD, Konrad HR (1975) Trigeminal neurinomas. Laryngoscope 85: 371–376
15. Findler G, Feinsod M, Sahar A (1983) Trigeminal neurinoma with unusual presentation. Report of a case with trigeminal somatosensory-evoked respose. Surg Neurol 19: 351–353
16. Genka S, Terao H, Matsutani M, Hori T, Ikeda A (1981) A choice of two-stage operation and the microsurgical anatomy for large trigeminal neurinoma. No Shinkei Geka 9: 747–751
17. Harris FS, Rhoton AL Jr (1976) Anatomy of the cavernous sinus. A microsurgical study. J Neurosurg 45: 169–180
18. Hedeman LS, Lewinsky BS, Lochridge GK, Trevor R (1978) Primary malignant schwannoma of the Gasserian ganglion. Report of two cases. J Neurosurg 48: 279–283
19. Hitchon PW, Graf CJ, Mc Cabe BF, Namba K (1979) Trigeminal neurilemmoma presenting as a sphenoid sinus mass. Surg Neurol 11: 305–307
20. Jefferson G (1955) Trigeminal neurinomas with some remarks on malignant invasion of the Gasserian ganglion. Proc Congr Neurol Surg 1: 11–54
21. Karmody CS (1979) Malignant schwannoma of the trigeminal nerve. Otolaryngol Head Neck Surg 87: 594–598
22. Kasantikul V, Brown WJ, Netsky MG (1982) Mesenchymal differentiation in trigeminal neurilemmoma. Cancer 50: 1568–1571
23. Katoh M, Kadoya S, Emori T, Kwak R (1985) Trigeminal neurinoma presenting abducens nerve palsy as initial symptom: a report of two cases. No Shinkei Geka 13: 555–560
24. Knudsen V, Kolze V (1972) Neurinoma of the Gasserian ganglion and the trigeminal root. Report of four cases. Acta Neurochir (Wien) 26: 159–164
25. Komatsu S, Sakurai Y, Mori T, Suzuki J (1979) Ten cases of trigeminal neurinoma. Neurol Med Chir (Tokyo) 19: 187–193
26. Kubota T, Hayashi M, Yamamoto S (1981) Subarachnoid hemorrhage due to trigeminal neurinoma. Surg Neurol 16: 157–160
27. Lebedev AN, Amirkhanian SE (1978) Diagnosis of neurinomas of the Gasserian ganglion. Zh Vopr Neirokhir 4: 43–49
28. Lechowski S, Majewski A, Slombowski Z (1974) Trigeminal nerve neurinoma situated in the posterior cranial fossa. Neurol Neurochir Pol 8: 135–137
29. Levinthal R, Benston JR (1976) Detection of small trigeminal neurinomas. J Neurosurg 45: 568–575
30. Levy WJ, Ansbacher L, Byer J, Nutkiewicz A, Fratkin J (1983) Primary

malignant nerve sheath tumor of the Gasserian ganglion: a report of two cases. Neurosurgery 13: 572–576

31. Miyagami M, Goto T, Sugawara T, Tsubokawa T, Moriyasu N (1974) Trigeminal neurinoma ganglion type and root type. Neurol Surg (Tokyo) 2: 63–70
32. Mornilori G (1970) Trigeminal neurinoma. Schweiz Arch Neurol Neurochir Psychiatr 107: 47–86
33. Mutsuga N, Kageyama N (1981) A case of neurinoma of the trigeminal root. No Shinkei Geka 9: 23–30
34. Nager GT (1984) Neurinomas of the trigeminal nerve. Am J Otolaryngol 5: 301–333
35. Newton TH, Potts DG (1974) Radiology of the skull and brain. In: Angiography, vol 2, book 4. Mosby, St. Louis, pp 2257–2285
36. Nilol'skiui VA, Temorov ES, Shakov TK (1974) Gasserian ganglion neurinoma in a child. Vopr Neirokhir 5: 55–56
37. Okudera T, Mihara K, Takahashi M, Soejima T, Fukui M (1975) Neuroradiologic diagnosis of trigeminal neurinoma originating from the Gasserian ganglion. Neurol Surg (Tokyo) 3: 835–848
38. Paillas JE, Grisoli F, Farnarier P (1974) Trigeminal nerve neurinomas. Report of 8 cases. Neurochirurgie 20: 41–54
39. Palacios E, Mc Gee EE (1972) The radiographic diagnosis of trigeminal neurinomas. J Neurosurg 36: 153–156
40. Parkinson D (1965) A surgical approach to the cavernous portion of the carotid artery. Anatomical studies and case report. J Neurosurg 23: 474–483
41. Patouillard P, Vanneuville G (1972) Walls of the cavernous sinus. Neurochirurgie 18: 551–560
42. Ross DL, Tew JM Jr, Benton C, Eisentrout C (1984) Trigeminal schwannoma in a child. Neurosurgery 15: 108–110
43. Schisano G, Olivecrona H (1960) Neurinomas of the Gasserian ganglion and trigeminal root. J Neurosurg 17: 306–322
44. Shimabukuro H, Masuzawa T, Miyagi K, Sato F (1983) Trigeminal neurinoma revealed by intratumoral hemorrhage following a minor head injury. Surg Neurol 19: 346–350
45. Sindou M, Szapiro J Jr (1986) Prognostic factors implicated in the microsurgical treatment of trigeminal neuralgia. In: Samii M (ed) Surgery in and around the brain stem and the third ventricle. Springer, Berlin Heidelberg New York Tokyo, pp 273–279
46. Tokunaga O, Shirabe S, Udamura Y (1972) Otoneurological study of a case of trigeminal neurinoma of the cerebellopontine angle. Otolaryngology (Tokyo) 44: 219–226
47. Trese MT, Fous RY, Hepler RS, Brown WJ (1979) Orbital embryonal rhabdomyosarcoma and intracranial schwannoma. Arch Ophthalmol 97: 1929–1930
48. Troijo A (1978) Infratentorial neurilemmoma of the trigeminal nerve in a child. Report of a case. Arq Neuropsiquiatr 36: 164–168
49. Vaquero J, Cabezudo JM, Leunda G, Carrillo R, Bravo G (1981) Simultaneous

posterior and middle cranial fossa neurinomas. Acta Neurochir (Wien) 55: 321–327
50. Vidovszky T, Benoist G (1979) Comparative study of trigeminal neurinomas and parasellar meningiomas. Acta Neurochir (Wien) [Suppl] 28: 397–401
51. Wullenweber R, Traupe H, Scharz G (1974) Angiographic demonstration of a trigeminal neurinoma. Neuroradiology 10: 225–229
52. Yamada H, Sakai N, Ando T, Nishimura Y, Kishimoto Y, Shimokawa K (1980) Trigeminal neurinoma with massive extracranial extension, report of a case. No Shinkei Geka 8: 469–473
53. Yamashita J, Asato R, Handa H, Nakao S, Ogata M (1977) Abducens nerve palsy as initial symptom of trigeminal schwannoma. J Neurol Neurosurg Psychiatry 40: 1190–1197
54. Yonas H, Jannetta PJ (1980) Neurinoma of the trigeminal root and atypical trigeminal neuralgia: their commonality. Neurosurgery 6: 273–277

Treatment of tumors invading the cavernous sinus

V. V. DOLENC, T. KREGAR, M. FERLUGA, M. FETTICH, A. MORINA

University Department of Neurosurgery, University Medical Centre, Ljubljana, Yugoslavia

A series of 140 patients with tumors of the skull base, excluding tumors of the eighth nerve and pituitary tumors confined to the sella, were treated by a direct microsurgical approach in the period from 1980 through 1985.

Most of the lesions were located in the medial portion of the sphenoid wing, the tuberculum, the diaphragm and the dorsum of the sella, the apex of the pyramid, the clivus and in the parasellar region in the cavernous sinus. Of the 63 intracavernous tumors, 48 invaded the cavernous sinus, while 15 originated in the cavernous sinus itself. In seven cases of intracavernous tumors, the lesion extended through the superior orbital fissure and/or the optic canal into the orbit. In eight cases, the tumor spread via the normal anatomical foramina, through the skull base and/or by direct destruction of the bone, below the cavernous sinus into the bony sinuses and to the compartments below the skull base.

Histology showed 40 out of the 63 intracavernous tumors to be benign meningiomas. 45 lesions were amenable to complete microsurgical removal, while in 18 cases, a part of the tumor, usually that around the ICA, had to be left in place.

There were four postoperative deaths; two patients died from pulmonary complications: one, and another 21 days after surgery. One patient succumbed to myocardial infarction 19 days postoperatively. One patient with a malignant lesion of the skull base and the cavernous sinus died three months after the operation. Fifty patients operated on for a parasellar intracavernous tumor recovered within six months after surgery; 37 showed a transient lesion of the cranial nerves three through six, while 12 had irreversible lesions of one or several cranial nerves three through six. Two patients were blind in the eye at the side of the lesion. In two cases, patency of the ICA could not be preserved: it was occluded proximally to the cavernous sinus in the petrous bone, and proximally of the ophthalmic artery in the cavernous sinus.

Five patients undergoing this type of surgery developed CSF leakage. The fistula closed spontaneously in three cases, while in two surgical intervention was required. Of the 59 patients operated on for a benign tumor of the cavernous sinus, 46 have resumed their previous occupation.

Introduction

In the past, cavernous sinus (CS) surgery used to be performed only exceptionally, but recently it has been growing more and more popular. Thanks to a deeper insight into the topographical anatomy of the CS, a direct operative approach is indicated in an increasing number of cases [4, 6].

It would be outside the scope of this report to deal with the normal and pathological anatomy of the CS; this subject has been largely explored in the literature [18].

The present indications for the CS surgery include tumors of the CS, as well as vascular lesions located inside the CS and medial to it [4, 5, 6].

In cases where the entire CS is filled with a tumor, all intracavernous structures in their entire course, from the apex of the petrous bone to the superior orbital fissure, should be explored. Needless to say, total exploration of the CS inflicts considerable additional damage to the venous flow through the CS. Since no viable solution has yet been found, we tackle this problem by making every effort to preserve at least the flow via the pterigoid plexus, which usually proves sufficient.

Problematic are tumors which encompass a long segment of the ICA in its entire circumference, or even impinge on the lumen of the artery. The eroded arterial wall is very likely to be damaged by dissection. The slightest operative trauma to such a wall may bring about rupture of the artery, which may occur even as late as two weeks postoperatively. Bearing in mind this potential hazard, we prefer to leave a part of the tumor on the wall and avoid in this way the risk of vascular traumatization.

Partial or complete loss of function of one or several ocular motor nerves, associated or not with pain in the area innervated by the ipsilateral trigeminal nerve, is usually due to a pathological process in the CS. Ipsilateral exophthalmos frequently results from such a lesion as well. At present, a definitive diagnosis is provided by a CT scan, but additional diagnostic techniques, such as angiography, venography, and neurophysiological studies are often employed in the diagnostic evaluation, and especially in the operative treatment of these lesions.

Recently, biopsy of the tumor, with the needle inserted through the orbit and the superior orbital fissure, has been introduced as a valuable diagnostic tool used before definitive therapy is undertaken.

The only successful therapeutic modality in benign tumors, including those located in the CS, is complete surgical excision.

Patients, methods, and results

In our series of 63 patients with an intracavernous tumor, there were 39 females and 24 males, ranging in age from 12 to 75 years. The time elapsed from the onset of symptoms to the establishment of definitive diagnosis ranged from several weeks in a malignant tumor, to 15 years in a cholesteatoma, the mean period being 2 years. In most cases the disease first manifested itself by a headache, which was most often retro-orbital in location (Table 1). Occasionally the pain occurred in the area supplied by the first and/or second branch of the trigeminal nerve. In many patients, the function of the ocular motor nerves was impaired even at an early stage. One third of cases only had exophthalmos and disturbances of drainage via the ophthalmic veins. Very few patients developed ophthalmoplegia before the establishment of ultimate diagnosis.

Table 1. Signs and symptoms due to intracavernous lesions

	No. of cases
Headache	27
Lesion of nerve(s) III through VI	25
Exophthalmos	17
Neuralgic pain in V/1 and/or V/2	5
Ophthalmoplegia	3

In the majority of patients, neurophysiological and neuroradiological studies were employed only at the stage when signs appeared in addition to clinical symptoms. The definitive diagnosis of intracavernous tumor was provided by a CT scan. Before undergoing intracavernous surgery, all our patients had patency of the communicating arteries (ACoA and PCoA) evaluated by carotid and vertebral angiography, including cross-circulation studies. The position of the ICA in the CS, as well as its shape and configuration, were considered most important too. Close examination of

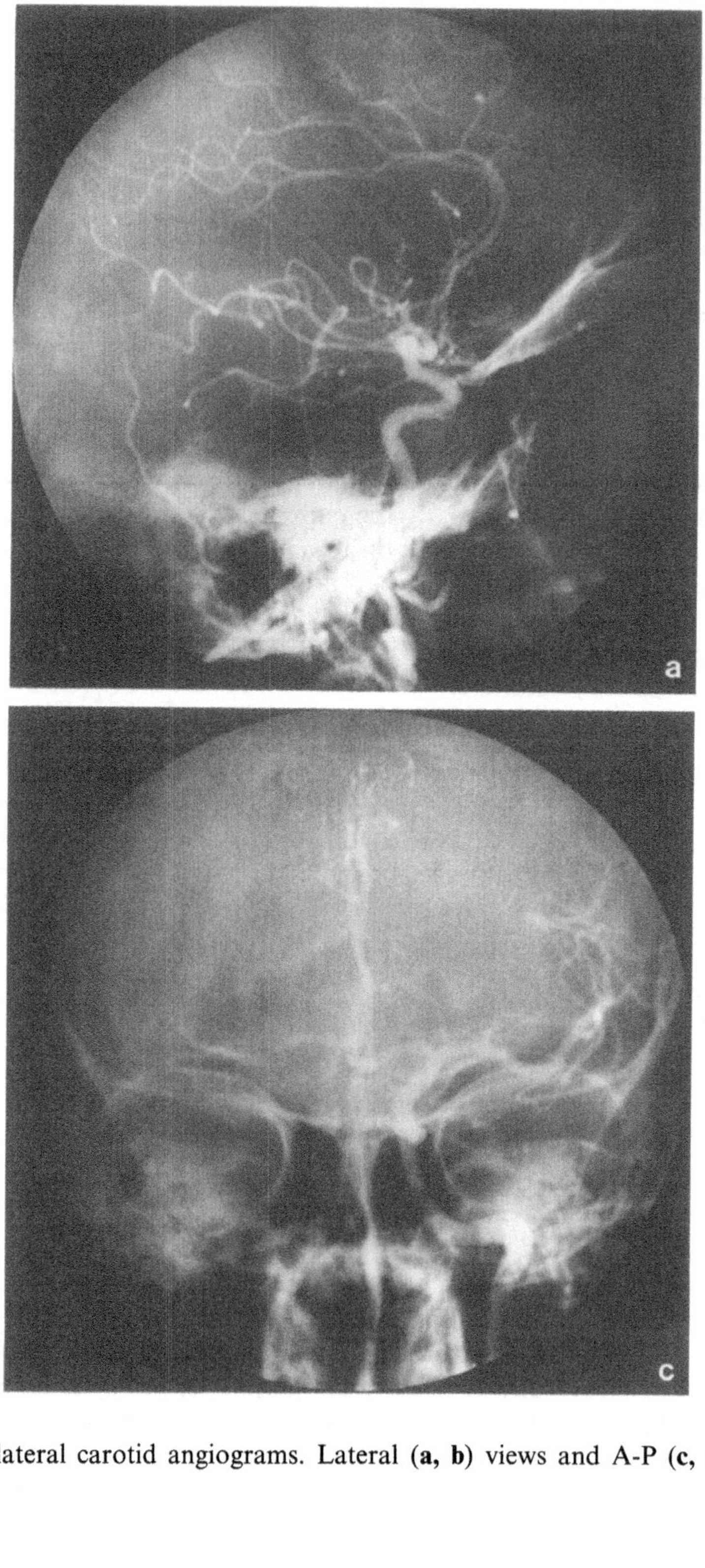

Fig. 1. Bilateral carotid angiograms. Lateral (**a, b**) views and A-P (**c, d**) views

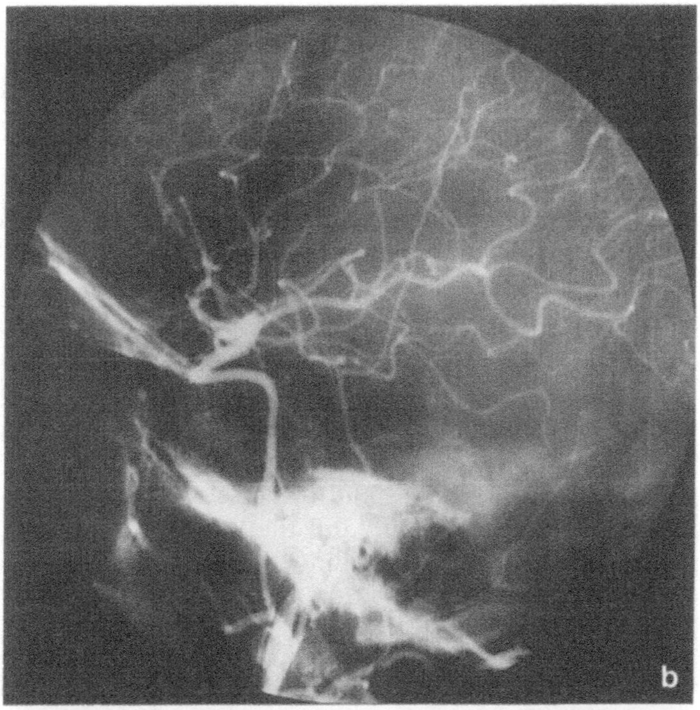

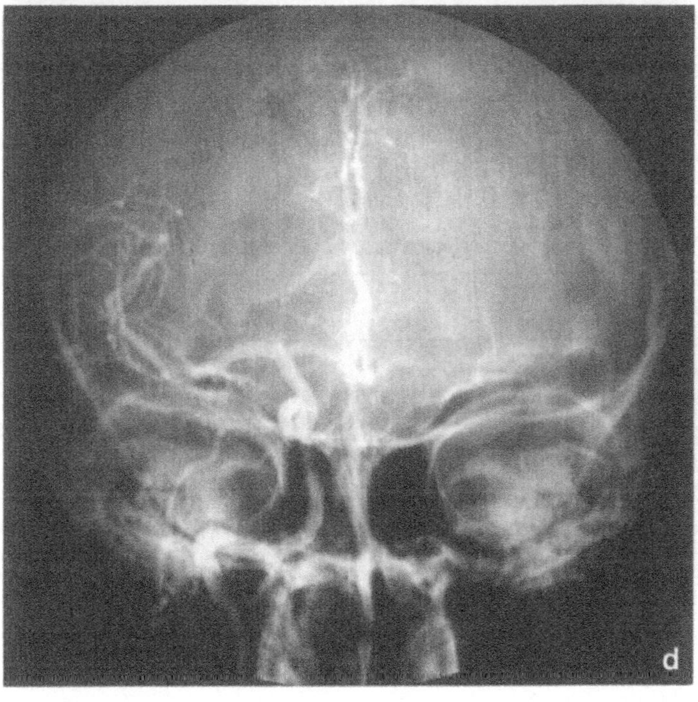

show significant displacement of the right intracavernous ICA (**b, d**) preoperative angiograms provided the ultimate answer as to the safety of complete excision of the intracavernous tumor (Fig. 1). Valuable information about the function of the ocular motor nerves was supplied by an EMG of oculomotor muscles. In a considerable number of patients, the preoperative diagnostic evaluation included evoked potentials of the optic nerves as well as classical perimetry. The findings obtained make possible a more objective estimate of changes which may occur after the operation. More than one third of our patients had had one or several previous operations done at other institutions before being admitted to this Department. Those surgical interventions did not include complete removal of the tumor; the intracavernous location of the lesion was namely revealed only on operation.

In 15 of our patients operated on for an intracavernous tumor, the lesion originated in the CS (Table 2). In the rest, the tumor invaded the CS, spreading either along the nerves and/or vessels, or directly via the dural wall of the CS. Only exceptionally did the tumor extend into the CS or outwards, through the foramen rotundum and the foramen ovale.

Table 2. Invasion of the tumor

	No. of cases
Along nerve(s) III through VI	27
Intracavernous origin	15
Direct invasion through the dura	12
From the sella	7
Along the ICA	2
Total	63

Tumors invading the CS from the outside produce displacement or compression of the ICA, depending on the point where they enter the CS. In cases where the entire CS is filled with a tumor, the point of its origin is generally difficult to establish. The origin of a tumor (usually a meningioma), its spread and invasion of the CS, are revealed by a CT scan, or, sometimes, by reconstruction of several CT images, in coronal and saggital sections.

Patients

It is of primary importance to determine whether the tumor originated in the CS (Fig. 2), or invaded the CS at a later stage.

Tumors originating outside the CS to invade the CS later on, most commonly arise from the following sites: the anterior clinoid, the medial part of the sphenoid wing, the superior orbital fissure (Fig. 3), and the apex of the pyramid, from where they spread to the CS forwards, and to the pontocerebellar angle backwards and downwards (Fig. 4). Tumors sometimes spread to the CS from the medial border (Fig. 5), or directly, through the lateral wall (Fig. 6). Whenever we managed to establish the origin and the direction of invasion of the intracavernous tumor before surgery, we found it much easier to make a plan of the operation and we succeeded in removing the entire tumor mass and preserving the CS structures. In spite of extensive preoperative studies regarding the origin, spread and nature of the intracavernous lesion, as well as the involvement of the intracavernous nervous and vascular structures, we accomplished complete excision of the tumor just in 45 cases, while in 18 cases partial removal only was possible for the following reasons: infiltration of the ICA wall by the tumor in nine cases, difficult dissection of nerve(s) three through six because of previous operations and scarring in seven cases, and malignancy of the tumor in two cases. Operative problems are listed in Table 3.

Excision of the tumor from the CS relieved headache in the majority of patients, as well as severe neuralgic pain in V/1 and/or V/2. The operation, however, was not successful in treating ophthalmoplegia which had occurred in three patients prior to surgery.

In most patients the operation succeeded in reducing exophthalmos, though it was completely abolished in only a very few cases. Improvement in the function of the cranial nerve(s) three through six was obtained just in cases showing partial involvement of these nerves. Patients with a complete loss of function prior to surgery showed no postoperative functional return.

Table 3. Complications associated with intracavernous tumor surgery

	No. of cases
None	10
Transient paresis of nerve(s) III through VI	37
Definite lesion of nerve(s) III through VI	12
Lesion of the optic nerve	2
Lesion of the ICA	2
Total	63

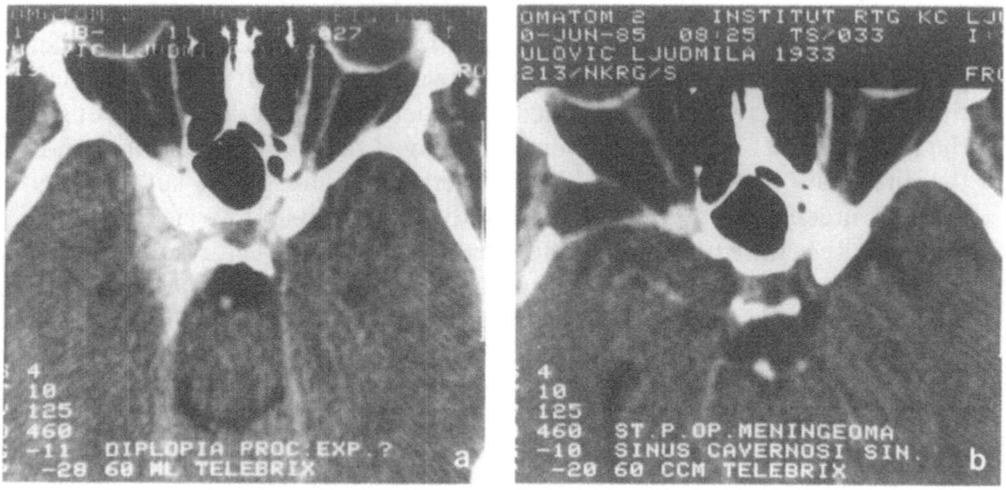

Fig. 2. a Preoperative CT scan shows an intracavernous tumor in the left CS. **b** Postoperative scan shows no tumor

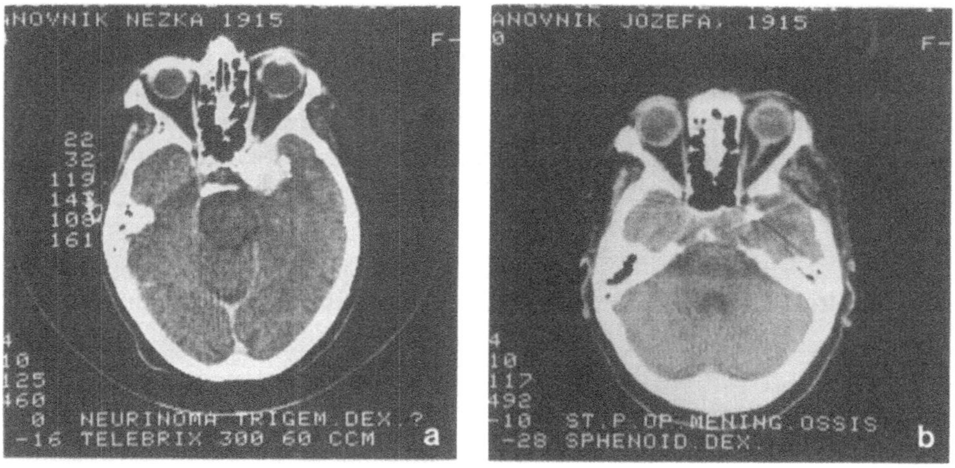

Fig. 3. a Preoperative CT scan shows a tumor located at the anterior clinoid, in the medial portion of the sphenoidal wing and in the superior orbital fissure, as well as in the CS. **b** Postoperative CT scan shows absence of tumor and normal situation

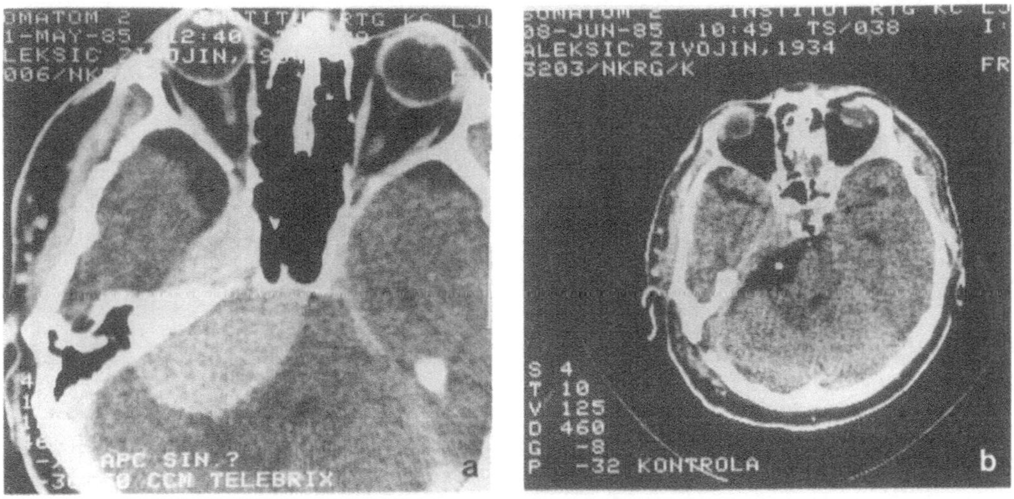

Fig. 4. a Preoperative CT scan shows a tumor at the left apex of the pyramid, extending to the CS and to the ponto-cerebellar angle (PCA). **b** Postoperative CT scan shows normal situation and no tumor

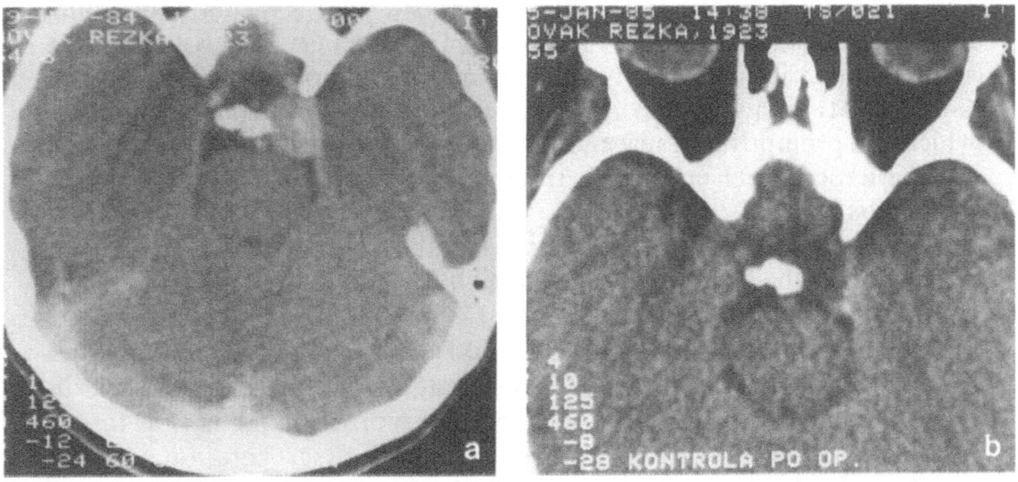

Fig. 5. a Preoperative CT scan shows a small tumor on the medial aspect of the right CS. **b** Postoperative CT scan shows normal situation on the medial aspect of the right CS

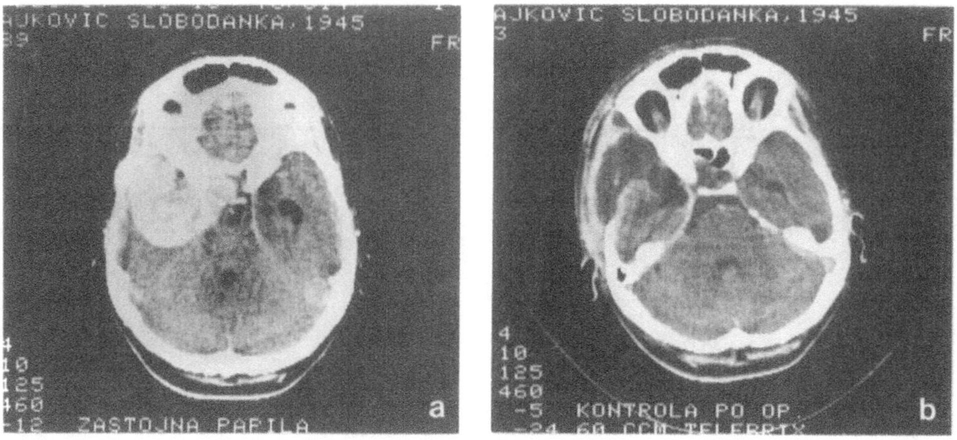

Fig. 6. a Preoperative CT scan shows a large tumor in the left middle cranial fossa, extending into the CS and in the sella, by direct invasion through the lateral wall of the CS. **b** Postoperative CT scan shows the situation after complete removal of the tumor

Four patients operated on for an intracavernous tumor died, the cause of death being pulmonary complication in two, myocardial infarction in one, and malignancy of the lesion in one patient. Five patients undergoing intracavernous tumor surgery developed CSF leakage. The fistula closed spontaneously in five patients, while two required operative treatment. In four patients with CSF leakage the course was complicated by meningitis, which was promptly and successfully treated. Closing of the fistula through scar formation which occurred in three patients is most likely attributable to meningitis itself.

Two patients requiring re-operation had the defect of the skull base filled with pieces of the temporal muscle, fixed by means of Tissucol sealant. The procedure proved very successful.

Three patients had to be re-operated on because of a residual tumor and recurrence, 2 to 3 years after the first operation. The presence of a scar in those patients made surgical re-interventions more demanding. The tumor histology, however, was unchanged from the first operation. Table 4 indicates the histological diagnosis of the intracavernous sinus tumors treated.

In four patients the extent of the tumor invasion required a two-stage surgical procedure using different operative approaches; one patient had to undergo three operations by three different approaches for the tumor to be completely removed (Fig. 7).

The combination of the pterional, subtemporal and petrosal approaches, described in our previous works [4, 5], was invariably used in all

Table 4. Histological diagnosis of intracavernous tumors

	No. of cases
Benign meningioma	40
Malignant meningioma	2
Chromophobe adenoma	7
Neurinoma of the fifth nerve	4
Neurofibromatosis	3
Fibrous dysplasia	2
Epidermoid	2
Cholesteatoma	1
Myxoma	1
Fibrosarcoma	1
Total	63

our patients. No special measures, such as hypotension, hypothermia, dehydration or lumbar puncture, were taken during surgery. In all patients enough space was available for the manipulation around the lesion, and no temporal lobe resection was required. Fifteen patients operated on for intracavernous tumors were placed on a 6 to 8 month course of antiepileptic treatment. The medication was not prescribed to treat epileptic seizures, but rather to control the EEG abnormalities which occurred at the site of operation. Manifest epilepsy has not yet been observed in any of our patients.

Discussion

Clinical features characteristic of various CS pathologies have been described in detail in previous works [8, 9, 10, 11, 13, 14, 15, 19]. It is well known that different pathological processes may present with a similar clinical picture [7, 20, 21].

Standard neuroradiological investigations, such as venography and angiography, provide information about the vascular portion of the CS only. A high-resolution CT scan has proved to be a valuable diagnostic tool, representing the basis for, at least, tentative diagnosis of a tumor [12]. The ultimate, histology-like diagnosis, however, cannot be made by means of the above-mentioned techniques. The recent introduction of a transorbital fine-needle aspiration biopsy [16] has unfolded a new chapter in the

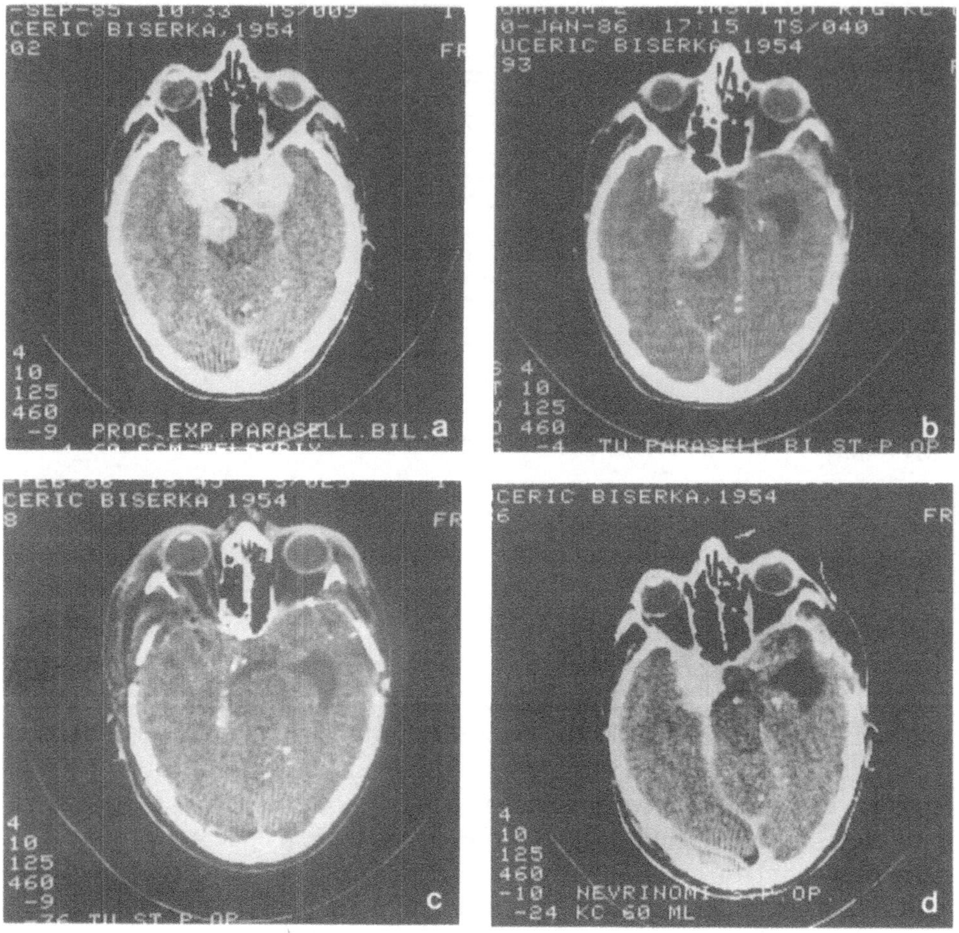

Fig. 7. CT scan shows the sequences of the three-stage surgery. **a** Tumors in both CSs: the left intracavernous tumor extends over the apex of the pyramid, down to the left PCA. **b** Situation following the first operation: complete excision of the lesion of the right CS. The lower part of the lesion exerts critical compression on the brain stem at the level of the PCA. **d** Situation following the second operation: excision of the lesion situated at the apex of the pyramid and in the PCA on the left by the left suboccipital approach. **c** Situation following the third operation: complete excision of the remaining part of the tumor from the left CS by the left pterional and subtemporal approach

diagnosis of intracavernous lesions. The latest discoveries in the field of pathological histology of the CS structures have considerably improved our understanding of meningiomas originating in the CS [2]. It is also essential to understand the normal and morbid anatomy of the CS, and to know the tendency of tumors to spread from the adjacent structures into the CS [1, 3, 18].

Careful dissection of individual structures in the CS, as well as in its immediate neighbourhood, allows complete opening of the CS and preservation of its vascular and nervous structures [4, 5, 6]. Recent studies have pointed to the possibility of abnormally copious venous flow from the brain to the saphenoparietal sinus, and through it to the CS. In such cases any interruption of these veins would seriously jeopardize drainage from the brain [17] and any extensive CS surgery would be most hazardous, and even impossible to accomplish. In our series of patients undergoing intracavernous sinus surgery, we have never encountered abnormally increased venous drainage to the CS, and therefore we had no difficulty sacrificing the veins without doing any harm to the patient.

Intracavernous tumors surgery has received increasing attention recently, and its proper value is finally being recognized. Radiotherapy of benign tumors has proven ineffectual, and currently complete removal of a benign tumor leading to full recovery of the patient is the generally accepted approach to the treatment of these lesions.

Thanks to many recent discoveries in the field of CS anatomy [18], a tumor can now be completely excised without damaging the function of the vascular and neural structures in the sinus. This aim is much easier to attain while a tumor is still small in size. Therefore, there is a need for the available diagnostic procedures to be further refined and developed in order to allow early detection of these lesions: early diagnosis is a basis for the successful complete surgical removal of intracavernous tumors. It is most difficult to remove completely a meningioma which has already spread over the base and invaded both CSs and the sella. A lesion of this extent is commonly associated with visual impairment, which additionally complicates the already serious situation. Intracavernous tumor surgery has its limitations, like any other kind of surgery; because of its duration it is restricted to younger age groups. It is therefore not in the interests of the patient to place him on conservative "treatment" for ten years or more. At the stage when unilateral or even bilateral loss of vision has occurred due to a benign meningioma of the CS, the patient will derive hardly any benefit from the operative treatment, and he will have no chance of having the quality of his life improved.

The fact that surgical removal of a tumor from the CS has become an attainable objective calls for a changed attitude towards this issue to be taken by conservative medicine, on the one hand, and on the other, it requires adequate preparation and training of the surgeon who is to undertake this kind of operation: a sine qua non for surgery of the CS is a high degree of competence in these operations, rather than merely the will to carry them out.

References

1. Bonnal J, Thibaut A, Brotchi J, Born J (1980) Invading meningiomas of the sphenoid ridge. J Neurosurg 53: 587–599
2. Bouchez B, Arnott G, Jomin M, Clarisse J, Delandsheer JM, Krivošić I, Woillez M, Lesoin F, Courteville-Delamarre V (1983) Les méningiomes primitivement issus du sinus caverneux. A propos de deux cas. Rev Otoneuroophthalmol 55: 251–262
3. Dolenc VV (1979) Microsurgical removal of large sphenoidal bone meningiomas. Acta Neurochir (Wien) [Suppl] 28: 391–396
4. Dolenc VV (1983) Direct microsurgical repair of intracavernous vascular lesions. J Neurosurg 58: 824–831
5. Dolenc VV (1985) A combined epi- and subdural direct approach to carotid-ophthalmic artery aneurysms. J Neurosurg 62: 667–672
6. Hakuba A, Nishimura S, Shirakata S, Tsukamoto M (1982) Surgical approaches to the cavernous sinus. Report of 19 cases. Neurol Med Chir (Tokyo) 22: 295–308
7. Ho KC, Meyer G, Garancis J, Hanna J (1982) Chemodectoma involving the cavernous sinus and semilunar ganglion. Human Pathology 10: 942–943
8. Hunt WE (1976) Tolosa—Hunt syndrome: one cause of painful ophthalmoplegia. J Neurosurg 44: 544–549
9. Julien J, Ferrer X, Drouillard J, Philippe JC, Desbordes P (1984) Cavernous sinus syndrome due to lymphoma. Short report. J Neurol Neurosurg Psychiatry 47: 558–560
10. King LW, Molitch ME, Gittinger JW Jr, Wolpert SM, Stern J (1983) Cavernous sinus syndrome due to prolactinoma: resolution with bromocriptine. Surg Neurol 19: 280–284
11. Kline LB, Galbraith JG (1981) Parasellar epidermoid tumor presenting as painful ophthalmoplegia. Case report. J Neurosurg 54: 113–117
12. Kline LB, Acker JD, Post MJD (1982) Computed tomographic evaluation of the cavernous sinus. Ophthalmology 89: 374–385
13. Koh CS, Tan CT, Alhady SF (1983) Cavernous sinus syndrome. A manifestation of non—Hodgkin's lymphoma of the ethmoid sinus. Med J Aust 2: 451–452
14. Lenzi GL, Fieschi C (1977) Superior orbital fissure syndrome. Review of 130 cases. Eur Neurol 16: 23–30
15. Mills RP, Insalaco SJ, Joseph A (1981) Bilateral cavernous sinus metastasis and ophthalmoplegia. Case report. J Neurosurg 55: 463–466
16. Slamovits TL, Cahill KW, Sibony PA, Dekker A, Johnson BL (1983) Orbital fine-needle aspiration biopsy in patients with cavernous sinus syndrome. J Neurosurg 59: 1037–1042

17. Sugita K, Kobayashi S, Yokoo A (1982) Preservation of large bridging veins during brain retraction. Technical note. J Neurosurg 57: 856–858
18. Taptas JM (1982) The so-called cavernous sinus: a review of the controversy and its implications for neurosurgeons. Neurosurgery 11: 712–717
19. Thomas JE, Yoss RE (1970) The parasellar syndrome: problems in determining etiology. Mayo Clin Proc 45: 617–623
20. Trobe JD, Glaser JS, Post JD (1978) Meningiomas and aneurysms of the cavernous sinus. Neuro-ophthalmologic features. Arch Ophthalmol 96: 457–467
21. Unsöld R, Safran AB, Safran E, Hoyt WF (1980) Metastatic infiltration of nerves in the cavernous sinus. Arch Neurol 37: 59–61

Pathological aspects in a series of 53 cavernous sinus tumors

I. Krivosic[1], M. Jomin[2], J. L. Christiaens[3], F. Lesoin[2], G. Combelles[3], J. P. Pruvo[4], M. Reyford[5], and A. Dupont[1]

[1] Laboratory of Neuropathology, Departments of [2] Neurosurgery B, of [3] Neurosurgery A, of [4] Neuroradiology, and of [5] Anaesthesia A, C.H.R.U., Lille, France

In the last ten years we have had the opportunity to study 53 oncological neurosurgical specimens of cavernous sinus among a total of 6000 (six thousand) neurosurgical specimens (Table 1). The first case was a classical patient who had Garcin's syndrome due to a pharyngeal cylindrome invading cavernous sinus. Later on we examined meningiomas around the cavernous sinus, meningiomas invading the cavernous sinus, tumors of nerves and metastasis. The question was raised which kind of tumor can appear in the cavernous sinus and how these tumors extend.

The aim of this study is to present a variety of oncological lesions observed in the cavernous sinus (Tables 1 and 2) in relation to the histoarchitecture of this region.

Meningiomas

The occurrence of primary meningiomas of the cavernous sinus can be explained by the existence of arachnoid tissue, especially clusters of meningo-epithelial cells from which meningiomas generally arise. Arachnoid tissue extends into the cavernous sinus from nerve sheaths, arachnoid around the pituitary stalk, as well as through the roof of the cavernous sinus. This arachnoid tissue then forms one interrupted network inside the cavernous sinus, and thus meningiomas can arise widely inside the cavernous sinus. Intracavernous meningiomas have as normal arachnoid tissue the capacity for dissue infiltration alongside the sheaths of intrasinusal connective tissue which exists as some sort of "skeleton" around the whole structure of the cavernous sinus (ICA, veins, nerves).

Table 1. Neurosurgical specimens studied in the Laboratory of Neuropathology, C.H.R.U. Lille, 1976–1986

Total of surgical neuropathological specimens		Cavernous sinus
Gliomas	1980	—
Meningiomas	1240	22
Nerves tumors	380	11
Metastasis	600	15
Connective tissue tumors	540	4
Others	1360	1
Total	6000	53

Table 2. Oncological lesions observed in the CS in the Laboratory of Neuropathology, C.H.R.U. Lille, 1976–1986

Tumors of cavernous sinus	
Nerves tumors	11
Meningiomas	22
Metastasis	15
Chondromas	2
Chordomas	2
Cylindromas	1
Total	53

The meningiomas will increase in size by two mechanisms:

a) by means of diffuse infiltration of connective tissue between the different elements. Contralateral extension is possible due to the existence of continuity of connective tissue sheaths. For these reasons the natural history of genuine and invading extracavernous sinus meningiomas is infiltration of both sinuses giving an aspect of a bridge (bridge meningioma) (Fig. 1);

b) by means of invading and collapse of the cavernous sinus venous pathway.

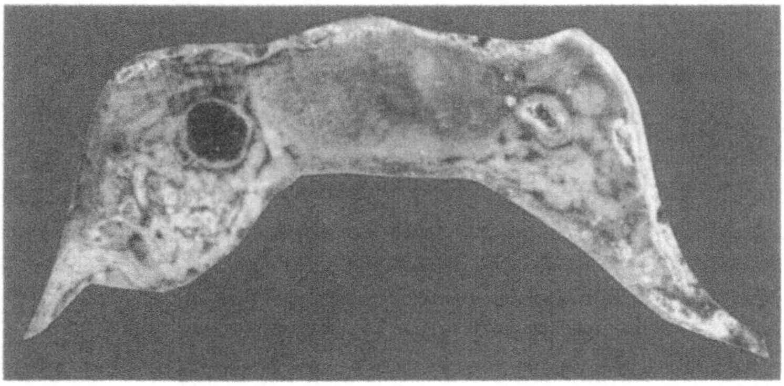

Fig. 1. Bridge cavernous sinus meningioma. Coronal section of the cavernous sinus. Postero-anterior view. The meningioma is bilateral. On both sides it extends by the ramified confluent by infiltrations around different cavernous sinus structures (infiltration follows the cavernous sinus connective tissue skeleton). Cavernous sinus veins are collapsed. The tumor extends from one side to the other in continuous connective tissue sheaths (periosteum and dura mater). The left internal carotid artery is thrombosed in this particular case

These two mechanisms give rise to the final compact aspect, which blads very little at surgery. The speed of growth and extension depends upon the degree of malignancy of the tumor and not of the histological varieties (Table 3). Evaluation of the grade of malignancy is of prognostic value.

Tumors of nerves

The nerves are localised in the lateral wall of the cavernous sinus except for nerve VI which initially, in the posterior aspect of the sinus, runs directly through the sinus. The nerves have their own dura mater sheaths separated

Table 3. Studied meningiomas (12 females, 10 males)

Histological type	Grade			
	I	II	III	IV
Meningotheliomatous	4	1		
Fibrous	2			
Mixed	8	2	1	
Hemangioblastic		1		
Anaplastic			2	1
Total	14	4	3	1

from the external sheath of the dura mater of the middle cranial fossa. Surgical approach of the nerve is therefore possible without entrance into the large cavernous sinus cavity by dissection of the external dura mater sheath and hemostatic control of veins found between the nerves. The variety of tumor was limited in this series to most common nerve tumors (Table 4).

Table 4. Studied tumors of nerves (6 females, 5 males)

Histological type	Grade			
	I	II	III	IV
Schwannoma	6			
Neurofibroma	2	2		1
Neuroblastoma				1
Total	8	1		2

Benign schwannomas

An accidental discovery of a microschwannoma showed us that this tumor arises by proliferation of schwann cells inside one nerve fascicle. During their evolution these tumors compress the rest of the fascicles without invading them, thus giving the theoretical possibility of preserving by microscopic dissection the nerves which are not invaded but simply compressed. The schwannomas are encapsulated; therefore their resection is possible.

Neurofibromas

They arise from the center of nerves and spread throughout the nerve up to the sheath, giving rise to a local bulging. From the beginning, the nerve is completly infiltrated and cannot be dissociated from the tumor. One of our cases originally presented with a neurofibroma of nerve III, then two years later cranial nerves IV, V, and VI were involved with separate neurofibromas.

Neuroblastomas

We have found one case—preoperatively a tumor invaded the Gasserian ganglion. It was only on histological examination that we were able to identify the existence of a tumor consisting of neuroblasts.

Metastasis

We observed two different conditions of metastatic invasion of the cavernous sinus, firstly as an accidental autopsy finding. Involvement of cavernous sinus appeared by CSF spread of meningeal carcinomatosis.

The second example was in a neurosurgical patient having an isolated limited involvement of the cavernous sinus by a tumor of unknown origin. Histological examination showed a metastasis of a carcinoma.

We can evoke two mechanisms for these metastasis, extension by contiguity from the neighbouring primary carcinoma as in a case of pharyngeal cylindroma extending into the cavernous sinus, or from bone metastasis. In cases without local bone metastasis direct implantation into the cavernous sinus ramified venous structures seem possible.

Chondromas

We had to examine two specimens of chondromas. Concerning the origin of chondromas, we can invoke the neighbouring skeleton of the base of the skull covered with cartilage. The question could be raised as to whether chondromas could grow from the cartilage of an Eustachian tube which is the most important cartilaginous structure in the vicinity.

The transnasal approach to the cavernous sinus

M. Loyo[1], J. F. Sanchez-Marle[2], R. Del Valle[1]3, and M. Mares[2]

[1] Department of Neurosurgery, National Medical Center, IMSS, and
[2] Department of Otorhinolaryngology, Military Central Hospital,
Mexico City, Mexico

Surgical treatment of the cavernous sinus lesions, which has long been neglected, has received new attention due to the diagnostic possibilities of computerized tomography, magnetic resonance and digital angiography. With these studies valuable information can be obtained as to whether a tumor is only adjacent to the wall of the sinus or is invasive; they also give accurate information about the position of the carotid artery in relation to the sinus, while perhaps the most important contribution is the early diagnosis of the tumors before their great size makes extirpation very difficult if not impossible.

Angiographic study also gives information regarding the need to practice a bypass procedure as a preliminary step to the surgical removal of a tumor with radiofluoroscopic control [4]. In this way the study of the anatomy of the region makes possible the direct approach to carotid cavernous lesions.

The pioneer work was done by Parkinson [11] in fistulas and Dolenc [2, 3] in the handling of tumors of the area.

The anatomical studies demonstrated that the carotid artery is situated medially in the cavernous sinus.

There are no nerves medial to the artery and the cavernous sinus has less trabeculations in this area, since the third, fourth, sixth and first division of nerve V are in the lateral wall of the cavernous sinus [5, 12, 13, 14].

We have observed during transsphenoidal surgery for pituitary tumors the relation of the sphenoidal sinus with the medial wall of the cavernous sinus [8, 9] (Fig. 1).

In this paper we describe a new way to inject * Tissuccol to treat a carotid

* Tissuccol—Immuno AG, Vienna, Austria

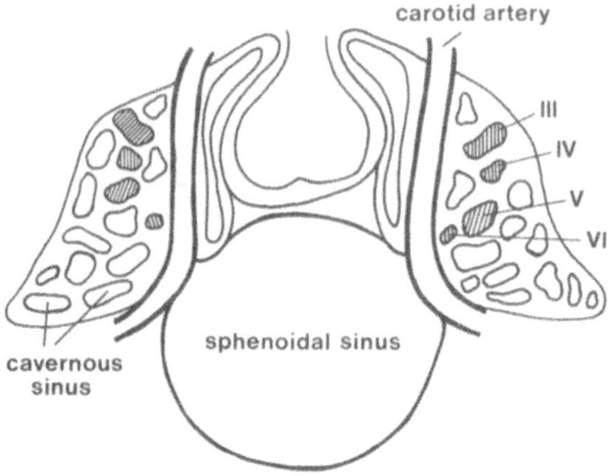

Fig. 1. The relationship of the sphenoidal sinus and the cavernous sinus are demonstrated

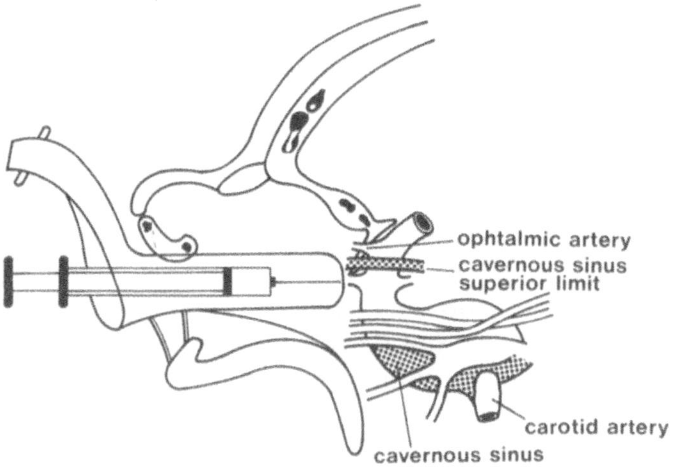

Fig. 2. The technique of injection to the cavernous sinus is demonstrated

cavernous fistula, through a transsphenoidal approach (Fig. 2). After exposing the anterior portion of the cavernous sinus, we can inject, between the carotid artery and the medial wall of the cavernous sinus, a sealing substance composed of fibrin and factor VIII, like that used by Isamat [6] who injects it through the transcranial approach.

We think that the transsphenoidal approach is less traumatic than the craniotomy.

Based on this technique and taking into consideration the anatomy of the region, we decided to use the direct transsphenoidal approach to the cavernous sinus.

The classic transsphenoidal surgery for pituitary tumors offers a limited field, so the handling of vascular or tumoral lesions of the area is almost impossible; for this reason we planned a modified approach that would give a better view of the area.

The sublabial approach used since the beginning of the century was abandoned because of the difficulty of visualization in a deep field.

However, with the use of the surgical microscope this approach was again used by Conley [1] and Maniglia [10], and this operation allows a wide access with good visualization of the medial wall of the cavernous sinus.

We used fresh cadavers to practice the necessary dissection and explore the possible use of this access to the area.

Technique

An horizontal incision is made in the sublabial gingiva from one maxillar tubercle to the other (Fig. 3).

The soft tissue is raised over both superior maxillar bones to expose the piriform opening and the nasal spine. The anterior part of the septum is dissected and then the dorsal portion.

The dissection is carried through the infraorbitary nerves without cutting them. Then the nasal cavity is entered after sectioning the mucosa below and laterally.

The lateral mucosa of the nasal fossa and the medial mucosa of the maxilla sinus are dissected leaving free the lateral bony wall of the nose that is removed with fast-cutting drills to the posterior portions. This maneuver allows the control of the sphenopalatine artery.

The nasal septum mucosa is dissected from the perichondrium to permit the total elevation of the mucosa in the superior portion. The cartilaginus septum is sectioned in the lower portion at the maxilla spine and displaced laterally to the same side of the sphenoidal rostrum which is clearly visualized and totally removed.

With this maneuver the sphenoidal sinus is totally exposed, and once the

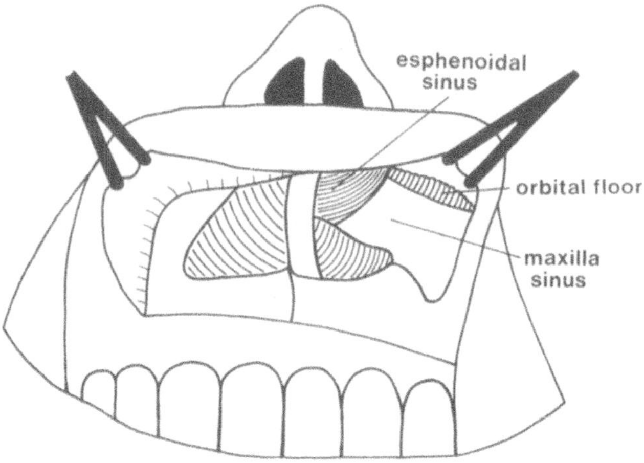

Fig. 3. Sublabial gingival incision

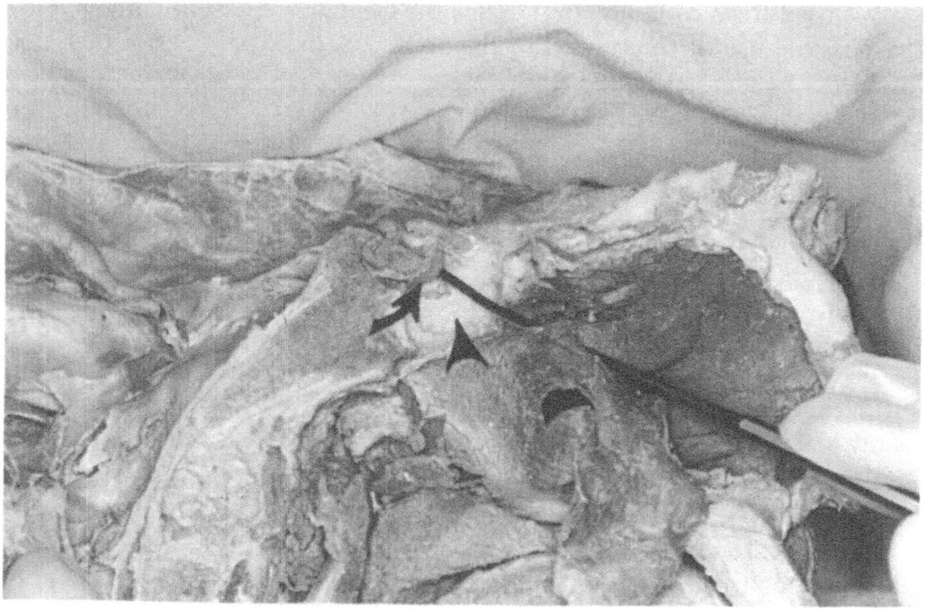

Fig. 4. The sphenoidal sinus (arrowhead) is exposed and the relations of the carotid artery (arrow) in the cavernous sinus can be observed. The probe shows the method of access

mucosa and bone are removed the medial dural wall, that is part of the cavernous sinus, is exposed (Fig. 4).

At this moment the use of the surgical microscope is initiated and a 3 mm incision is made in the dura mater and the sinus packed with * Surgicel to control the venous bleeding; the carotid artery is exposed step by step to reach the origin of the ophthalmic artery (Fig. 5).

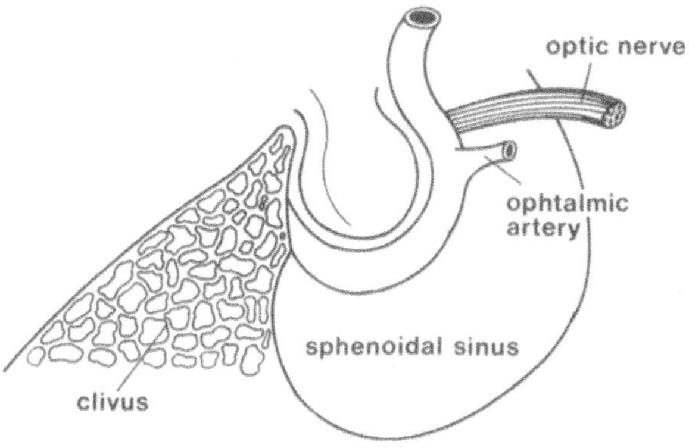

Fig. 5. Exposure of the carotid and ophthalmic arteries

The meningohypophyseal arteries may be encountered as well as the oculomotor nerves. As the carotid siphon is exposed with this technique, we believe intracavernous aneurysms and meningiomas of the area can be handled. To close the field, the sphenoidal sinus is filled with muscle and fat, the nasosinusal structures are set in place, and with the use of a Foley catheter and gauze they are stabilized.

We have already used this technique successfully to operate tumoral lesions located in this area, as can be seen in Figs. 6 and 7.

We believe this technique will have a lower mortality and morbidity rate that the transcranial route.

* Surgical—Ethicon Ltd., Somerville, New Jersey, U.S.A.

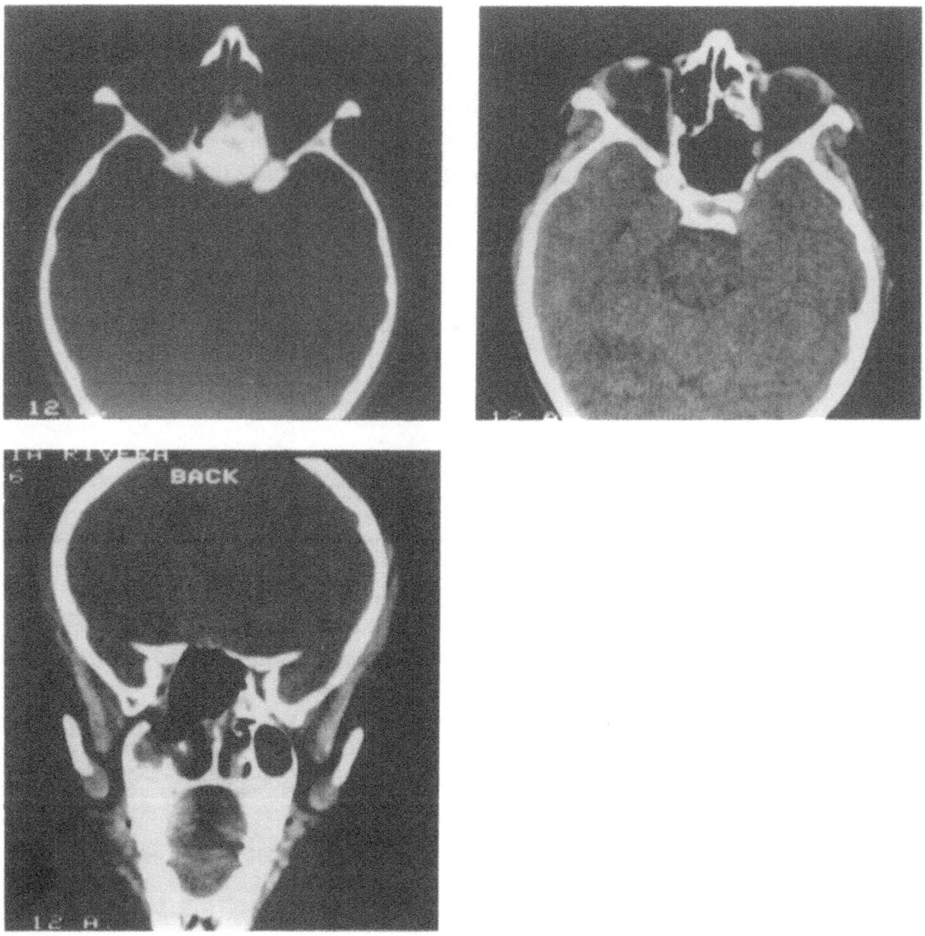

Fig. 6. Pre- and postoperative CT scans of the removal of a fibrous displasia of the sphenoidal bone

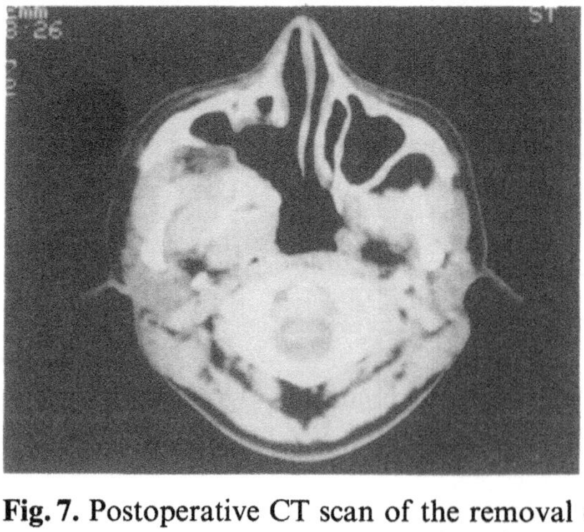

Fig. 7. Postoperative CT scan of the removal of a fibroma that was invading the sphenoidal bone

References

1. Conley J, Price J (1979) Sublabial approach to the nasal and the nasopharyngeal cavities. Am J Surg 138: 615–618
2. Dolenc V (1983) Direct microsurgical repair of intracavernous vascular lesions. J Neurosurg 58: 824–831
3. Dolenc V (1985) A combined epi- and subdural direct approach to carotid ophthalmic artery aneurysms. J Neurosurg 62: 667–672
4. Hardy J (1963) Televised radiofluoroscopic control in intracranial surgery. Union Med Can 92: 907
5. Harris FS, Rhoton AL Jr (1976) Anatomy of the cavernous sinus. A microsurgical study. J Neurosurg 15: 169–180
6. Isamat F (1986) Direct intracavernous obliteration of high flow carotid-cavernous fistulas. Presented at the int symp on cavernous sinus in Ljubljana, Yugoslavia
7. Kaplan HA, Browder J, Kvieger AJ (1976) Intracavernous connections of the cavernous sinuses. J Neurosurg 45: 166–168
8. Loyo M et al (1986) Transsphenoidal microsurgery for the treatment of hypophyseal adenoma. Rev Med IMSS 24: 189–193
9. Loyo M et al (1984) Combined supra-infrasellar approach for large pituitary tumors. Neurosurgery 14: 485–488
10. Maniglia AJ (1986) Indications and techniques of midfacial degloving. Arch Otolaryngol Head Neck Surg 112: 750–752
11. Parkinson D (1973) Carotid-cavernous fistula: direct repair with preservation of the carotid artery. J Neurosurg 38: 106
12. Rhoton AL, Harris S, Reen H (1978) Microsurgical anatomy of the sellar region and cavernous sinus. Neurosurgery 8: 54–58
13. Taptas JN (1982) The so-called cavernous sinus: a review of the controversy and its implications for neurosurgeons. Neurosurgery 5: 712–717
14. Wallace S, Goldberg HI, Leeds NE, Mishkin M (1976) The cavernous branches of the internal carotid artery. Am J Roentgenol 101: 34–46

Transsphenoidal surgery of pituitary adenomas developed towards the cavernous sinus

M. Buchfelder and R. Fahlbusch

Department of Neurosurgery, University Erlangen — Nürnberg, Erlangen, Federal Republic of Germany

Today various therapeutic surgical approaches are available for the treatment of pituitary adenomas. Modern radiology provides an excellent image of the localization and extent of tumors extending towards the cavernous sinus and the topographical pathology of the adjacent anatomical structures. Particularly the information gained by thin-collimation computerized tomography [1, 7], angiography [9] and nuclear magnetic resonance (NMR) scanning [5] is helfpul in the preoperative evaluation of parasellar tumors and facilitates the decision making between the transcranial and transsphenoidal approach. It is not so much the total size of the adenoma but the delineation and the connection between the intra- and parasellar tumor parts which influence the indication for the "upper" or "lower" approach [2, 4, 12]. Since the introduction of computerized tomography we have learned that only a small minority of those pituitary adenomas displacing or invading the cavernous sinus cause a cavernous sinus syndrome as described in the past [14]. Mostly endocrine symptoms due to hormone oversecretion in functioning adenomas or hypopituitarism in hormonally inactive adenomas lead to the diagnosis of these intra- and parasellar tumors. Cranial nerve palsy, although providing clinical information about the tumor site, occurred in only 8/77 in this series. This report is focused on the endocrinological results and the prognosis of extraocular nerve muscle palsy.

Patients

We herein report on our experience with transsphenoidal surgery of parasellar pituitary adenomas in 77 patients operated on in a 3-year-period

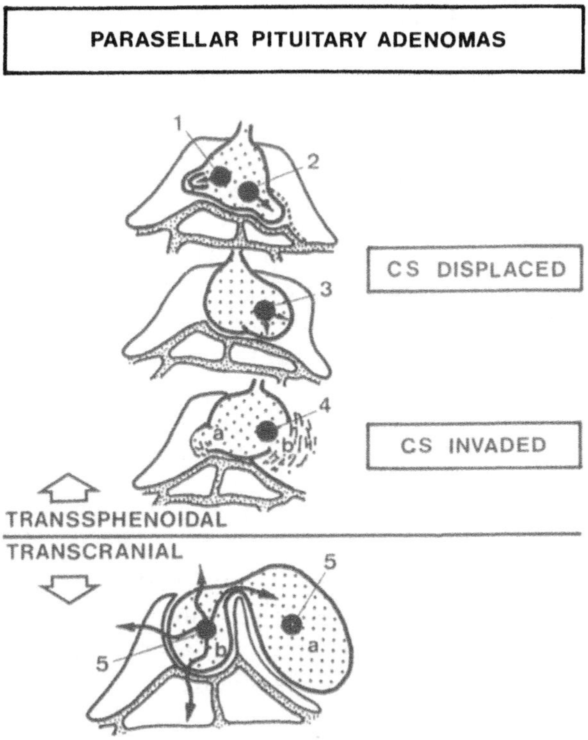

Fig. 1. Classification of parasellar tumor extension: *1* circumscribed displacement of the medial wall of the cavernous sinus; *2* subcavernous tumor extension along the basal dura; *3* massive lateral tumor extension with displacement of the cavernous sinus as a whole *4a* localized invasiveness, *b* generalized invasiveness; *5a* supracavernous parasellar and subtemporal extension, *b* extrasellar extension with generalized invasiveness

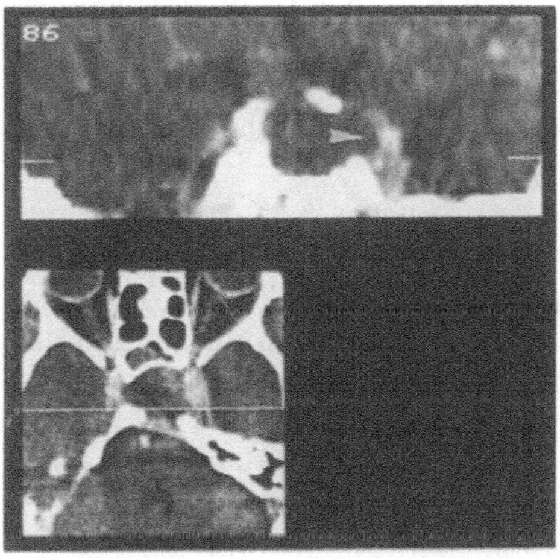

Fig. 2. Thin-collimation coronal CT reconstruction of a pituitary adenoma with displacement of the cavernous sinus (arrow)

from December 1982 until February 1986. During this interval 435 operations for pituitary adenomas were performed in the Department of Neurosurgery, University of Erlangen — Nürnberg. The transsphenoidal approach was used 404 times. Parasellar pituitary adenomas accounted for 19% of the pituitary adenomas operated on via this route. Apart from the patients reported herein, 8 other patients with parasellar and subtemporal tumor extension had transcranial surgery performed in our unit. Lateralized intrasellar adenomas, although often found adjacent to the cavernous sinus, were not included in this series.

Surgical pathology

We have classified tumor localization and extension on the basis of radiological and surgical findings. In 44 patients the tumors extended only towards the cavernous sinus without any suprasellar component, in 18 patients there was additional suprasellar tumor extension without visual compromise, and in 15 other patients a chiasma syndrome was present. Seventy patients had macroadenomas (diameter > 10 mm), while in only 7 cases microadenomas (diameter < 10 mm) were found.

The cavernous sinus was displaced but not invaded in the majority of our patients (Fig. 1). Localized lateral extension of the adenoma causing a circumscribed displacement in the medial wall of the cavernous sinus (type 1) was found in 12 of our patients.

Tumor extension along the basal dura into the subcavernous area (type 2) was recently described by Ahmadi et al. [1] in a radiological report and we stress that it deserves special attention. It was found in 3 cases in this series.

In most cases of these parasellar pituitary adenomas (46/77) the cavernous sinus was displaced laterally as a whole by a massive lateral tumor extension (type 3).

Localized (type 4 a) or generalized (type 4 b) invasiveness which was found in 7 and 8 cases, respectively, was signalized intraoperatively by tumor perforation into the medial wall of the cavernous sinus and visualization of the trabecular system during and after tumor removal.

There is general agreement among neurosurgeons that large adenomas with parasellar or subtemporal extension (type 5 a) which are massively developed lateral to the sella either by supracavernous or subcavernous extension, as well as generally invasive adenomas (type 5 b), have to be treated by a transcranial, intradural approach [2, 4, 12]. Figure 3 shows the CT scan of such a tumor which must not be operated on via the transsphenoidal route.

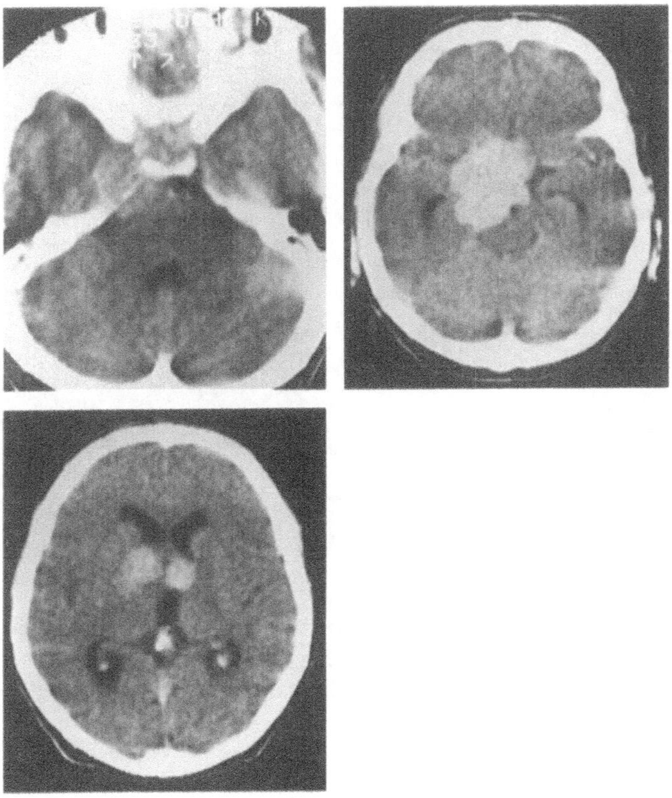

Fig. 3. CT scan of a giant pituitary adenoma with parasellar and subtemporal as well as suprasellar extension. This case is a classical indication for the transcranial-intradural approach

Operative technique

The transsphenoidal operation was carried out as described previously [3] with the patient positioned supine and the surgeon standing at the patient's head. A medial sublabial incision was made and the nasal mucosa was detached unilaterally from the cartilaginous and bony nasal septum by blunt dissection. The osseous septum was partly resected and the sphenoid sinus was opened with the aid of rongeurs or the air drill. As soon as the sphenoid sinus was entered, the operating microscope was applied. The mucosa of the sphenoid sinus was removed. The opening of the sellar floor ranged from 8–10 × 10–12 mm in intrasellar microadenomas but was considerably larger in parasellar adenomas. Curettes and microforceps were used for tumor removal. Adenomas with extensive lateral displacement of the cavernous sinus needed a lateral curettage which was commonly performed as far as 2–

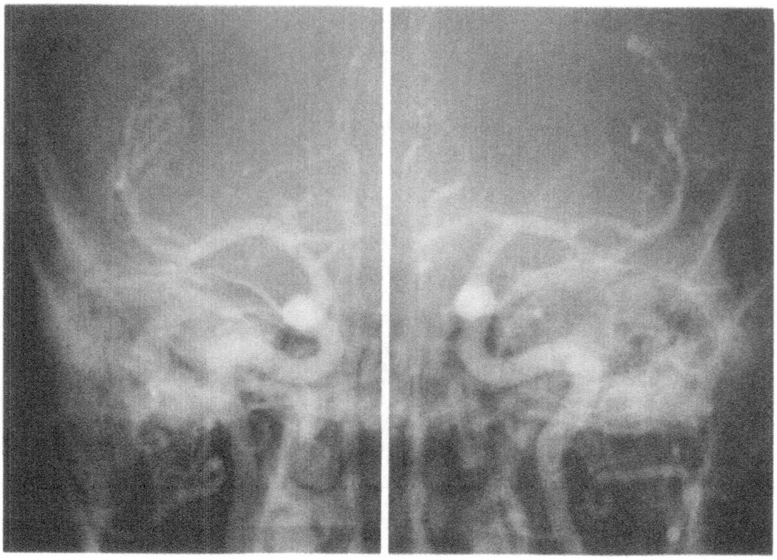

Fig. 4. Angiography provides information about the degree of lateral displacement of the carotid artery (and thus, indirectly about the cavernous sinus). The left carotid artery is shifted laterally as compared to the right side

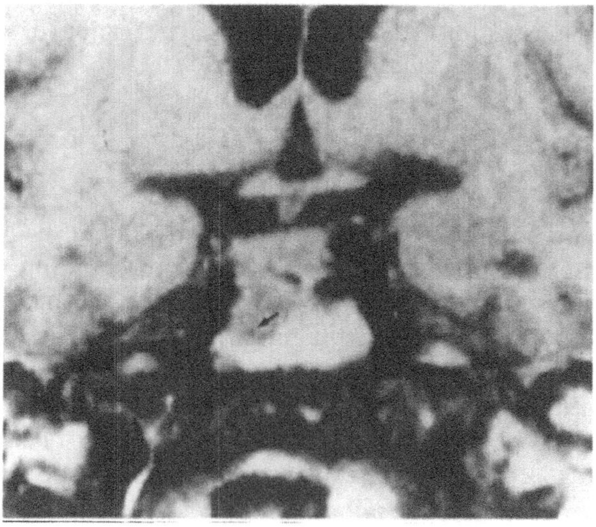

Fig. 5. Nuclear magnetic resonance image of subcavernous lateral adenoma extension (arrow). This corresponds to type E of parasellar tumor development (in Fig. 1)

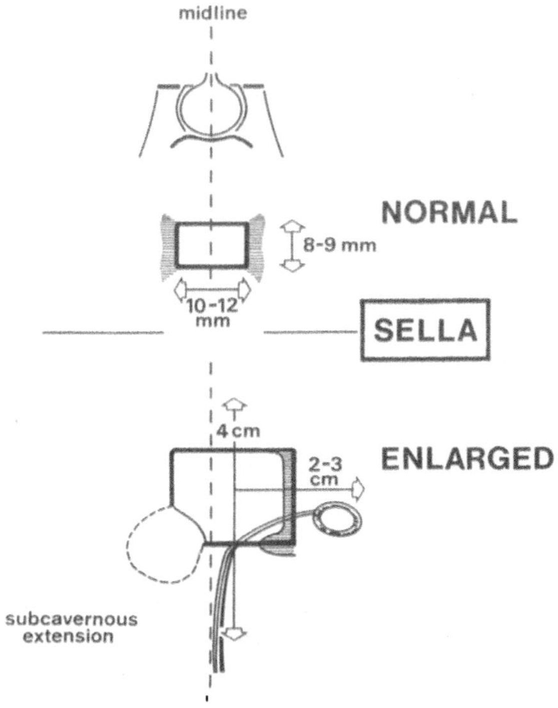

Fig. 6. Comparison of sella floor resection and lateral tumor curettage in cases of intrasellar microadenomas and in cases with considerable parasellar extension of pituitary macroadenomas

3 cm from the midline and even further in some cases (Fig. 6). Adequate exposure of the enlarged sella by sufficiently opening the sphenoid sinus is mandatory for a safe surgical procedure. Bleeding from lacerations in the medial wall of the cavernous sinus was commonly encountered but generally did not represent a serious surgical problem. In most cases it was easily controlled by compression with gelfoam. Usually, packing of the sella was not necessary. In cases of invasive tumors the cavernous sinus was entered following the tumor spread. Bleeding was not so severe as one would expect. Suction was applied to remove the adenoma from the trabecular system which could be visualized. Care must be taken not to damage the carotid artery which sometimes is in contact with the intrasellar dura [13] and may be palpated. Complete hemostasis was achieved after satisfactory removal of the tumor. A small piece of fascia lata from the thigh was used to cover the diaphragm and was fixed by fibrin glue. In the event of CSF leaking intraoperatively, a lumbar drainage was performed and 45–60 ml of CSF were drained daily for 4–5 days. In cases of invasive adenomas postoperative radiation therapy with doses of approximately 50 Gray in fractions of 2 Gray over 4–5 weeks was performed.

Endocrinological results

In hormonally active tumors the most sensitive tool available for the detection of tumor remnants is monitoring of the hormone oversecretion. While in prolactin-, in growth-hormone- and in ACTH-secreting adenomas causing Nelson's syndrome basal serum levels of prolactin (normal range: below 500 μU/ml), growth hormone (normal range: below 5 ng/ml) and ACTH (normal range: 20–50 pg/ml) are usually considered sufficient by neurosurgeons, the decision about remission in Cushing's disease is based on the results of dynamic endocrine testing. Here, basal serum cortisol levels are expected to be suppressed to below 2 μg/100 ml after oral administration of 2 mg dexamethasone overnight [3].

It is generally observed that the best results of transsphenoidal surgery for hormone-secreting pituitary tumors are achieved in intrasellar microadenomas [2, 3, 4, 15]. However, the hormone-excess was also normalized in all 5 microadenomas extending extraglandularly towards the cavernous sinus (Table 1). Among macroadenomas the best results were achieved in acromegalic patients. In this group oversecretion of GH could be normalized in 13 out of 20 patients with non-invasive and in 1 out of 6 of the invasive macroadenomas. In all the other hormone-secreting parasellar macroadenomas the hormone excess persisted. These cases require further treatment, either medically by dopamine-agonists in prolactinomas or somatostatin analogues in acromegaly or by irradiation in all cases not sufficiently controlled by medical therapy and in cases of invasive tumors. Medical therapy with dopamine-agonists also seems to show a new perspective in the management of prolactinomas developed towards the cavernous sinus. We could shrink 5 parasellar macroprolactinomas by a short-term medical preoperative treatment with dopamine agonists and thus diminish the lateral extension of the tumors. After 2–6 weeks transsphenoidal surgery was considerably facilitated. While normoprolactinemia was not achieved despite these effects, in only one of these tumors there is evidence for residual tumor in the postoperative CT scan. This seems to be an acceptable result in a group of tumors difficult to treat. None of our prolactinoma patients had optomotoric nerve lesions. However, resolution of a cavernous sinus syndrome caused by a prolactinoma by administration of bromocriptine has been described in the literature [6] and is clinical evidence of tumor size reduction.

Optomotoric nerve function

Paresis of optomotoric nerves preoperatively was present in 8 out of 77 patients. The oculomotor nerve was affected 4 times, the abducens nerve 3 times and in addition there was total ophthalmoplegia in another case. Duration of the extraocular muscle paresis ranged from one day to three

Table 1. Normalization of the hormone excess by primary transsphenoidal surgery in functioning parasellar pituitary adenomas

Endocrinological classification	Secreted hormone	Criteria for normalization	Total no. of patients	Normalization Rate		
				Micro-adenomas	Macro-adenomas non invasive	Macro-adenomas invasive
Acromegaly	Growth-hormone (GH)	Basal serum growth-hormone level < 5 ng/ml	27	1/1	13/20	1/6
Prolactinoma	Prolactin (PRL)	Basal serum prolactin level < 500 μU/ml	17	2/2	0/13	0/2
Cushing's disease	Adrenocorticotropic hormone (ACTH)	Suppression of serum cortisol levels to < 2 μg/100 ml after 2 mg dexamethasone	3	2/2		0/1
Nelson's syndrome	Adrenocorticotropic hormone (ACTH)	Basal serum ACTH level < 50 pg/ml	2		0/2	

months. An apoplectiform, sudden onset of optomotoric nerve palsies is generally considered suggestive of pituitary tumor infarction or hemorrhage [10]. In three cases the history indicated such an event, but during surgery signs of a recent or old hemorrhage were found in 5 cases. As demonstrated in Table 2, the overall outcome was favorable. Complete

Table 2. Influence of transsphenoidal surgery for parasellar pituitary adenomas on optomotoric nerve palsies (n = 8)

	Unchanged	Improved	Normalized
Total ophthalmoplegia	—	—	1
Oculomotor nerve palsy (N III)	1[a]	—	3
Abducens nerve palsy (N VI)	—	1	2[b]

[a] Including one patient with concomitant Wernicke's encephalopathy
[b] Including one patient with latent N IV palsy and transitory diplopia

recovery was seen in 6 out of the 8 patients when they had a follow-up between 3 months and one year after transsphenoidal surgery. In 5 of these cases some improvement was already noted one week after the operation. We would like to emphasize that preoperative duration of these nerve palsies did not influence the tendency of the extraocular nerve recovery.

In this series no patient acquired extraocular nerve palsies following tanssphenoidal adenomectomy, but transitory palsies have been described after transsphenoidal surgery [8]. Results from the literature confirm the favorable prognosis for optomotoric nerve lesions following transsphenoidal surgery for pituitary adenoma. Wilson and Dempsey [15] report on 5 out of 12 patients who fully recovered from preoperative abnormalities of ocular motility. Schäfer et al. [11] observed a complete recovery of extraocular nerve paresis in 2 cases and a partial recovery in the third after transsphenoidal removal of pituitary adenoma.

Complications

In this series there was no mortality or serious morbidity. The overall mortality in our whole series of 434 patients treated in Erlangen was 0.2% for all transsphenoidal and 0.7% for all transsphenoidal and transcranial operations put together. In transsphenoidal surgery major complications like meningitis or CSF fistulas occur in about 1% cases [2, 3]. In one of our cases, a lady with a large macroprolactinoma, treated several years previously by transcranial surgery, both a meningitis and a CSF fistula occurred. She fully recovered after antibiotic treatment and a reoperation. Deterioration of anterior pituitary function and a permanent diabetes isipidus are rare, as well as acquired optomotoric nerve palsies or a deterioration of vision. Their frequency is much less than 1%.

Conclusions

We have introduced a practical classification of pituitary adenomas for the neurosurgeon.

The prognosis for optomotoric nerve lesions is favorable after transsphenoidal resection of pituitary adenomas and functional recovery is independent of the preoperative duration of the palsy.

Surgical "cures" in functioning macroadenomas are uncommon and further treatment—either medical or by irradiation—is usually required to obtain normal hormone levels.

Since intra- and parasellar pituitary adenomas can be approached by the transsphenoidal route with low morbidity and mortality, this method of surgery should be primarily considered. It is also suitable for invasive adenomas provided that, in respect to surgical tumor removal, a sufficiently large connection between the intrasellar and parasellar tumor portions exists. We highly recommend this surgical technique also for the operative treatment of large pituitary adenomas developed towards the cavernous sinus, particularly to those who have already gained some experience with the operative treatment of intra- and suprasellar tumors by this approach.

References

1. Ahmadi J, North CM, Segall HD, Zee CS, Weiss MH (1985) Cavernous sinus invasion by pituitary adenomas. AJNR 6: 893–898
2. Fahlbusch R (1981) Surgery of pituitary adenomas. In: Beardwell C, Robertson GL (eds) Clinical endocrinology. The pituitary. Butterworths, London, pp 76–105
3. Fahlbusch R, Buchfelder M, Schrell U (1985) Neurochirurgische Therapie neuroendokrinologischer Störungen. Internist 26: 293–301
4. Guiot G, Derome P (1976) Surgical problems of pituitary adenomas. In: Krayenbühl H et al (eds) Advances and technical standards in neurosurgery, vol 3. Springer, Wien New York, pp 3–33
5. Huk W, Fahlbusch R (1985) Nuclear magnetic imaging of the region of the sella turcica. Neurosurg Rev 8: 141–150

6. King LW, Molitch ME, Gittinger JW, Wolpert SM, Stern J (1983) Cavernous sinus syndrome due to prolactinoma: Resolution with bromocriptine. Surg Neurol 19: 280–284
7. Kline LB, Acker JD, Post MJD, Vitek JJ (1981) The cavernous sinus. A computed tomographic study. AJNR 2: 299–305
8. Laws ER, Kern EB (1976) Complications of transsphenoidal surgery. Clin Neurosurg 23: 401–416
9. Rao KC, Allen HA, Haney PJ, Yu R, Levine H (1981) Vascular studies in the preoperative evaluation of pituitary adenomas before transsphenoidal surgery. Surg Neurol 21: 175–181
10. Reid RL, Quigley ME, Yen SS (1985) Pituitary apoplexy—a review. Arch Neurol 42: 712–719
11. Schäfer M, Steudel WI, Grau H (1981) Paralysis of the extraocular muscles in tumours of the sella turcica. In: Samii M, Jannetta PJ (eds) The cranial nerves. Springer, Berlin Heidelberg New York Tokyo, pp 264–268
12. Sekhar LN, Møller AR (1986) Operative management of tumors involving the cavernous sinus. J Neurosurg 64: 879–889
13. Taptas JN (1982) The so-called cavernous sinus: a review of the controversy and its implications for neurosurgery. Neurosurgery 11: 712–717
14. Weinberger LM, Adler FH, Grant FC (1940) Primary pituitary adenoma and the symptom of the cavernous sinus. Arch Ophthalmol 97: 1197–1246
15. Wilson CB, Dempsey LC (1978) Transsphenoidal neurosurgical removal of 250 pituitary adenomas. J Neurosurg 48: 13–22

Subject index